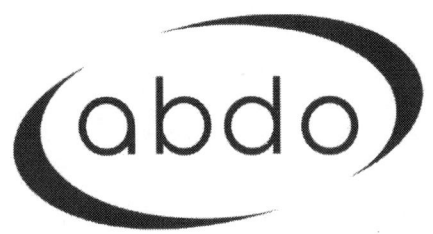 **Association of British Dispensing Opticians**

**ABDO
199 Gloucester Terrace
London
W2 6LD**

© A H Tunnacliffe

ISBN 0-900099-30-5

Printing history
First edition	1995
Second edition	1998
Third edition	2003
Reprinted	2007 with updated single vision lens index

Association British Dispensing Opticians
Other publications

Abnormal Ocular Conditions	D.M. Pipe & L.J. Rapley
British Standards Extracts	B.S.I & ABDO
Introduction to Visual Optics	A.H Tunnacliffe
Low Vision – An inter-professional approach	N. Andrew, R. Harsant & C. Lawrence
Low Vision Assessment	J. Macnaughton
Ocular Anatomy and Histology	D.M. Pipe & L.J Rapley
Ophthalmic Lenses Availability	P. Gilbert
Optics	A.H Tunnacliffe & J.G Hirst
Practical Dispensing	A.I. Griffiths
Practical Ophthalmic Lenses	M. Jalie & L. Wray
The Principles of Ophthalmic Lenses	M. Jalie
Worked Problems in Ophthalmic Lenses	A.H Tunnacliffe & G.D Janney
Worked Problems in Optics	A.H Tunnacliffe
Worked Problems in Visual Optics	A.I. Griffiths

Contents

Dispensing Single Vision Lenses

Patient's age, prescription and the choice of lens

Pre-presbyopia 1
Early presbyopia — 1
Table 1   Range of clear vision for some ages, Adds and working distances — 1
Established presbyopia — 2

Factors involved in the choice of lenses

1 Lens materials — 2
  1.1   Refractive index — 2
        Table 2 Optical properties of glass and plastic ophthalmic lens materials — 3
        Optical properties of white mid- and high-index glasses — 3
  1.2   V-value — 4
  1.3   Density and Specific Gravity — 4
  1.4   Relative Curvature — 4
        Table 3 Relative curvature values and thickness reduction — 5
  1.5   Plastic lens materials — 5

2 Lens forms and lens thickness — 5
        Table 4   Advantages of aspheric design plus lenses — 6
        Availability of single vision aspherics — 6

3 Dispensing minus lenses — 7
  3.1   Oblique visual performance of minus lenses — 7
  3.1.1   Oblique astigmatism and best form minus lenses — 7
        Table 6   Minimum Tangential Error Best Form Minus Spheric Lenses — 8
  3.1.1.1 Pantoscopic tilt and vertical centration — 9
  3.1.2 The effect of transverse chromatic aberration — 9
  3.1.3 The form of toric lenses — 10
  3.2   Checking surface powers with the lens measure — 12
  3.3   Determining the refractive index of a minus lens — 12
        Table 10   Estimating an unknown refractive index — 14
  3.4   Full aperture and reduced aperture lenses — 14
  3.4.1 Field of view in minus lenses — 14
  3.4.2 Edge thickness in minus lenses — 15
  3.4.2.1 Lenticulars — 16
        Fitting lenticulars — 16
  3.4.3 Power rings and coatings — 17
        Table 11   Reflectance from lenses of different indices — 17
        Hard Coat and Hard Coat and AR Coat combination — 17
  3.5   Minus lenses in near vision — 18
  3.6   Choice of lenses and frames — 18
  4   Dispensing plus lenses — 21
  4.1   Effect of form and diameter on lens thickness — 21
  4.2   Uncut sizes, finished lenses, and lens thickness — 22
  4.3   Plus aspherics have a shallow back curve — 22
  4.4   Centration of single vision lenses — 22
  4.5   Prescribed prism — 23
  4.6   Single vision lenses solely for near vision — 24
  4.7   High plus lenses in near vision — 25
  4.8   Field of view in high plus single vision lenses — 26

Vertex distance consequences

Summary of effects of keeping the vertex distance small — 27
Vertex distance measurement — 29
Empty frame and minus lens Rx – the vertex distance — 29
Empty frame and plus lens Rx – the vertex distance — 30

Ordering single vision spectacles — 31

The dispensing optician's rôle — 31

Availability of Full Aperture Single Vision Lenses — 32

Dispensing Progressive Addition Lenses

Advantages of Progressive Addition Lenses   35
Disadvantages of Progressive Addition Lenses   35

(A) Specifying progressive addition lenses

Isocylinder lines   39
Hard, soft and ultrasoft design PALs   40
Vector plots   40
Isopower lines   41
Distance and reading widths   41
The power profile   41

(B) Features of PAL design

Second generation PALs   42
Asymmetric and symmetric designs   42
Mono and multi-designs   43
Aspherisation and PALs – the Fourth Generation   44
Through the lens design – the Fifth Generation   44
OPALs – lenses for intermediate and close-work   45
The effect of increasing Addition   46
Short corridor PALs   47
A simple method of classifying PALs   47
Limit of isocylinder plot usefulness   47

(C) Dispensing progressive lenses

Choosing the patient   48
Choice of progressive lens   48
Other considerations in PAL selection   48
Fitting progressive addition lenses   49
Customised progressive lenses   50
Frame selection   50
Checking glazed PALs   51
Prism thinning   52
Prescribed Prisms   53

(D) Patient acceptance of PALs

The patient's visual requirements   53
Table 5 Procedure for dealing with problems with PALs   54
Incorrect dispensing   54
Effect of pupil size   54
Faulty lenses   55
Summary   55
Essential fitting measurements   56

Occupational Progressive Addition Lenses

Introduction   57
Properties of the lenses   58
Personal comments on OPALs   61
Dispensing OPALs   61
Introduction   62

Table of Contents

Dispensing Bifocal Lenses

Advantages of bifocals	63
Disadvantages of bifocals	63
Important optical principles of bifocals	63
Segment diameter	64
Lateral and vertical placement of the segment	65
Segment inset for coincident fields of view	65
Geometrical inset of the bifocal segment	66
Vertical placement of the bifocal segment	66
Definition of segment height	68
Near Vision Effectivity Error (NVEE)	68
Position of the distance optical centre in bifocals	68
Vision around the segment top zone	69
Bifocals in Anisometropia	69
Prism adaptation	69
Bifocal spectacle correction	70
Finding the patient who needs prism compensation	70
Prism compensated lenses and other approaches	70
Trial prism compensation with Fresnel prisms	71
Prism compensation with unequal segments	71
Dispensing Bifocal Lenses	72
Choice of Patient for First-time Bifocals	72
Established wearers of bifocals	73
Choice of Conventional Bifocal	73
Jump and no-jump at the segment top	74
Aspheric Bifocals in the low to medium power range	74
Lenticular and high powered aspheric bifocals	74
Occupational and Special Bifocals	75
Bifocals with high Adds	75
Front and Back Surface Segments	76
The Smart Seg Progressive Bifocal	76
Segment Top Positioning vis-à-vis the Eye	76
Conventional fitting	77
VDU use	77
Juvenile Stress Myopia and Accommodation Control	78
Double D Segments	78
Upcurve bifocals	78
Head and eye position during measurements	78
Ordering Bifocals	78
Verification of Bifocals	81
Measurement of the Addition in Bifocals	81
Power, axis, centration, and prism tolerances	81
Tolerances on lens positioning and optical centration	83
Pairing of Tolerances on all Lenses	83
Planos and plano-cylinders	83
Prism Base Setting Tolerances	83
Prism Power Tolerances	84
Segment dimension and positioning tolerances	84
Subjective Characteristics of Spectacle Lenses	84
Glazing	84
Listing of British Standards Publications	85

Dispensing Trifocal Lenses

Introduction	86
The need for an intermediate correction	87
General Purpose and Occupational Trifocals	88
The Intermediate Add on Trifocals	88
Fitting trifocals	88
The Smart Seg alternative	88
Split trifocals for different prismatic effects	89
Occupational Progressive Addition Lens alternatives	89

The Principles of Spectacle Frame Fitting

1 The forces retaining the frame in place	90
1.1 Pad bridges and the reaction forces	91
1.2 The reaction forces behind the ears	92
1.3 Minimising pressure	92
2 Matching the frame to the head	93
3 Head and facial asymmetries	94
3.1 Asymmetrical frontal and splay angles	94
3.2 Head width considerations	94
3.3 Unequal ear heights	95
3.5 Hyper-brow and hyper-eye	95

Dispensing Tints

Introduction	97
Tints and filters	97
1 Terminology	97
Reflectance, transmittance and absorptance	97
Luminous transmittance	98
Classification of tints by material and form	99
2 Properties of tinted lenses	100
Transmittance properties	100
Where is the ultraviolet radiation cut-off?	100
Photochromic lenses and driving	103
Polarising lenses	103
Is the colour of a tinted lens significant?	103
3 Uses of tinted lenses	105
Cosmetic, fashion and comfort tints	105
Sunglass tints 107	
Tints for dyslexia and migraine	107
Contrast filters for sports and driving	108
Industrial filters	110
Filters for medical conditions	110
Special occupational filters	112
Visual Display Unit (VDU) and fluorescent light filters	113
Filters to assist colour deficiency	114
4 Prescribing and dispensing tints	114
UV blockers	114
Light tints for cosmesis only	115
Light tints which have some other purpose	115
Dark tints	115
Fixed versus photochromic tints	116
Special purpose tints	117
Replacing a damaged tinted lens	117

Dispensing Single Vision Lenses

The term *single vision lens* refers to the fact that the lens aperture is designed to have the same power over its entire area. This area may be the so-called full eye-size or a half-eye, as illustrated in figure 1. Primarily, one thinks of single vision lenses being used to correct the focus in patients with ametropia. That is, the pair of lenses in a spectacle frame render the eyes artificially emmetropic, which means that the unaccommodated[†] eye is then focused for distant objects. However, perhaps at least as many single vision spectacles are used solely for reading, and some are used solely for intermediate tasks beyond the reading distance but not further away than about 2 metres.

Patient's age, prescription and the choice of lens

For the purpose of deciding on the optimum lens type for a patient it is convenient to consider three age groups: the **pre-presbyope**[‡], the **early presbyope**, and the established presbyope. In a somewhat oversimplified but fairly practical classification, these groupings might be categorised by age as under 40, 40 to 50, and over 50. The pre-presbyope, under 40 years of age, will have sufficient amplitude of accommodation to be able to manage all but extremely near visual tasks with a single vision pair of lenses which correct his/her ametropia.

Dispensing for the **pre-presbyope** is relatively simple since in the majority of cases the patient will be able to focus at all distances from far to reasonably near. The dispenser must however be aware that the prescriber may in some cases give some extra plus power to a pre-presbyope in order to reduce the accommodation demand for prolonged close-work. In this latter case the single vision lenses will not be suitable for distance vision since the extra plus power produces a far point of distinct vision which is relatively near. For example, with an addition of +1.00 DS onto the distance prescription, the far point of distinct vision will be only 1 metre from the spectacle plane.

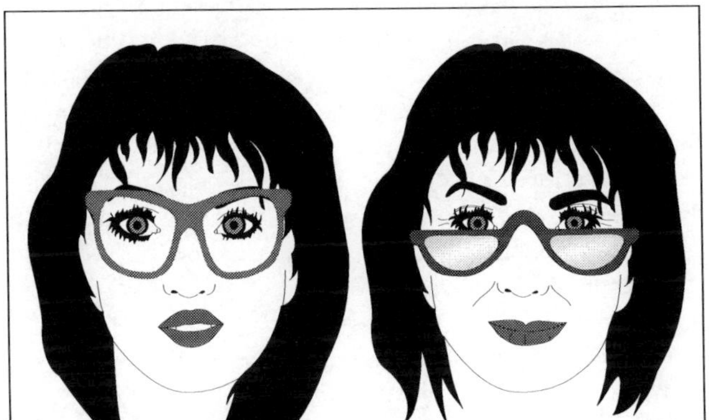

In the early **presbyopic case**, aged 40 to 50 years, the amplitude of accommodation reduces to such an extent that prolonged close work causes ocular discomfort (asthenopia) and a reading addition (Add) becomes necessary for near vision tasks. This Add, the addition of spherical plus power to the distance Rx, will depend on the patient's amplitude of accommodation and on the working distance for the task. With single vision lenses the far point of distinct vision (also called the far point of accommodation) will be a distance 1/*Add* in front of the spectacle plane, and when this limitation interferes with the patient's normal conduct of his/her activities then bifocals or multifocal lenses will have to be considered. It should be noted that the far point of distinct vision with a reading Add will become less remote as the Add increases. Table 1 indicates the range of clear vision*, the distance between far and near points with spectacles incorporating a reading Add, and it is evident that this aspect of close-work spectacles must be explained to patients during the discussion about lens types.

Table 1 Range of clear vision for some ages, Adds and working distances (WD)

Age	Add	W.D. (cm)	Range of clear vision (cm)
45	+0.50	40	200 to 29
	+1.00	35	100 to 25
	+1.25	30	80 to 24
50	+1.00	40	100 to 33
	+1.50	35	67 to 29
	+2,00	30	50 to 25
55	+1.50	40	67 to 33
	+2.00	35	50 to 29
	+2.25	30	44 to 27
60	+1.75	40	57 to 36
	+2.25	35	44 to 31
	+2.75	30	36 to 27
70	+2.50	35	40 to 33
	+3.00	30	33 to 29
	+3.75	25	27 to 24

Fig. 1 Full eye-size and half-eye style spectacle frames. Note that the term *eye-size* is used in practice although the term *lens size* would be more appropriate since frames do not have eyes.

[†] *Accommodation* — the act of changing the eye's power.
  Unaccommodated — the eye has its weakest power.
[‡] *Presbyopia* — ageing sight: the amplitude of accommodation has reduced to such an extent that close-work is uncomfortable and/or blurred.

* The distance between the artificial far and near points whilst wearing the near vision correction. These are the furthest and nearest points of distinct vision with the spectacle lenses. The term *artificial* indicates the patient is wearing spectacle lenses.

As the Add increases we see from Table 1 that the range between the (artificial) far and near points of distinct vision decreases, and this can be of considerable irritation to a patient. When this reduced range of clear vision becomes a handicap, say to an elderly patient who likes to play cards and therefore needs to be able to see the centre of the table, or for any other visual task beyond the artificial far point with single vision lenses, then bifocal or multifocal lenses will need to be considered, unless half-eye single vision spectacles would suffice. This latter solution would definitely be a possibility if the patient were slightly myopic so that the true far point (the far point without spectacles) was somewhere around the correct focus for the intermediate task.

In **established presbyopia**, over 50 years of age, the Add gradually increases with advancing age, and intermediate tasks become more difficult with just a single focus lens. For example, consider a 53 year old patient with no distance correction (emmetropia) who has previously been wearing a +1.00 Add. From Table 1 we see that the artificial far point is 1 metre from the spectacles and the artificial near point is at 33 cm. Assuming these spectacles were prescribed at say 48 years of age and he now needs a +1.50 Add for reading, then the artificial far point will be brought closer to a distance of only two-thirds of a metre. With a higher Add, the effect is worse. If he requires a +2.00 Add for reading, then his artificial far point will only be $1/2.00 = 0.5$ metres away. If this proves too close he will have to consider other forms of spectacle lens which offer him an increased range of focus. In this context, it cannot be stressed too strongly that it is both the prescriber's and the dispenser's function to determine the patient's visual requirements by systematic questioning about the visual tasks the patient undertakes. It is most important to question the patient about occupational and hobby visual activities.

Factors involved in the choice of lenses

The dispenser must advise the patient on a range of variables when helping a patient to decide on the most suitable lenses. We are here assuming that single vision lenses are deemed optically suitable for the patient's needs, but one must always be aware that financial contraints may limit a patient to less expensive lenses than optical considerations alone would suggest as the best solution. However, given that we are discussing optimum single vision lenses here, the factors involved in dispensing them will be discussed under the headings:

1 **Lens materials**
2 **Lens forms and lens thickness**
3 **Dispensing minus lenses**
4 **Dispensing plus lenses.**

1 Lens materials

There are two groups of materials, glass and plastic. Glass lenses historically came first, glass being manufactured in Egypt more than 4000 years ago. Spectacles[†], also referred to as glasses or eyeglasses, defined as two lenses in a frame, date back to the 14th Century in Europe, although they appeared earlier in China. The first lenses were of naturally occurring silicon compounds quartz and beryl, but in 1885 Ernst Abbe and Otto Schott, two now famous names in lens manufacture, demonstrated that the optical properties of glass could be much improved by the addition of new elements to the glass melt, and a century of further research has produced the variety of glass types available today.

Plastic lenses are also referred to as organic, resin, or hard resin lenses, these latter names being offered as less disparaging designations than plastic. However, plastic is now recognised as a fundamental, important, and technologically advanced product in society and, as a result, the term plastic lens is rarely thought of as referring to a second-rate material nowadays. Indeed, where plastic lenses overlap the range of glass lenses, they have optical properties every bit as good as glass.

Comparing glass and plastic lenses, the essential difference in these materials is in the density. Plastic has a lower density than glass and if two lenses are made with the same volume then the plastic one will be lighter than the glass one. However, it is not quite this simple; there are a number of variables to be taken into account. Besides lens materials needing to be physically durable and resistant to atmospheric attack, factors which we assume to be inherent, the choice of material depends on *refractive index*, *V-value*, and *density*, and not to be forgotten, cost. Table 2 lists the available white glass and plastics materials at the time of writing (April, 1995). Note that the term white refers to untinted material, a white surface appearing uncoloured when viewed through a white lens. Further consideration needs to be given to the fact that plastic lenses are more prone to scratching since these materials are not as hard as glass. We shall mention anti-scratch coatings in section (3).

1.1 Refractive index

Symbolised by n, refractive index is probably the first property of optical media met by students of the subject. It soon becomes apparent that, as a general rule, the higher the refractive index then the thinner the spectacle lens can be made. Hence, without further consideration one would think that because a thin lens has a better cosmesis, we should go for the highest refractive index each time. But, when we refer to Table 2 we see that there is a general trend for glass higher refractive index materials to have a higher density and to be consequently heavier, and in both glass and plastic the higher refractive index material is usually accompanied by a lower V-value[‡]. This is undesirable because the quality of vision through the periphery of the lens is better if the V-value is high.

For thin, lightweight lenses, with good vision over the field of view, we ideally need high index, high V-value, and low density materials. It is evident from Table 2 that some judgement and compromise is going to be necessary on the part of the dispenser, since if he/she goes for a high index to obtain a thin lens, the V-value is going to be less, not to mention the higher density with glass lenses. This again raises the ever-present need of the dispenser to advise the patient of the choices and indicate the compromises being made: one generally compromises vision when choosing a high index material to reduce lens thickness.

[†] Alessandro di Spina of Florence, Italy. is credited with their introduction in Europe. The first portrait illustrating glasses was of Hugh of Provence by Tommaso da Modena at Treviso in 1352.

[‡] Also known as constringence, Abbe number, Abbe value, V-number, v-value, and v-number. (v is the Greek letter nu.)

Table 2 Optical properties of glass and plastic ophthalmic lens materials

Optical properties of white mid- and high-index glasses compared with spectacle crown

Supplier or manufacturer	Glass	Refractive index	V-value	Specific gravity	Relative curvature
All	Crown	1.523	58.9	2.54	1.00
Corning	UV Clear	1.523	59.7	2.48	1.00
Corning	1.6/41 Blanc TC	1.601	41.5	2.63	0.87
Schott	S.1018	1.601	42.2	2.67	0.87
DESAG	Hi-Crown	1.604	43.8	2.67	0.87
Corning	1.7/42 Blanc	1.700	41.6	3.21	0.75
Schott	Highlite	1.701	31.0	2.99	0.75
Schott	Tital 40	1.701	39.5	3.20	0.75
Hoya	LHI	1.702	40.2	2.99	0.75
DESAG	Lantal	1.800	35.4	3.62	0.65
Corning	1.8/35 Blanc	1.802	34.6	3.65	0.65
Hoya	THI-II	1.806	33.3	3.47	0.65
Nikon	Pointal	1.835	31.5	3.59	0.63
Corning	1.9/31 White	1.885	30.6	3.99	0.59

RC is relative curvature where $RC = (1.523 - 1)/(n_m - 1)$. If n_m, the material refractive index, is greater than 1.523, RC gives the relative thickness compared with the same lens in 1.523 index. For example, if $n_m = 1.700$, then $RC = 0.75$ and the lens will be 0.75 or 75% of the thickness of the equivalent lens in 1.523 material.

Optical properties of white plastic lenses (Relative Curvature is compared with spectacle crown glass)

Supplier or manufacturer	Plastic	Refractive index	V-value	Specific gravity	Relative curvature
PPGI[†]	CR 39	1.498	58.0	1.32	1.05
PPGI (see Taylor)	Trivex	1.53	45.0	1.11	0.99
Sola	Spectralite	1.537	47.0	1.21	0.97
Signet Armorlite	RLX Lite	1.555	36.0	1.24	0.93
Younger	Youngerlite	1.556	37.7	1.22	0.93
Essilor	Ormex	1.561	37.0	1.23	0.93
Signet Armorlite	Kodak Thin & Lite	1.562	36.0	1.24	0.93
Nikon	Nikon Lite DXII	1.560	41.0	1.17	0.93
Gentex	Polycarbonate	1.586	30.0	1.20	0.89
UK (AO)	Alphalite	1.592	36.0	1.42	0.88
Essilor	Ormil	1.595	36.0	1.36	0.87
Rodenstock	Perfalit 1.6	1.597	40.5	1.30	0.87
Zeiss	Clarlet 1.6	1.600	42.0	1.30	0.87
Pentax		1.600	42.0	1.30	0.87
Hoya	Eyas 1.6	1.600	41.0	1.32	0.87
Norville	Norlite	1.600	37.0	1.34	0.87
Nikon	Nikon Lite III	1.600	36.0	1.34	0.87
Sola	Sola Six	1.600	35.0	1.26	0.87
Seiko	Super 16	1.600	34.0	1.38	0.87
Signet Armorlite	1.6	1.594	32.0	1.34	0.87
Zeiss	Clarlet 1.66	1.664	32.0	1.36	0.79
Pentax, Rodenstock		1.67	32.0	1.35	0.79
Nikon	Nikon Lite IV	1.67	32.0	1.35	0.79
Hoya	Eyry	1.70	36.0	1.41	0.75
Hoya	Teslalid	1.71	36.0	1.40	0.75
Nikon, Seiko, WLC	Very high index	1.74	33.0	1.46	0.71

[†] Pittsburgh Plate Glass Industries

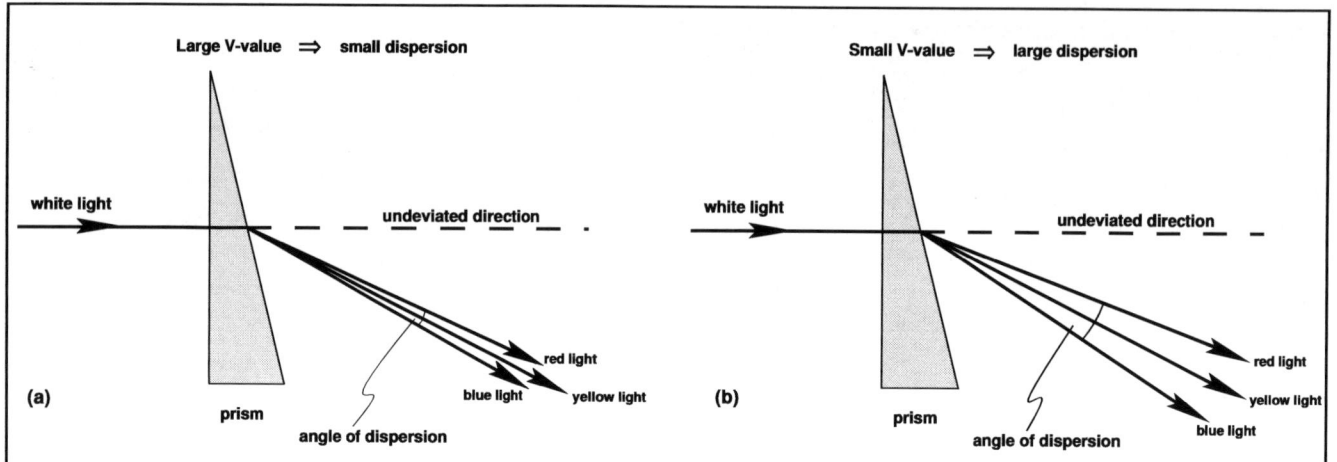

Fig. 2   Illustration of the effect of (a) high and (b) low V-values. The spread of light, dispersion, by a prism with a low V-value is greater than with a high V-value. When the colours are dispersed the image formed by the spectacle lens is not as sharp as it would be with less dispersion, hence vision is better with high V-value materials. Since the prismatic effect of a spectacle increases away from the optical centre, the quality of vision in oblique gaze is adversely affected by low V-value materials.

1.2 V-value

V-value[†] is a function of refractive index, which in turn is a function of the wavelength of light used to measure it. For example, if the refractive index of spectacle crown glass is measured with three wavelengths which give rise to the sensation of a red (656.3 nm), a yellow (587.6 nm), and a blue (486.1 nm), then the V-value turns out to be

$$V = \frac{n_d - 1}{n_F - n_C}.$$

The letters d, F, and C are Fraunhofer's letter scheme for labelling various wavelengths, where C, d, and F refer to the red, yellow, and blue wavelengths quoted above. The effect of V-value on the dispersion or spread of light is illustrated in figure 2. Because an image in an optical system will be more sharply defined if there is little dispersion of the colours upon refraction, higher V-values are preferable.

The lower the V-value, the greater is the risk that a patient will reject lenses on the grounds that the vision in oblique gaze is 'blurred', due to dispersion. With the multiplicity of lens materials now available, it is incumbent upon the dispenser to be familiar with these effects. Although occasionally a patient will complain of blurring due to a low V-value material, it is not often encountered with values of 40 or more. However, higher power lenses have greater prismatic effects away from the optical centre, and these lenses are just the ones where a higher refractive index combined with a low V-value is likely to be used. Knowing the effect of low V-value on vision, it is therefore the dispenser's duty to advise the patient on this matter when the lenses are being chosen.

1.3 Density and Specific Gravity

Density is a physical property of a material related to mass and volume. It is defined as

$$density = \frac{mass}{volume}$$

so that $mass = density \times volume.$ Now weight is proportional to mass, so weight is therefore proportional to density: double the density means double the weight for a given volume. Hence, we prefer low density materials in order to keep down the weight spectacle lenses. The lens volume is kept down by keeping the thickness down and this is usually achieved in high power lenses by using high refractive index materials, subject, of course, to the compromise on V-value.

In the ophthalmic industry, density is measured in the convenient units grams per cubic centimetre (g/cm^3). Some manufacturers quote specific gravity rather than density where specific gravity is a relative density measurement, the density of the material divided by the density of water. Because water has a density of 1 g/cm^3 at 4°C, the specific gravity of a substance has the same numerical value as its density if we use the units quoted, the units for specific gravity cancelling as shown below.

$$specific\ gravity\ of\ material = \frac{density\ of\ material}{density\ of\ water} \quad \frac{g/cm^3}{g/cm^3}$$

The units, shown on the right hand side above, obviously cancel since the numerator and denominator are identical. Hence, specific gravity has the advantage that no unit need be quoted, which is also true of refractive index and V-value.

1.4 Relative Curvature

The last column of Table 2 lists relative curvature values determined from the expression

$$RC = \frac{1.523 - 1}{n_m - 1}.$$

1.523 is the refractive index of spectacle crown for yellow light of wavelength 587.6 nm, according to the convention in the UK[‡]. It can be shown that relative curvature is a quite accurate indicator of relative lens thickness. That is, compared with spectacle crown glass, a lens of the same power and size in some material of refractive index n_m will have a relative edge thickness given by the relative curvature. For example, 1.7 index glass has a relative curvature $RC = 0.75$, so the edge thickness of a minus lens,

---

[†] Just how the V-value is determined is covered in *Optics*, by Tunnacliffe and Hirst, page 163 et seq.

[‡] Note that in Germany they use green light of wavelength 546.1 nm to designate spectacle crown glass (also known as ophthalmic crown). Thus, German companies quote spectacle crown as having a refractive index of 1.525.

say, will be only three-quarters as thick in 1.7 index material compared with the same lens power and size in spectacle crown. Table 3 gives the relative curvatures of the range of materials currently available.

Table 3 Relative curvature values and thickness reduction

Refractive Index	Relative Curvature	% thickness reduction (compared with 1.523 glass)
1.6	0.87	13%
1.7	0.75	25%
1.8	0.65	35%
1.9	0.58	42%

For practical use, the last column may be conveniently remembered as 15, 25, 35, and 45, without sensible loss of accuracy.

1.5 Plastic lens materials

Several plastics are used for ophthalmic lenses, although not all are used with the same frequency. Lenses made from polymethyl methacrylate (PMMA or acrylic) are still available but not commonly used nowadays. Polycarbonate is mainly used for protective lenses. CR 39 (Columbia Resin), and more recently polyurethane, are the commonly used plastics for ophthalmic lenses. Polyurethane can be made in flexible and rigid forms, the latter being used for spectacle lenses, but in one flexible form it is well known as the clothing material Lycra.

PMMA was the first plastic used for ophthalmic lenses. It became available shortly after World War II but, because of its easily scratched surfaces, it was soon replaced by CR 39, especially since this latter material could be surface tinted by dyeing.

Polycarbonate has a low V-value (30.0) and because of its comparatively soft nature lenses must be given an anti-scratch or hard-coat. It is available as prescription lenses but it tends to be used mainly in protective goggles and industrial standard impact resistant spectacle lenses.

Polyurethane lenses have been available for about a decade. They were initially available in mid-index (1.55 to 1.64) values, but latterly they have been produced in the high index range (1.65 to 1.74). All the polyurethane lenses have a somewhat lower V-value than CR 39's. Besides having a higher refractive index than CR 39, polyurethane lenses can be made thinner in minus form. It is not possible to make minus CR 39 lenses with a centre thickness less than 1.8 mm, but polyurethane minus lenses are available with centre thicknesses between 1.0 and 1.5 mm. Coupled with the higher refractive index, this has made them an attractive alternative to CR 39. Some polyurethane materials also have a lower density than CR 39, so they can be considerably lighter. Nikon's Nikon Lite DXII material has the lowest density of any lens at 1.17 g/cm^3. Sola's Spectralite, classed as a cross-linked acrylate copolymer, is an interesting material, having a reasonable compromise between its refractive index (1.537) and its V-value (47.0). Since 1997, 1.6 index plastics with V-values of 40 have become available.

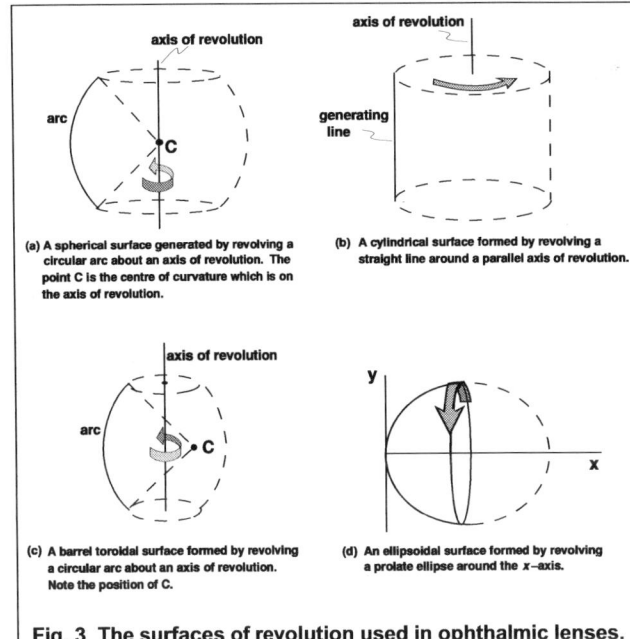

Fig. 3 The surfaces of revolution used in ophthalmic lenses.

2 Lens forms and lens thickness

With respect to lenses, the term *form* refers to the lens shape and thickness. Both the shape and the thickness depend on the surfaces used to make the lens, and the thickness also varies with the lens diameter and lens power. Surface shapes commonly used in single vision ophthalmic lenses are shown in figure 3.

Currently, the most common forms of single vision lenses are the meniscus form, a curved lens with a convex spherical front surface and a concave spherical back surface, and the toric form with one spherical and one toroidal surface. Cross sections of plus and minus versions of these lenses are shown in figure 4. In 1986, the more complex aspherical surface was introduced into the low to medium power plus range. The ellipse is one of a group of curves called conicoids or conic sections from the fact that they can be derived from plane sections of a double cone. Based on the prolate ellipsoid of figure 3(d), plus lenses actually use a deformed conicoid as shown in figure 5

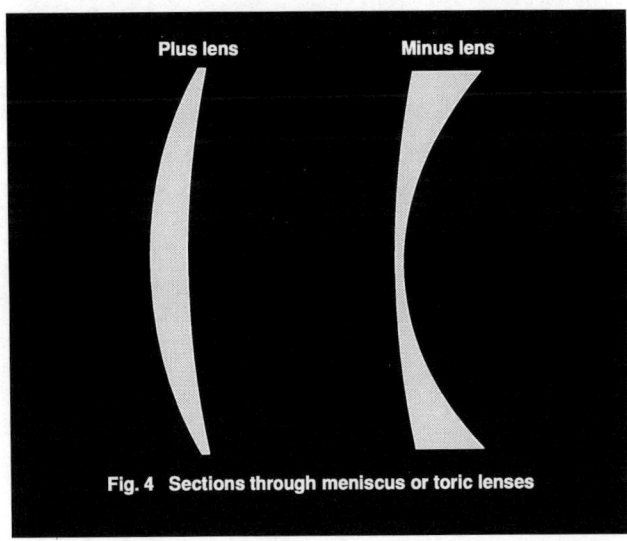

Fig. 4 Sections through meniscus or toric lenses

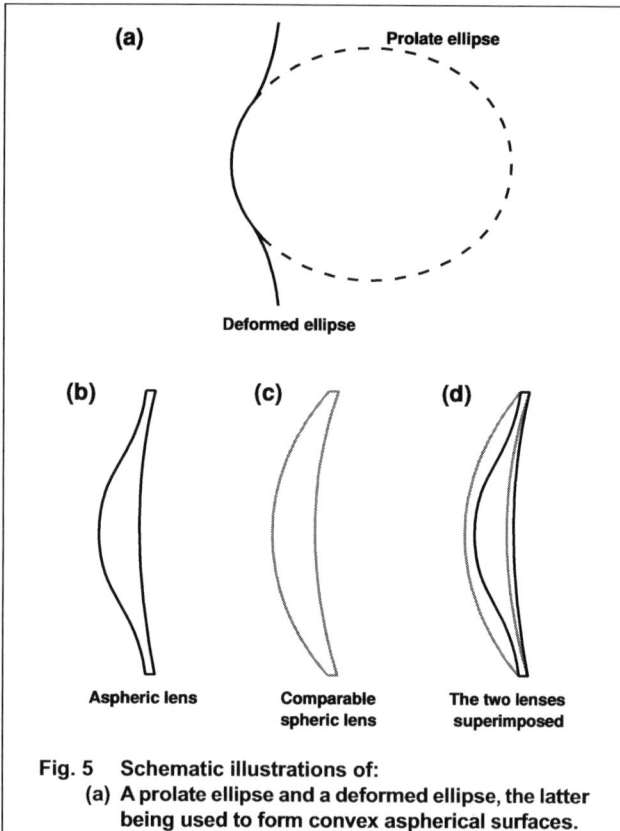

Fig. 5 Schematic illustrations of:
(a) A prolate ellipse and a deformed ellipse, the latter being used to form convex aspherical surfaces.
(b) Comparison of an aspheric and a spheric lens to show the reduced thickness and mass.

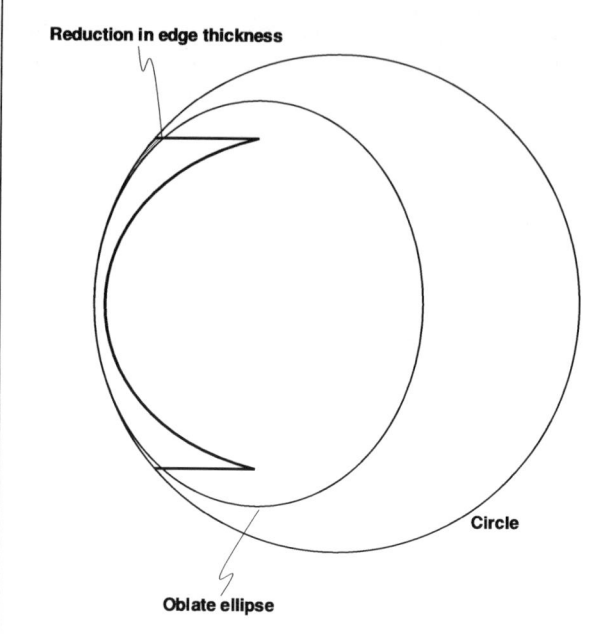

Fig. 6 A schematic illustration of a minus aspheric lens with a front aspherical surface. The shaded area indicates the reduction in edge substance obtained by using an oblate aspherical front surface. Table 4 indicates that the saving in edge thickness is not exactly dramatic for the extra financial outlay the patient will have to find.

This allows a thinner flatter lens to be made in the same power. However, with plus lenses, the main thrust of aspheric lens design is to provide very good oblique visual performance across the whole range of powers, something which is not possible beyond about +7.00 D with spherics. In the process of improving the optical performance of medium to high plus power lenses, aspherics also incorporate some additional benefits; see Table 4.

Table 4 Advantages of aspheric design plus lenses

Good oblique power
No more distortion than spherics
Less oblique astigmatism
Little sensitivity to fitting distance
Slightly less spectacle magnification
Thinner, lighter lens
Noticeably flatter lens with consequently better cosmesis

Aspheric minus lenses became available in low to medium powers shortly after the introduction of plus aspherics. Again the front surface is aspherical and the only reason for going the aspheric route in minus lens design was to produce slightly thinner lens edges. Although useful, the thinning effect with minus aspheric lenses is not very great. Consider, for example, a −6.00 DS lens in spheric and aspheric forms as detailed in Table 5. The saving on a 75 mm diameter uncut is 1.2 mm, which is appreciable. This saving becomes less as the lens power increases because the front surface becomes increasingly flatter with minus spheric lenses in order to accord with best form design for good oblique visual performance. As lenses become flatter they become thinner and so one might expect less saving. For example, with a −10.00 DS lens power the saving would only be 0.5 mm with refractive index and centre thickness the same as in Table 5.

Table 5 Edge thickness of spheric and aspheric −6.00 DS lenses. $n = 1.56$, Ø75mm and $t = 1.5$mm.

Lens	Front surface power	Edge thickness
Spheric	+3.00	10.30 mm
Aspheric	+1.25	9.10 mm

Summary

Aspheric single vision lenses do produce thinner, lighter, and obviously flatter lenses in plus powers, but the saving in edge thickness is not very dramatic in minus aspheric lenses.

Availability of single vision aspherics

Over the period since the introduction of Rodenstock's plus powered Cosmolit CR 39 single vision lens in 1986 virtually all manufacturers have introduced at least one aspheric lens into their range. In the plus range, aspheric lens prices have fallen compared with spheric lens prices and we might be seeing the day when aspherics become the standard single vision lens. They are now available in CR 39, mid-index, and high index plastics, and in a limited range of glass lenses, including 1.6 index photochromic material.

All single vision lenses available in the UK are listed at the end of this paper and the full information is drawn together annually in the *Ophthalmic Lens Availability* file, compiled by Dr A H Tunnacliffe and available from the ABDO.

3 Dispensing minus lenses

The form of a lens affects the oblique visual performance and, although proprietary branded lenses will generally have the correct form, there are occasions when it is essential for the dispenser to have access to lens form data. So, for this reason this section will commence by looking at oblique visual performance of minus lenses. The subsection layout will be as follows:

3.1 Oblique visual performance of minus lenses
    3.1.1   Oblique astigmatism and best form minus lenses
    3.1.1.1 Pantoscopic tilt of the lens
    3.1.2   The effect of transverse chromatic aberration
    3.1.3   The form of toric lenses

3.2 Checking surface powers with the lens measure

3.3 Determining the refractive index of a minus lens

3.4 Full aperture and reduced aperture lenses
    3.4.1   Field of view
    3.4.2   Edge thickness
    3.4.3   Power rings and coatings

3.5 Minus lenses in near vision

3.6 Choice of lenses and frames

3.1 Oblique visual performance of minus lenses

Oblique gaze through spectacle lenses chiefly involves consideration of two aberrations, namely oblique astigmatism and transverse chromatic aberration. Oblique astigmatism is minimised or eliminated by judicious choice of the lens form, whilst transverse chromatic aberration is dependent on V-value.

3.1.1 Oblique astigmatism and best form minus lenses

Oblique astigmatism arises from the asymmetry of refraction of narrow tangential and sagittal fans of rays in oblique gaze. The idea is to choose that form of lens where the oblique astigmatism introduced by the first surface is neutralized by that at the second surface. The theory has been dealt with in many papers over the years and is fully covered in standard texts. Spheric lenses (two spherical surfaces) can be used to produce good oblique performance, although an aspheric lens will have a thinner edge. Table 6 gives the minimum tangential error best form spherics for refractive indices 1.498, 1.523, 1.600, 1.700, and 1.800. The design criteria are that the lenses

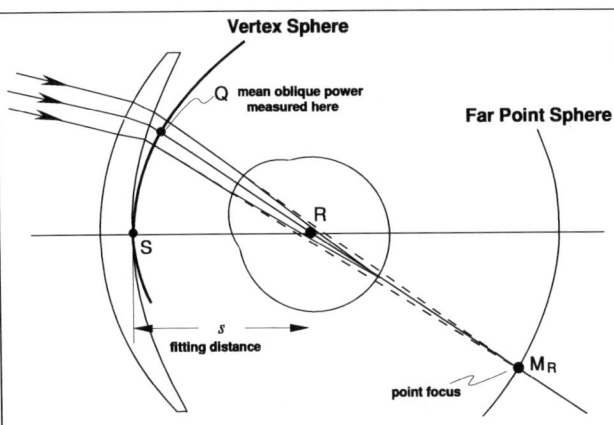

Fig. 7 Illustration of an ideal best form plus lens in which a point focus forms on the far point sphere in oblique gaze. The Oblique Astigmatic Error (*OAE*) and the Mean Oblique Error (*MOE*) are both zero. In this case, after refraction at the eye the rays focus at the foveola. The distance QM_R is equal to the back vertex focal length of the lens, hence the oblique power is measured at Q. R is the eye's centre of rotation.

should be relatively insensitive to fitting distance change and should have acceptably small amounts of oblique astigmatic error (*OAE*) and mean oblique error (*MOE*). Zero *OAE* means that the astigmatism is corrected and zero *MOE* means that the power is corrected for oblique gaze. *MOE* is a power error and states the difference between the Mean Oblique Power (*MOP*) and the back vertex power. If both were zero then the lens would be optically ideal as far as power is concerned, but usually compromises have to be made in lens design and small amounts of these errors are found to be tolerable. Note that the fitting distance is the distance from the back vertex of the lens to the eye's centre of rotation, 27 mm being taken as the average value. See figure 7 for an illustration of fitting distance and far point sphere (shown for a plus lens).

If the *OAE* = 0, then the lens is a **point focal form**, and if the *MOE* = 0 it is called a **Percival design** where the disc of least confusion is on the far point sphere in oblique gaze. A **minimum tangential error design** has the tangential image shell as close as possible to the far point sphere. The latter design is usually less sensitive to the fitting distance, performing well for different patients' varying cornea to eye centre of rotation distances. Because we do not know this distance when dispensing, lenses should have a good oblique gaze performance over a wide range of fitting distances. The principles of the three design philosophies mentioned above are illustrated schematically in figure 8.

Table 6, on page 8, shows Minimum Tangential Error best forms for spheric lenses across the range of refractive indices from 1.498 to 1.8. The calculations for the results in Table 6 were done with computer programs and are exact ray traces with Coddington's equations for oblique astigmatism. In the computations for Table 6, the fitting distance was taken as:
    27 mm for lens powers up to -8.00
    28 mm for lens powers from -9.00 to -14.00
    29 mm for lens powers from -15.00 to -20.00
    30 mm for lens powers from -21.00 to -26.00
    and 31 mm for those powers -27.00 and over.
The reasoning behind this is not a hard and fast rule but that

Dispensing Single Vision Lenses

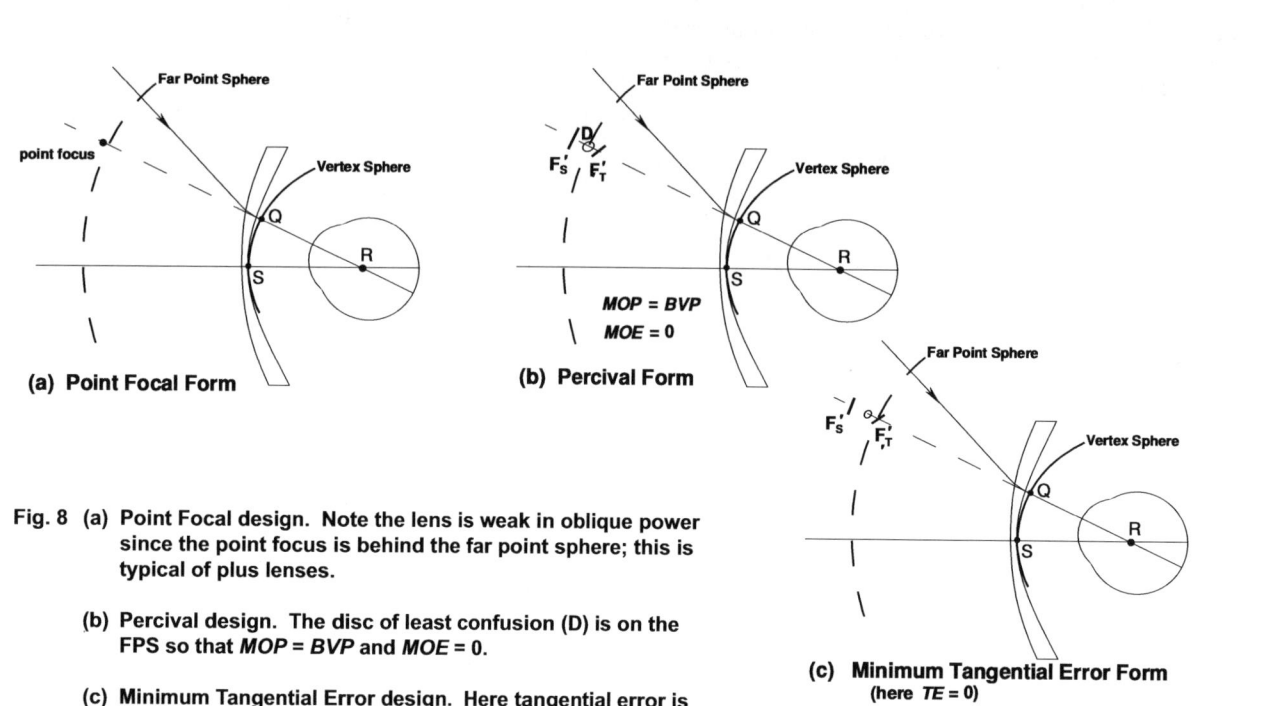

Fig. 8 (a) Point Focal design. Note the lens is weak in oblique power since the point focus is behind the far point sphere; this is typical of plus lenses.

(b) Percival design. The disc of least confusion (D) is on the FPS so that MOP = BVP and MOE = 0.

(c) Minimum Tangential Error design. Here tangential error is shown at its ideal value TE = 0.

Table 6 Minimum Tangential Error Best Form Minus Spheric Lenses.
The table can be used to specify the design when ordering a non-proprietary lens.

Lens Power	Front surface sphere power for the refractive indices below				
	1.498	1.523	1.600	1.700	1.800
−1.00	+5.00	+5.00	+7.00	+8.50	+9.67
−2.00	+4.25	+4.25	+6.00	+7.25	+8.50
−3.00	+3.75	+3.75	+5.25	+6.37	+7.67
−4.00	+3.25	+3.25	+4.50	+5.75	+6.87
−5.00	+2.62	+2.75	+4.00	+5.25	+6.12
−6.00	+2.37	+2.37	+3.50	+4.75	+5.50
−7.00	+2.00	+2.00	+3.00	+4.25	+4.87
−8.00	+1.62	+1.75	+2.50	+3.62	+4.37
−9.00	+1.00	+1.25	+2.12	+3.00	+3.87
−10.00	+0.75	+1.00	+1.75	+2.62	+3.50
−11.00	+0.62	+0.75	+1.50	+2.25	+3.00
−12.00	+0.50	+0.50	+1.12	+1.75	+2.62
−13.00	+0.25	+0.37	+0.75	+1.50	+2.25
−14.00	+0.12	+0.25	+0.62	+1.12	+1.87
−15.00	0.00	0.00	+0.37	+0.87	+1.62
−16.00	0.00	0.00	+0.12	+0.50	+1.12
−17.00	0.00	0.00	0.00	+0.25	+0.75
−18.00	+0.12	+0.12	0.00	+0.12	+0.50
−19.00	+0.50	+0.50	0.00	0.00	+0.25
−20.00	+0.75	+0.75	0.00	0.00	0.00
−21.00	+1.00	+1.25	0.00	0.00	0.00
−22.00		+2.00	+0.50	0.00	0.00
−23.00			+1.50	0.00	0.00
−24.00				0.00	0.00
−25.00				+0.50	0.00
−26.00				+1.00	0.00
−27.00				+2.00	0.00
−28.00				+3.00	0.00
−29.00				+2.00	+0.50
−30.00				+1.50	+0.75

27 mm is about the mean fitting distance for eyes with axial lengths of 24 mm ±2 mm, and that over 8 D error the axial length increases by roughly 2 mm for each 6 D increase of myopia. The centre of rotation probably moves backwards by half this amount, that is, 1 mm for every 6 D increase in myopia.

The higher powers are near enough point focal in performance. At the top end of each power range the power error is less than 0.50 D and there is less than 0.25 D of oblique astigmatism. Powers beyond the indicated ranges have errors outside these amounts. As the power increases in the table, the ocular rotation was reduced to maintain about 35° fixation (macular) half-field of view in object space (on one side of the lens' optical axis).

Beyond the ranges shown and in the absence of computer analysis, it is best to order a plano front surface. The author has seen an example of poor lens form in a very high minus lens where a −31.00 D lens was made in CR 39 material with the front surface −11.00 DS. The oblique performance of this lens for an object half-field of 35° is −34.30 DS / −4.00 DC. Made in 1.7 index glass with a plano front surface, the performance is −31.54 DS / −0.34 DC ! Both lenses were in lenticular form. This illustrates the need for a dispenser to have access to computer analysis, either personally or in the form of published results, in order to specify the form for the laboratory.

3.1.1.1 Pantoscopic tilt and vertical centration

When designing spectacle lenses the optical axis of the lens is taken to pass through the eye's centre of rotation, as indicated in figure 8(a). The reason for this is that there will then be a symmetry of focus for eye rotations in any direction from the optical axis. In that diagram the 'plane of the lens' is vertical, but in practice the spectacle frame, and therefore the lenses, will be tilted in some 10° at the bottom rim. This ensures that the patient does not look under the lenses when looking downwards, but rather sees through them. This tilt is called the *pantoscopic tilt*, the word pantoscopic being derived from *pan=all, scope=view*. Incidentally, this tilt has a useful fitting consequence: the frontal angle of the nose is larger in a plane tilted in towards the cheeks. This increases the vertical component of the reaction force on the spectacle frame bridge and helps to hold up the spectacles more easily. The optical consequence of the pantoscopic tilt is that the optical centres of the lenses must be moved to make the optical axis pass through the eye's centre of rotation, as required in the lens design. Figure 9 illustrates the situation and from this figure we can derive a rule about the vertical centration of spectacle lenses. In the upper part of the diagram, from the situation in the lens design calculations where the plane of the lens is vertical, the lens is tilted to a pantoscopic angle of τ in the lower part of the diagram as a result of fitting the frame. From the triangle shown, the optical centre must be moved downwards by a vertical decentration c_v to ensure the optical axis passes through R. Suppose the pantoscopic angle is 10°, a typical value, and the fitting distance $s = 27$ mm, then

$$c_v = s \tan \tau = 27 \tan 10° = 4.8 \approx 5 \text{ mm}.$$

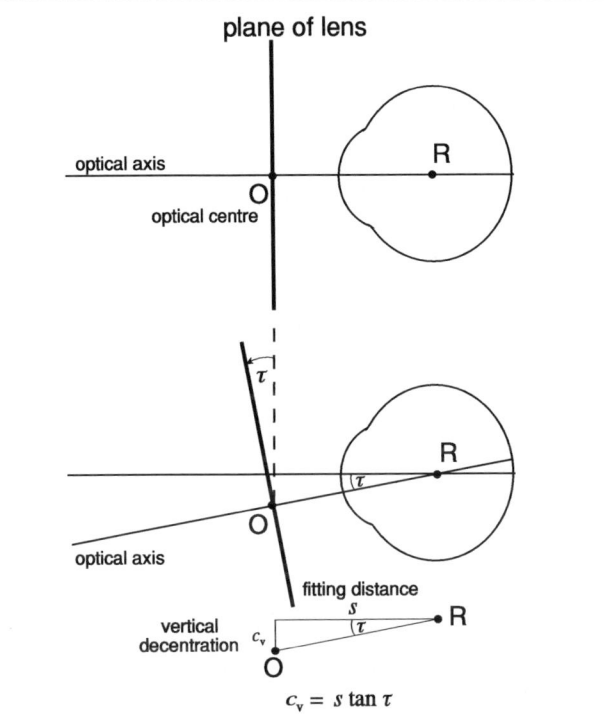

Fig. 9 Relationship between the pantoscopic tilt (τ) and the vertical centration of the spectacle lens. For each 1° of tilt as shown, the optical centre should be moved 0.5 mm downwards from the pupil centre position in the upper part of the diagram, thus ensuring the optical axis passes through eye's centre of rotation R.

That is, the optical centre should be placed 5 mm below the pupil centre with the head erect and the eyes looking straight ahead (the *primary position of gaze*). This leads to the vertical centration rule:

For each degree of pantoscopic tilt the optical centre should be moved 0.5 mm downwards from the pupil centre position in the primary position of gaze.

An exception to this rule occurs with snooker spectacles where the optical centre should be moved upwards because the spectacle frame front is tilted in the opposite sense. This rule ensures that the lens performs to its design criteria and the patient experiences the best possible vision in oblique gaze.

3.1.2 The effect of transverse chromatic aberration

Transverse chromatic aberration (TCA) is the angular dispersion of the colours of the spectrum as depicted in figure 2, where it was called the angle of dispersion. In order to maintain best form performance, inspection of Table 6 shows that the refractive index of the lens should increase as we reach very high powers. In addition, we must not forget the increasing prismatic effect in peripheral gaze with increasing lens powers. This leads to increasing TCA and immediately draws our attention to the need for the highest possible V-value to minimise TCA. V-values can be obtained from Table 2. It is generally advisable to use values not less than 40, although this will not be possible if one opts for a refractive index greater than 1.7 in glass or 1.6 in plastic.

The extra chromatic aberration with lower V-values causes an asymmetrical spread of light in the image of a point object, this spread being in the tangential meridian; that is, in the base-apex line direction of the prismatic effect. This results in tangential blur. High contrast achromatic objects may be seen with coloured fringes in oblique gaze, but more often a patient objecting to lenses with a low V-value will complain of poor vision (blurring) when viewing more typical low to medium contrast objects. This is due to the image contrast being reduced by the tangential blur. The blur is normally reported with oblique distance vision and not with near vision. With single vision lenses, most near vision is undertaken within zones close to the principal axis of the lens where the prismatic effects are smaller. Thus, in near vision, even high contrast objects such as black print on a white background do not generally elicit complaints of poor vision from this source.

TCA is given by the expression $TCA = P/V$ where P is the prismatic effect at the point on the lens and V is the V-value. Since the prismatic effect is $P = cF$, to a very close approximation from Prentice's Rule, then $TCA = cF/V$, from which we see the well-known facts that tangential blur is proportional to the distance c from the optical centre and to the lens power, and inversely proportional to the V-value. That is, in English, the tangential blur is worst in the periphery of high powered lenses, but can be kept to a minimum by using a high V-value material. Also, if the spectacles are fitted as close as possible to the eyes, which minimises the power in the case of minus lenses, the patient will not use a point on the lens quite as far from the optical axis and this therefore helps to minimise the TCA effect.

There is little evidence to suggest how much TCA is tolerable before a patient will complain of blur from this cause. Some authors opt for a threshold of 0.1^Δ, which is an angle of 3.4 arcminutes between the red and blue rays (C and F in Fraunhofer notation). On a -10.00 D lens, this will occur only 3 mm from the optical centre if the V-value is 30, and 6 mm if the V-value is 60. In terms of angular rotation of the eye, these distances on the lens are approximately 6° and 12°, respectively. If the lens power were -5.00 D, and the V-value 60, this would allow a 24° eye rotation without TCA becoming noticeable. This is a fairly reasonable eye rotation so, in practical terms, *over -5.00 D and with lower V-values than that for CR 39 and spectacle crown, the patient ought to be warned of the potential problem of blurring due to TCA*, if they did not already know of it from their present spectacles. The problem might only be expected to cause a patient complaint when changing to a higher index material with its consequent reduction in V-value. This latter well-known relationship is evident when one scans the refractive indices and the V-values in Table 2.

The normal practice of glazing single vision spectacles with the optical centres about 5 mm below the pupil centre position means that the patient is looking above the optical centre in distance vision. The author has come across one patient with -4.00 DS lenses who changed from CR 39 to a mid-index plastic with a V-value of 40 and subsequently noticed slight blur when viewing distant signs. This was entirely due to TCA since it was not present when he tilted his head backwards and looked more nearly through the optical centres. In such cases it may be necessary to glaze the lenses with the optical centres a little higher than usual, and adjust the pantoscopic tilt of the frame accordingly.

Dispensing points from sections 3.1.1 and 3.1.2

1 Over -5.00 D lens power, and with V-values below 58, it is advisable to warn first time wearers of such materials that they may experience some blur in oblique gaze.

2 To optimise oblique vision, the dispenser should ensure that the lens is supplied in best form and the pantoscopic tilt rule is applied.

3.1.3 The form of toric lenses

Jalie has pointed out that minus lenses with a cylindrical element in the prescription give a better oblique performance if the back surface is toroidal. There is also a slight advantage with a barrel surface compared with a tyre form. Nowadays, most lenses, including plus ones, are made with a back toroidal surface.

The aim with best form toric design is to choose that form which produces the same oblique power astigmatism along the base and cross curve meridians. To illustrate this point, consider the example -5.00 DS / -2.00 DC. We would like the oblique power to be the same as the paraxial power stated in the prescription, but if this is not possible then we shall accept equal cylinders and a spherical power as close to -5.00 as possible. Table 7 shows the performance of the four forms; plus barrel and tyre forms, and minus barrel and tyre forms. Inspection shows that the minus barrel form has oblique sphere and cylinder powers most nearly equal to the back vertex power of -5.00 DS / -2.00 DC. The minus barrel form is slightly undercorrected (0.29 D) in the oblique sphere power for the 30° zone along the cross curve, but this would be deemed acceptable. In any case, the minus barrel form is the best of the four. The minus barrel forms for the minus power range of lenses are shown in Tables 8(a) and (b). These tables are for refractive indices 1.523 and 1.700, respectively. The form is given with the front surface sphere curve shown in the table. Such tables enable the dispenser to tailor medium and high powered minus prescriptions for the patient, thus ensuring the best oblique performance. With very high powers, the dispenser may not be able to obtain the exact best form lens; they may be impractical, especially in lenticular form. Also, the prescription laboratory will have a range of semi-finished lenses with base curves (finished sphere curves) only in certain powers. It may be necessary to contact the laboratory to discuss the form in a particular case.

In both Table 8(a) and (b), notice the general pattern of flattening form as both the sphere and the cylinder increase in power. That is, the front surface curve flattens on going from top to bottom of the table, or from left to right. This mimics the general tendency of best form spherics to flatten as the minus power increases. This is a bonus because flatter forms of minus lenses mean thinner edges. Suppose a dispenser were to order a -15.00 DS / -3.00 DC lens in a glass with refractive index 1.700. More often than not, the form would not be specified and the prescription house would be expected to make the lens in 'best form'. What would happen if the lens were made, not untypically, with a minus cylindrical front surface instead of the back toroidal

Table 7 The oblique performance of −5.00DS / −2.00DC lenses made in plus and minus barrel and tyre forms. Ocular rotation 30° and refractive index 1.600.

Form	Oblique Power along base curve	along cross curve
Plus barrel with −11.50 sphere curve	−4.53 DS / −2.17 DC	−4.67 DS / −2.17 DC
Plus tyre with −11.33 sphere curve	−4.57 DS / −2.17 DC	−4.70 DS / −2.17 DC
Minus barrel with −9.62 base curve	−4.93 DS / −1.97 DC	−4.71 DS / −1.97 DC
Minus tyre with −10.25 base curve	−4.84 DS / −1.96 DC	−4.60 DS / −1.96 DC

surface form in Table 8(b)? Computation in the 25° zone shows the lens would have oblique powers of

−14.88 DS / −4.62 DC and −15.26 DS / −2.90 DC

along the cyl power and axis meridians, respectively.

Compare this with the best form with front surface +1.00 DS:

−14.78 DS / −2.93 DC and −14.93 DS / −2.93 DC.

A plus cylinder on the front surface gives the result:

−14.42 DS / −3.62 DC and −14.36 DS / −3.48 DC.

The need for the dispenser to know the best form is immediately evident and Tables 7 and 8 should be consulted in these categories of dispensing.

Table 8(a) Distance best form minus torics for n = 1.523. All lenses have a minus base barrel toroidal surface and the numbers shown in the table are the front surface sphere powers (to the nearest 0.12 D).

Rx sphere	Rx cylinder −1.00	−2.00	−3.00	−4.00	−5.00	−6.00
	Front surface sphere power					
0.00	+7.00	+5.75	+5.00	+3.75	+3.00	+2.50
−1.00	+6.37	+5.50	+4.75	+4.00	+3.37	+2.75
−2.00	+5.62	+5.00	+4.37	+3.75	+3.25	+2.75
−3.00	+5.00	+4.50	+4.00	+3.50	+3.00	+2.50
−4.00	+4.50	+4.00	+3.50	+3.12	+2.62	+2.50
−5.00	+4.00	+3.50	+3.12	+2.75	+2.25	+2.00
−6.00	+3.37	+3.00	+2.62	+2.25	+2.00	+1.75
−7.00	+3.00	+2.50	+2.25	+1.87	+1.62	+1.37
−8.00	+2.50	+2.12	+1.87	+1.50	+1.37	+1.12
−9.00	+1.87	+1.62	+1.37	+1.00	+0.87	+0.62
−10.00	+1.50	+1.25	+1.00	+0.75	+0.62	+0.37
−11.00	+1.25	+1.00	+0.75	+0.50	+0.37	+0.25
−12.00	+0.87	+0.75	+0.50	+0.25	+0.12	0.00
−13.00	+0.62	+0.37	+0.25	0.00	0.00	0.00
−14.00	+0.37	+0.25	0.00	0.00	0.00	0.00
−15.00	0.00	0.00	0.00	0.00		
−16.00	0.00	0.00	0.00			
−17.00	0.00	0.00	0.00			
−18.00	0.00	0.00				
−19.00	0.00					

Table 8(b) Distance best form minus torics for $n = 1.700$.
All toric lenses have a minus base barrel toroidal surface and the numbers shown in the table are the front surface sphere powers (to the nearest 0.12 D).

Rx sphere	Rx cylinder 0.00	−1.00	−2.00	−3.00	−4.00	−5.00	−6.00
	Front surface sphere power						
0.00	+8.50	+9.00	+8.25	+7.25	+6.50	+5.75	+5.00
−1.00	+8.50	+9.00	+8.25	+7.25	+6.50	+5.75	+5.00
−2.00	+7.25	+8.50	+7.75	+7.00	+6.25	+5.62	+5.00
−3.00	+6.37	+8.00	+7.25	+6.50	+6.00	+5.37	+4.75
−4.00	+5.75	+7.25	+6.62	+6.12	+5.50	+5.00	+4.50
−5.00	+5.25	+6.62	+6.00	+5.62	+5.12	+4.62	+4.25
−6.00	+4.75	+6.12	+5.62	+5.12	+4.75	+4.25	+3.87
−7.00	+4.25	+5.62	+5.12	+4.75	+4.25	+3.87	+3.50
−8.00	+3.62	+5.00	+4.62	+4.25	+3.87	+3.50	+3.12
−9.00	+3.00	+4.25	+3.87	+3.50	+3.12	+2.75	+2.50
−10.00	+2.62	+3.75	+3.37	+3.00	+2.75	+2.37	+2.12
−11.00	+2.25	+3.25	+3.00	+2.62	+2.37	+2.12	+1.87
−12.00	+1.75	+2.87	+2.50	+2.25	+2.00	+1.75	+1.50
−13.00	+1.50	+2.50	+2.12	+1.87	+1.62	+1.25	+1.12
−14.00	+1.12	+2.12	+1.75	+1.50	+1.25	+1.12	+0.87
−15.00	+0.87	+1.50	+1.25	+1.00	+0.75	+0.62	+0.50
−16.00	+0.50	+1.25	+0.87	+0.75	+0.50	+0.37	+0.25
−17.00	+0.25	+0.87	+0.62	+0.50	+0.25	+0.12	0.00
−18.00	+0.12	+0.62	+0.50	+0.25	+0.12	0.00	0.00
−19.00	0.00	+0.37	+0.25	0.00	0.00	0.00	0.00
−20.00	0.00	+0.25	0.00	0.00	0.00	0.00	0.00
−21.00	0.00	0.00	0.00	0.00	0.00	0.00	
−22.00	0.00	0.00	0.00	0.00	0.00		
−23.00	0.00	0.00	0.00	0.00			
−24.00	0.00	0.00	0.00				
−25.00	+0.50						

3.2 Checking surface powers with the lens measure

The lens measure, figure 10, is an essential tool if the dispenser is to ensure that lens forms are correct, especially in medium to high powered lenses where poor form can mean poor vision. It may be simply that the dispenser needs to ensure that new lenses match the form of previous prescription lenses, or it may be that he/she needs to check the glazed lenses comply with the order.

The lens measure is calibrated to read surface power when the refractive index is 1.523. For other refractive indices, although the calculation is simple, it is quicker and more convenient to consult a surface power conversion table. Table 9 gives the surface power values for a range of refractive indices. Intermediate values can be found by a linear interpolation.

3.3 Determining the refractive index of a minus lens

It is not unusual nowadays to be confronted in practice with a pair of spectacles with medium to high power lenses and with no previous record of the lenses, as when a patient visits the practice for the first time. It is highly likely that such minus lenses will not be made in a low refractive index material and one needs to estimate the refractive index to be able to order something similar in a new pair. Because minus lenses are so thin in the centre, we can use thin lens theory and state that the lens power is equal to the sum of the surface powers: $F = F_1 + F_2$. However, surface power readings will only be true if we have converted them in a case where the refractive index is not 1.523.

Dispensing Single Vision Lenses

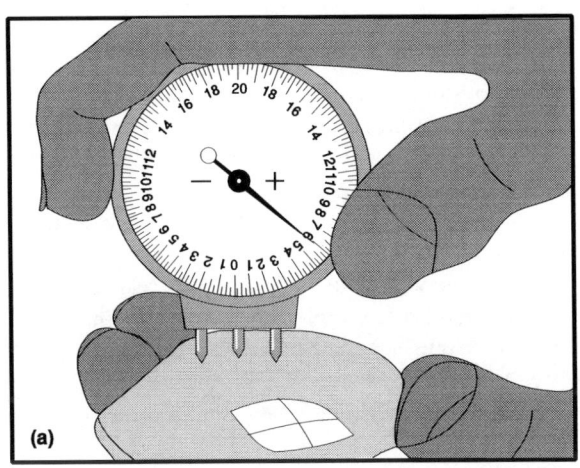
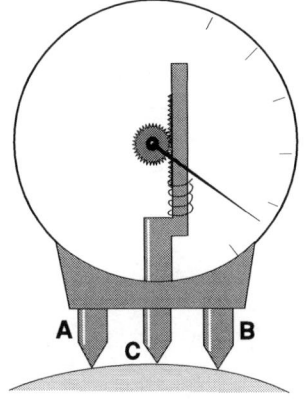

Fig. 10 (a) The lens measure in use on a spectacle lens surface. It is calibrated to read surface powers on 1.523 refractive index material. For other refractive indices a conversion table or a calculation is required.
(b) A schematic illustration of the mechanical workings of the lens measure. The instrument actually measures the sag by the movement of the central leg.

Table 9 Lens measure conversion table. Surface powers on lenses with refractive indices differing from 1.523

Lens Measure Reading	Powers for the refractive indices below					
	1.498	1.560	1.580	1.600	1.700	1.800
0.00	0.00	0.00	0.00	0.00	0.00	0.00
0.50	0.48	0.54	0.55	0.57	0.67	0.76
1.00	0.95	1.07	1.11	1.15	1.34	1.53
1.50	1.43	1.61	1.66	1.72	2.01	2.29
2.00	1.90	2.14	2.22	2.29	2.68	3.06
2.50	2.38	2.68	2.77	2.87	3.35	3.82
3.00	2.86	3.21	3.33	3.44	4.02	4.59
3.50	3.33	3.75	3.88	4.02	4.68	5.35
4.00	3.81	4.28	4.44	4.59	5.35	6.12
4.50	4.28	4.82	4.99	5.16	6.02	6.88
5.00	4.76	5.35	5.54	5.74	6.69	7.65
5.50	5.24	5.89	6.10	6.31	7.36	8.41
6.00	5.71	6.42	6.65	6.88	8.03	9.18
6.50	6.19	6.96	7.21	7.46	8.70	9.94
7.00	6.67	7.50	7.76	8.03	9.37	10.71
7.50	7.14	8.03	8.32	8.60	10.04	11.47
8.00	7.62	8.57	8.87	9.18	10.71	12.24
8.50	8.09	9.10	9.43	9.75	11.38	13.00
9.00	8.57	9.64	9.98	10.33	12.05	13.77
9.50	9.05	10.17	10.54	10.90	12.72	14.53
10.00	9.52	10.71	11.09	11.47	13.38	15.30
10.50	10.00	11.24	11.64	12.05	14.05	16.06
11.00	10.47	11.78	12.20	12.62	14.72	16.83
11.50	10.95	12.31	12.75	13.19	15.39	17.59
12.00	11.43	12.85	13.31	13.77	16.06	18.36
12.50	11.90	13.38	13.86	14.34	16.73	19.12
13.00	12.38	13.92	14.42	14.91	17.40	19.89
13.50	12.85	14.46	14.97	15.49	18.07	20.65
14.00	13.33	14.99	15.53	16.06	18.74	21.41
14.50	13.81	15.53	16.08	16.63	19.41	22.18
15.00	14.28	16.06	16.63	17.21	20.08	22.94
15.50	14.75	16.60	17.19	17.78	20.75	23.71
16.00	15.24	17.13	17.74	18.36	21.41	24.47
16.50	15.71	17.67	18.30	18.93	22.08	25.24
17.00	16.19	18.20	18.85	19.50	22.75	26.00
17.50	16.66	18.74	19.41	20.08	23.42	26.77
18.00	17.14	19.27	19.96	20.65	24.09	27.53
18.50	17.62	19.81	20.52	21.22	24.76	28.30
19.00	18.09	20.34	21.07	21.80	25.43	29.06
19.50	18.57	20.88	21.63	22.37	26.10	29.83
20.00	19.04	21.41	22.18	22.94	26.77	30.59

A minus lens made in 1.523 refractive index material

It is a simple matter to decide whether a minus lens is made in spectacle crown material or not. If the sum of the surface powers gives the same result as the power reading on the focimeter, then the lens is made in 1.523 index material.

A minus lens made in a higher refractive index material

Here the back vertex power reading from the focimeter will not agree with the sum of the surface powers. For example, a lens in 1.7 index material and reading -12.00 on the focimeter will have a sum $F = F_1 + F_2 = -9.00$ using the lens measure surface power readings F_1 and F_2. The reasoning behind this result is met by students in their first year, and the problem will not be laboured here. Suffice it to say that there is a relationship between the true refractive index of the material, the focimeter power reading, and the lens power obtained by summing the surface powers obtained by the lens measure. The method is not applicable to plus lenses because they cannot be considered by thin lens theory, but this is not too troublesome since it is mainly with minus lenses where the problem of determining the refractive index of a lens occurs.

Given the assumption that thin lens theory is sufficiently accurate, and that one can attempt to read the lens measure to the nearest 0.06 D, then it is possible to determine the refractive index sufficiently accurately to be able to distinguish between 1.5, 1.6, 1.7, 1.8, and 1.9 index materials. One cannot however distinguish between 1.56 and 1.58, say. The method is not that accurate.

The calculation results in the formula:

$$\frac{n_{TRUE} - 1}{1.523 - 1} = \frac{\text{lens power by focimeter}}{\text{lens power by lens measure}}$$

If we put 1.6, 1.7, 1.8, and 1.9 for n_{TRUE} in this expression, we arrive at the values in Table 10. Thus, in the example above, the ratio is $-12 / -9 = 1.3$, to one decimal place, and from Table 10 we obtain the refractive index 1.7.

Table 10 Estimating an unknown refractive index

Lens power by focimeter / Lens power by lens measure	Refractive index
1.1	1.6
1.3	1.7
1.5	1.8
1.7	1.9

3.4 Full aperture and reduced aperture lenses

The choice of lens size is influenced by the power of the lens and the decentration required. With minus lenses, it is the temple edge thickness of the lens which most concerns both practitioner and patient, since this is likely to be thicker than the nasal edge. This effect is illustrated in figure 11. The patient does not like to see a thicker edge on new spectacle lenses compared with that on the previous pair. Besides being less cosmetically acceptable, it suggests the eyes are 'getting worse'. Even quite small, seemingly innocuous powers can produce edge thicknesses which are objectionable. For example, one man who purchased a frame in the United States and had it (correctly) glazed over here with his -2.25 spheres failed to understand why the edge thickness came out at an apparently massive 7.5 mm. He had chosen an 80 mm diameter lens size which required 10 mm decentration. The maximum edge thickness in his previous pair had been barely more than 5 mm. Naturally, he objected. This case is a perfect illustration why people should not buy frames without professional advice.

The problem then is to produce spectacles with the best cosmetic appearance. This means minimising edge thicknesses and 'power ring' reflections as much as possible, whilst obtaining a satisfactory field of view. The problem of weight has already been mentioned in connection with the density of the lens material, but lens size and lenticulation[†] also have a bearing on this. The problems will be discussed under the headings of *field of view*, *edge thickness*, and *power rings*.

3.4.1 Field of view in minus lenses

Whether one considers entrance pupil fields of view or the fixation field of view, minus lenses produce an overlap of the fields through and around the lens margin. Figure 12(a) is a standard fixation field of view diagram indicating the overlapping fixation fields at the edge of the lens[‡]. It is apparent that there is an overlap of the field seen through the

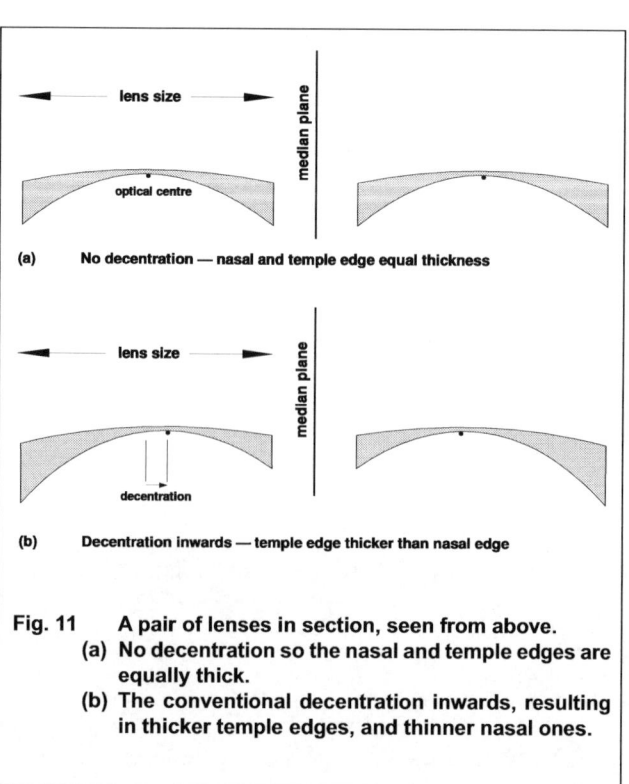

Fig. 11 A pair of lenses in section, seen from above.
(a) No decentration so the nasal and temple edges are equally thick.
(b) The conventional decentration inwards, resulting in thicker temple edges, and thinner nasal ones.

[†] Reducing the optic zone of the lens by thinning the edge. This will be considered shortly.
[‡] The eyes have a maximum field of fixation of 50°, so ocular rotations beyond this amount are impossible, and even this is very uncomfortable. So, the illustration in figure 12(a) is specious. Nonetheless, it is schematically true.

lens and that seen around the edge of the lens. This overlap accounts for the name *ring diplopia*, suggesting the potential for double vision near the edge of the lens. However, it is no exaggeration to say that this is never noticed by patients, at least, not in the author's experience. The reasons are easy to understand. With low myopia and a full aperture lens, the rim is so far from the primary line of sight that it is impossible to turn the eye through the angle required to fixate outside the edge of the lens. Also, with rimmed frames, the rim obstruction would be more noticeable than any ring diplopia. With a 25 mm semi-diameter lens size, the eye would need to make about a 45° duction which is so close to the 50° limit as to be very uncomfortable. In the case of lenticulars, figure 12(b), the margin power is so different from the optic zone power that any vision around the sighted portion is very blurred and diplopia is not therefore noticed. Thus, ring diplopia is unlikely to be observed and is therefore more a theoretical problem.

Incidentally, notice how with minus lenses the field of view is increased in object space, caused by the prismatic effect bending the light round into the eye.

3.4.2 Edge thickness in minus lenses

The strategies for obtaining cosmetically acceptable edge thicknesses are:
Small lens size.
High index lenses.
Aspheric lenses.
Lenticulars, including blended and continuous curve forms.

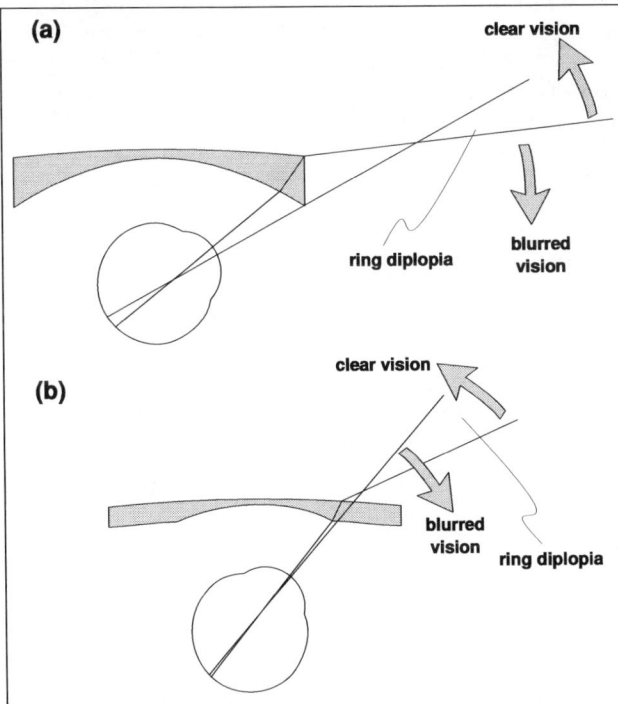

Fig. 12 (a) Ring diplopia at the edge of a minus lens — a theoretical problem. It does not seem to be noticed with large lens sizes, and with lenticulars the difference between clear and blurred vision is so great as to make the blurred vision easily ignored.
(b) A lenticular lens. This is only used for high myopia so the blurred vision through the margin of the lens is easily ignored. In fact, it is of such low contrast that it almost certainly fails to stimulate the retinal contrast detectors.

We have briefly mentioned the edge thickness / refractive index relationship in section 1.1, on page 2. Figure 13 is a diagrammatic representation which immediately illustrates this effect of refractive index. The lenses are accurately drawn cross sections of −10.00 best forms. So, stating the obvious, for technically trained persons, for a given lens diameter *a higher refractive index produces a thinner edge*. It hardly needs stating that smaller lens sizes will produce thinner edges, but in this day of large apertures in spectacle frames it should be emphasised that it is the dispenser's responsibility to warn myopic patients about the edge thickness effect of large lenses. Occasionally, dispensers must be prepared to tell a patient that they will not dispense certain lenses in unsuitably large lens sizes, even if it means the patient (customer?) goes elsewhere.

The first two strategies in the preceding list need no more discussion vis-à-vis edge thickness. But, controlling lens size is also one way of controlling the weight. Another is by choosing materials with a lower density. Figure 14, overleaf, shows some lens weights computed with best forms. The main conclusions to be drawn from these graphs are that:

1. High index glass lenses are not significantly different in weight from spectacle crown lenses.

2. CR 39 lenses are about 40% lighter than glass lenses.

3. Mid-index polyurethane lenses are about half the weight of glass lenses.

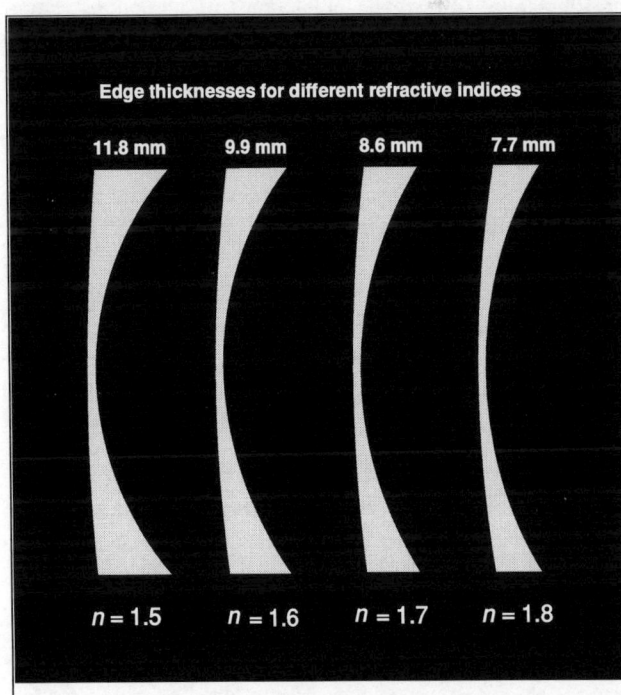

Fig. 13 Computed best form −10.00 D lenses, Ø60 mm, drawn to actual size. The effect of refractive index on edge thickness is vividly apparent. Several manufacturers produce samples like this, which graphically illustrate the point to patients.

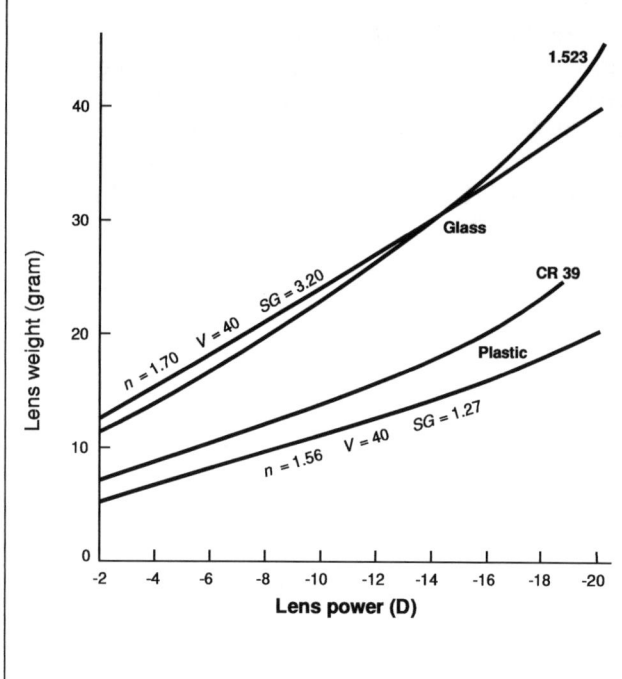

Fig. 14 Lens weights compared for 50 mm diameter lenses. All centre thicknesses are 1.5 mm except for CR 39 which is 2.0 mm. The centre thickness of minus lenses is made thicker in CR 39 material to obtain sufficient stability.

3.4.2.1 Lenticulars

Another way of controlling the edge thickness of minus lenses is the well-known use of *lenticulars*, see figure 15. Round, oval, and profile lenticulars have been with us for a long time. The older types of lenticular design have an unsightly demarcation between the optic zone and the margin. This is obviated by the more recent 'blended' lenticular design. Here, the back surface of a high minus lens is actually made as a continuous surface which still has optic and margin portions, but the two are made to 'blend' together. Several types are available: the Wrobel Super Lenti, the Myodisc, and the Lentilux.

There are three cosmetic advantages of blended lenticulars. Firstly, the edge thickness is much reduced, improving the appearance of the spectacles, reducing the lens weight, and lessening power reflections from the edge. In the case of the Lentilux, the margin is plane, or nearly so, and has a maximum edge thickness not exceeding 5 mm. The mean edge thickness across the power range is only 3.5 mm.

The second advantage of blended lenticulars is that the lens appears very much like a relatively weak powered full aperture lens. Larger lens sizes can be dispensed. Close inspection, unlikely by an observer, is required to notice the change in curvature from the optic zone to the margin. The third advantage is that the minification of the wearer's cheeks and temples is almost totally absent. Figure 16 illustrates this improvement where the right lens is a −15.00 Lentilux and the left one is a full aperture 1.7 index lens of the same power.

There is another, not so apparent advantage of the Lentilux lens. Its rear surface is aspherical over the optic zone and this produces a good optical performance in oblique gaze. Also, the use of an aspherical surface allows a larger optic zone than that obtained with a spherical surface, before blending into the plane margin.

One should be careful to discuss the form of these lenses with the supplier, especially in the higher powers. A cylindrical correction is generally incorporated as a minus or plus cylinder on the front surface, rather than a back toroidal surface. A plus cylindrical front surface gives a better oblique optical performance than a minus cylinder on the front surface of a flat lens (see the example on page 12).

A patient changing from visible lenticulars to one of the blended variety should be warned of some slight adaptational problems. More head movement is required because the usable area may be less than in some visible lenticulars, and certainly less than in full aperture lenses. The author has come across one patient who could not "ride his bicycle as well as in his full aperture lenses", he had to turn his head further to look at traffic behind! Nonetheless, he admitted that this one small disadvantage was outweighed by the markedly improved cosmesis.

Fitting lenticulars

As with lenticulars in general, it is suggested that the optical centre be fitted about 3 mm below the pupil centre (eye in the primary position) which would require a 6° pantoscopic tilt. Fitting the optical centre not too far below the pupil centre reduces the effect of transverse chromatic aberration in distance vision; the patient spends most of his/her time looking through lenses at a slightly lower position than the primary

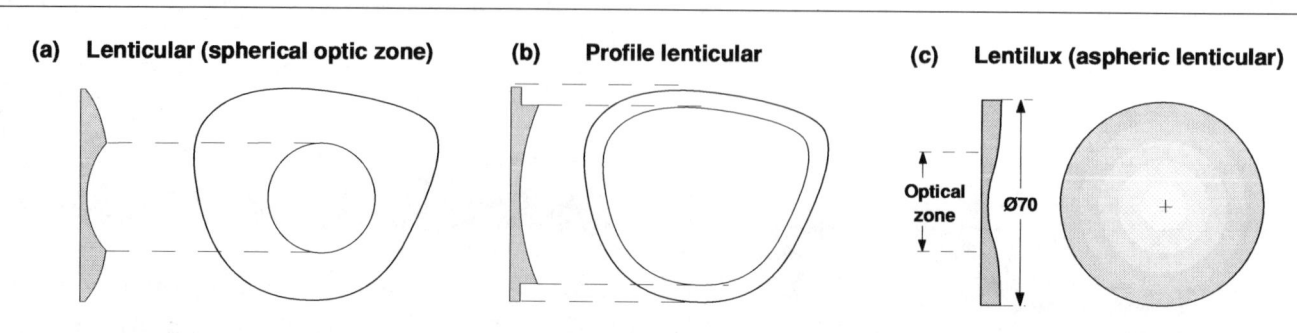

Fig. 15 Forms of lenticular lenses which are designed to reduce edge thickness in minus lenses. Type (c), the aspheric 'blended' type, is the most modern and has certain cosmetic advantages considered in the text.

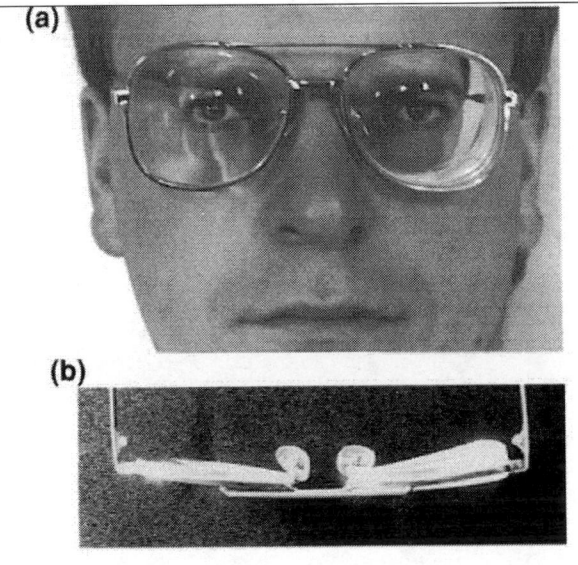

Fig. 16 (a) Comparison of the cosmetic appearance with aLentilux aspheric blended lenticular (RE) and a full aperture 1.7 index lens. Note that the 'minification' of the face with the full aperture lens, and the complete absence of this effect with the Lentilux. Both lenses are multi-AR coated. Glazed samples like this are useful in demonstrating the improved cosmesis to patients; the dispenser can put on the sample to show the effect to the patient.

(b) Edge-on view of the thicknesses.

position of gaze, so the recommended optical centre position is a reasonable compromise for distance and near vision use.

3.4.3 Power rings and coatings

Formed by internal reflections from light arising from and near the edge of the minus lens, these are less troublesome now than in the days prior to the availability of anti-reflection coatings. Figure 17 shows the improved cosmesis with

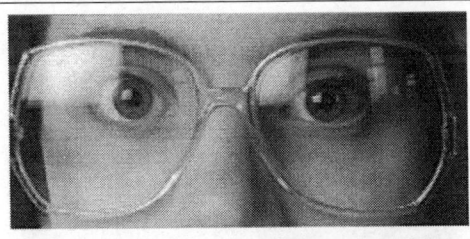
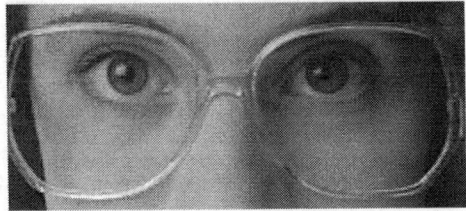

Fig. 17 Demonstration of the advantage of antireflection coating from the observer's point of view: the wearer's eyes are more easily seen and communication via eye contact is more satisfactory. Removal of reflections also prevents this sort of stray light reaching the wearer's retina and reducing his/her retinal image contrast.

Photographs from Siltint's entry in the Ophthalmic Lens Availability File.

antireflection coating. Antireflection coating is advisable for all distance corrections and with close-work spectacles where reflections from the back surface may be troublesome, say from bright walls or windows behind the subject. Nowadays it should be routine to demonstrate the advantages of AR coating during dispensing, especially for myopes. Additional procedures to reduce power rings even further are:

1. Edge coating.
2. Edge painting.
3. Tinting the lens.
4. Mini-bevel (peak bevel, hide-a-bevel).
5. Dark, thick rims for the frame.
6. Blended lenticulars.

All these methods are designed to reduce the amount of light coming from the edge of the lens, and in the case of blended lenticulars, to reduce the extent of the light source, the edge itself.

It is worth reminding ourselves that all **high index lenses should be AR coated** since the surface reflectance is increased compared low index materials. Indeed, for optimum cosmesis and visual performance, all materials should be AR coated. The fraction of normally incident light reflected from both surfaces of lenses of various refractive indices is shown in Table 11. It is evident that uncoated high index lenses reflect a considerable proportion of the incident light.

Table 11 Reflectance from lenses of different indices

Index	Reflectance (%)
1.498	7.8
1.523	8.4
1.600	10.4
1.700	13.0
1.800	15.7
1.900	18.3

The benefits of antireflection coatings are noticeable with the low index materials, so the near absence of reflections in high index materials is appreciated both by the patient and observers alike.

Hard coating

Whilst dealing with AR coating it is worth mentioning hard coating on plastic lenses, both with CR 39 and mid-index plastics. Note that it is inadvisable to refer to these coatings as scratch resistant coatings since they can still be scratched! They can be obtained alone or in combination with AR coatings and tints.

Hard Coat and AR Coat combination

Several manufacturers offer this on their own lenses, although Siltint and Norville can do it on either uncuts or cut lenses. Note that any ***tinting must be done before AR coating***. Table 12 lists the available combinations of hard coat and multi-layer AR coating (MAR).

Table 12 Hard and AR Coat combinations (MAR = multi-AR coating)

Coating		Transmittance (%)	Manufacturer	Application
Crizal	Reflection Free + Hardcoat + water repellent	99.2	Essilor	Most Essilor CR 39 and Ormex Lenses
XARE	Hard/MAR and Cleancote (water repellent)	99.0	Norville	CR 39
SARE	MAR and Cleancote	99.0	Norville	CR 39 and mid-index plastic
HV99	MAR + Hard + water repellent coating	99.0	Hoya	All Hoya plastic lenses
Hard HM	MAR + Hard + water repellent coating	98.6	Hoya	CR 39
HCC	Hard Clear Coat with water repellent layer	98.5	Nikon	All Nikon plastic lenses except 1.74 index
DHCC99		99.0	Nikon	1.74 index lenses
Solitaire	Hard coat, MAR and Clean Effect	99.2	Rodenstock	1.5 and 1.6 index plastics
RLX Plus	Tintable and AR coatable		Signet Armorlite	In-the-mould hardcoat on CR 39 and 1.557 index
CleAR	Multi-AR, hard and water repellent coating	99.6	Signet Armorlite	All Signet Armorlite plastic lenses
Safire	MAR, hard and water repellent coatings	99.2	Silting	All single vision and multifocal plastic lenses
UTMC	Ultra Tough Multicoat with water repellent layer	99.0	Sola	CR 39, Spectralite, Polycarbonate and Transitions
Carat	MAR, hard and water repellent coatings	99.2	Zeiss	Zeiss plastic lenses

3.5 Minus lenses in near vision

Oblique performance in near vision with minus spheric lenses is generally best with a slightly flatter form than for distance vision. When the distance form has reached a plane front surface, in the high minus region, the near vision best form is then slightly minus on the front surface. So why do we not dispense these biconcave forms for reading? The reason is fairly simple; an object space field of view of 20° is generally large enough and it is found from computer analysis that minus distance best form lenses perform adequately for near vision within this zone, so they can be used for both distance and near vision. Consider Table 13, in which the near vision performance of a −6.00 DS lens is shown in the distance and near vision best forms. In this table, the Mean Oblique Image Vergence (MOIV) is the mean of the tangential and sagittal vergences measured on the chief ray at the vertex sphere. The accommodation is measured at the vertex sphere also. Notice that slightly less accommodation is required in oblique gaze than in paraxial use of the lens. This effectivity phenomenon increases with ocular rotation and lens power, so that with a −15.00 lens power and 30° ocular rotation the oblique accommodation is 0.67 D less than the paraxial accommodation. The lens behaves like a Progressive Lens with a weak Addition. The author has seen one patient, a typist aged 48 years, with −8.00 DS right and left, who had old upswept lenses glazed with the optical centres at the pupil centre position. On looking down and to the left she gained a 0.27 D 'Addition' from this oblique effectivity. When fitted with new spectacles with the optical centres in the conventional position, about 5 mm below the pupil centre position, she complained that she could not manage this close work task as well as in the old glasses. So, beware. Occasionally you will find knowledge of this reduced accommodation requirement in oblique gaze with minus lenses will enable you to solve otherwise seemingly insoluble problem cases. You should remember from Visual Optics, that the accommodative requirement of spectacle wearing myopes is less than for emmetropes and corrected hypermetropes along the optical axis of the lens in any case. This oblique effectivity is in addition to that and further accounts for medium and high power minus lens wearers not needing a reading addition as soon as their hypermetropic cousins.

In Table 13, the near vision lens form has zero oblique astigmatic error (OAE) and is 0.37 D flatter. The difference in performance though is hardly noticeable and, together with a similar analysis over the minus range of lens powers, confirms that distance design minus lenses perform well for near vision. Similarly, distance design aspherics perform extremely well for near vision at 20° ocular rotation.

Hence, the only unusual near vision consideration one might occasionally have to make concerns the slight reduction of oblique accommodation, as illustrated in the −8.00 DS example above.

3.6 Choice of lenses and frames

Frame choice is usually simple with low powered lenses. There is little edge thickness problem to worry about unless overlarge lens sizes are used and/or the decentration is excessive. Nonetheless, it is possible to make drastic errors if either the lens size or the decentration is too large, even with very low powers like the −2.25 example on page 14. Table 14 should be helpful, giving edge thicknesses at various semi-diameters for a range of powers and refractive indices. Of course, the table refers to full-aperture lenses. It does not extend into the very high power range since lenticulars are likely to be the only option considered then. The power range is also smaller for the lower refractive indices since it is expected that the dispenser will prefer to use higher index materials beyond the power ranges chosen. In fact, *the choice of index is often determined by the manufacturer limiting the range of certain lenses.*

Table 13   Near vision performance of distance and near vision best form −6.00D lenses.
1.523 index glass, fitting distance 27mm, ocular rotation 20°, object distance 35 cm.

Lens	Front surface power	MOIV	OAE	Paraxial accommodation	Oblique accommodation
Distance design	+2.37	−8.77	+0.03	2.86	2.77
Near design	+2.00	−8.80	0.00	2.86	2.80

For example, the Hoya HL-II 1.56 index spheric plastic lens is only made up to −10.00 (with cyl to +4.00). At this power and 75 mm diameter, with a +1.25 DS front surface, the edge thickness is almost 17 mm! There is little point in producing lenses beyond this power; the need to transfer to a higher index is evident. In Table 14, the centre thickness is assumed to be 1.5 mm for all materials, except for 1.498 (CR 39) where a 2 mm centre thickness was chosen.

Table 14 can be used to estimate the edge thickness of a lens made in different refractive indices. Suppose the distance from the centration point to the furthest point on the rim is 34 mm, as nearly as one can measure, and the lens power is −6.00 D. Then one should choose the −6.00 lenses, move across to the 34 mm semi-diameter column, and read down the edge thicknesses for the refractive indices stated:

Lens power	Refractive index	34 mm semi-diameter edge thickness (mm)
−6.00	1.498	9.9
−6.00	1.523	8.9
−6.00	1.600	8.0
−6.00	1.700	7.1
−6.00	1.800	6.3

Linear interpolations between powers give excellent results since, if the tables were graphed, the graphs would be nearly linear. For example, the table does not give edge thicknesses for −7.00 lenses. By calculation, a −7.00 in 1.700 index material would have an 8.1 mm edge at 34 mm semi-diameter. From the table in the 34 mm column, in 1.700 index material the −6.00 has an edge thickness of 7.1 mm and the −8.00 an edge thickness of 9.0 mm. Halfway between for the −7.00 we predict 8.1 mm!

A further type of interpolation can be made when a lens has a *different refractive index* from those listed in the table. For example, if the refractive index required is 1.56, which is near enough midway between 1.523 and 1.600, and taking the −6.00 D lens power at 34 mm semi-diameter, the interpolated result is

$$\frac{\text{edge thickness for } 1.523 + \text{edge thickness for } 1.600}{2}$$

$$= \frac{8.9 + 8.0}{2} = 8.5 \text{ mm}$$

to one decimal place. The actual result is 8.5 mm!

Edge thicknesses of 16 mm and over were not recorded. It is highly unlikely that neither this thickness nor anything even near it would be acceptable and it is advisable to consider blended lenticulars well before this thickness is reached. The table should be used to decide when it is advisable to change up to a higher refractive index or when to change to lenticulars. The edge thickness criterion used must be the practitioner's decision, helped by looking at the patient's previous spectacles to decide what may be an acceptable limit.

Choice of frame and lenses are somewhat interdependent and revolve around the need to keep lens weight and thickness down whilst satisfying the patient's desire for large modern lens shapes in many cases. It behoves the dispenser to limit the choice of frame to a relatively small lens size when Table 14 suggests the outcome would be too thick a lens edge with full aperture lenses.

Other factors affecting frame choice are the rim thickness, the optical density of the rim material, and the bearing surface of the bridge. The latter simply implies that the area of the bearing surface should be as large as possible to minimise the pressure on the nose. Whilst dealing with this topic it is worthwhile mentioning that display frames should be set-up so that they have an approximately 10° pantoscopic tilt on the face. In this plane the facial frontal angle of the nose is larger than in a fronto-parallel plane so the fitting should be judged with the correct pantoscopic tilt; see figure 18. If a display frame is chosen, and the fitting determined with a zero pantoscopic tilt say, then when the tilt is applied later the frontal angle of the frame will not match the facial frontal angle, being too small and the frame will rest on the corners at the junction of the nasal and lower rims. The result will be a reduced area of frame bridge contact with the nose and a greater than necessary pressure on the nose. Of course, in any individual case, display frames can be tilted more or less than the set-up value to check that the frontal angle alignment will be correct in a finished pair of spectacles. It would be helpful cosmetically, where the lens edge thickness is 6 mm

Dispensing Single Vision Lenses

Table 14   Edge thickness of full aperture minus meniscus spectacle lenses at various semi-diameters. Centre thickness 1.5 mm, except for CR 39 (1.498) material lenses, where 2 mm was chosen.

Lens Power	Refractive index	\multicolumn{9}{c}{Semi-diameters of lens (mm)}
		24	26	28	30	32	34	36	38	40
−2.00	1.498	3.2	3.4	3.7	4.0	4.3	4.6	4.9	5.3	5.7
−2.00	1.523	2.7	2.9	3.1	3.3	3.6	3.9	4.3	4.6	5.0
−2.00	1.600	2.5	2.7	2.9	3.2	3.4	3.7	4.0	4.3	4.7
−2.00	1.700	2.4	2.5	2.7	2.9	3.1	3.4	3.6	3.9	4.3
−2.00	1.800	2.3	2.4	2.6	2.7	2.9	3.2	3.4	3.6	3.9
−4.00	1.498	4.4	4.9	5.4	5.9	6.5	7.2	7.9	8.7	9.5
−4.00	1.523	3.8	4.2	4.7	5.2	5.8	6.4	7.0	7.7	8.6
−4.00	1.600	3.5	3.9	4.3	4.8	5.3	5.8	6.4	7.1	7.8
−4.00	1.700	3.2	3.6	3.9	4.3	4.7	5.2	5.7	6.3	6.9
−4.00	1.800	3.0	3.3	3.6	4.0	4.3	4.8	5.2	5.7	6.2
−6.00	1.498	5.7	6.4	7.1	8.0	8.9	9.9	11.0	12.3	13.6
−6.00	1.523	5.0	5.6	6.3	7.1	8.0	8.9	10.0	11.1	12.3
−6.00	1.600	4.5	5.1	5.7	6.4	7.2	8.0	8.9	9.9	11.0
−6.00	1.700	4.1	4.6	5.1	5.7	6.4	7.1	7.9	8.8	9.7
−6.00	1.800	3.8	4.2	4.7	5.2	5.7	6.3	7.0	7.7	8.5
−8.00	1.498	7.0	7.9	8.9	10.1	11.4	12.8	14.5		
−8.00	1.523	6.2	7.1	8.1	9.2	10.4	11.7	13.2	14.9	
−8.00	1.600	5.6	6.3	7.2	8.1	9.2	10.3	11.6	12.9	14.5
−8.00	1.700	5.0	5.6	6.4	7.2	8.0	9.0	10.1	11.2	12.5
−8.00	1.800	4.5	5.1	5.7	6.4	7.2	8.0	8.9	9.9	10.9
−10.00	1.498	8.3	9.5	10.8	12.3	14.1				
−10.00	1.523	7.5	8.6	9.9	11.3	12.9	14.7			
−10.00	1.600	6.7	7.6	8.7	9.9	11.3	12.8	14.5		
−10.00	1.700	5.9	6.7	7.6	8.6	9.7	11.0	12.3	13.8	15.5
−10.00	1.800	5.3	6.0	6.8	7.7	8.6	9.7	10.8	12.1	13.5
−12.00	1.498	9.8	11.3	13.1	15.2					
−12.00	1.523	8.8	10.2	11.9	13.7	15.9				
−12.00	1.600	7.8	9.0	10.3	11.9	13.6	15.6			
−12.00	1.700	6.8	7.8	8.9	10.2	11.5	13.1	14.8		
−12.00	1.800	6.1	7.0	7.9	9.0	10.2	11.4	12.9	14.5	
−14.00	1.498	11.4	13.4	15.7						
−14.00	1.523	10.3	12.1	14.3						
−14.00	1.600	9.0	10.4	12.1	14.1					
−14.00	1.700	7.7	8.9	10.3	11.8	13.5	15.4			
−14.00	1.800	6.9	7.9	9.1	10.3	11.8	13.3	15.1		
−16.00	1.498	13.3								
−16.00	1.523	12.0	14.4							
−16.00	1.600	10.2	12.0	14.1						
−16.00	1.700	8.7	10.2	11.8	13.6	15.7				
−16.00	1.800	7.7	8.9	10.3	11.8	13.5	15.4			
−16.00	1.498	15.9								
−18.00	1.523	14.3								
−18.00	1.600	11.7	14.0							
−18.00	1.700	9.8	11.5	13.4	15.7					
−18.00	1.800	8.6	10.0	11.5	13.3	15.3				
−20.00	1.600	13.5								
−20.00	1.700	11.0	13.1	15.5						
−20.00	1.800	9.5	11.1	12.9	15.0					
−22.00	1.700	12.4	15.0							
−22.00	1.800	10.5	12.4	14.7						
−24.00	1.700	14.1								
−24.00	1.800	11.7	14.0							
−26.00	1.800	13.0	15.8							

or more, say, to consider covering some of this thickness with the frame rim, rather than supplying rimless or thin metal rims. Also, a dark, opaque rim has the advantage of preventing some light reaching the lens margin and so reducing power ring reflections. No hard-and-fast rules can be made, but the practitioner's judgement must be used and the patient advised accordingly.

4 Dispensing plus lenses

Of patients attending for an optometric examination, if we exclude ametropia between −1.00 and +1.00, hypermetropia accounts for almost three-quarters of the cases[†]. So, we might expect to be dispensing three times as many plus lenses as minus ones. With the virtual demise of aphakia since the intraocular lens became *de rigeur* following cataract surgery, we dispense far fewer high plus powered lenses nowadays. Nevertheless, we still have some aphakic patients and naturally occurring high hypermetropic and reading corrections do occur, although in probably fewer than 5% of dispensings. For discussion purposes, the author will define low, medium, high, and very high plus power ranges as follows:

	Hypermetropia		
Low	Medium	High	Very high
0.25 to 2.75	3.00 to 6.00	6.25 to 9.00	over 9.00

4.1 Effect of form and diameter on lens thickness

As with minus lenses, plus lenses have the same problem with regard to weight and thickness, except here it is the centre thickness rather than the edge thickness which is the problem. The larger the lens, the greater the thickness and the weight. From the cosmetic point of view, plus lenses become more bulbous as they increase in power and diameter. Figure 19 illustrates the effect of lens form on lens thickness with three best form spherics and an aspheric, all +6.00 D in power. The improved cosmesis with a plus aspheric lens is evident from this figure. So, *plus aspherics allow us to reduce weight, thickness, and the bulbousness of lenses compared with spherics.*

Further reduction in centre thickness and sagittal height is possible with higher refractive indices. For example, with 1.56 index plastic, there is a reduction in centre thickness of about 1 mm, compared with the CR 39 lenses in figure 19. Computed figures for such a lens give

Aspheric ($n = 1.56$) **Sagittal height** **Centre thickness**
    8.6 mm   6.2 mm

So it is worth going down the higher refractive index route. There are now several 1.6 index materials with 40 to 42 V-values available.

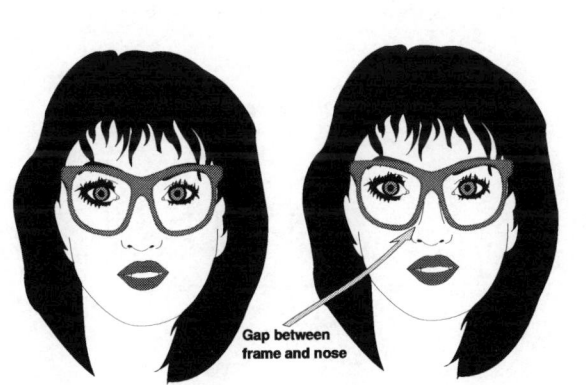

Fig. 18 In those cases where the pantoscopic tilt is determined solely by the need to prevent the patient looking under the lower rim, then the frame fitting should be determined with the correct tilt. This ensures a match is obtained between the nasal bearing rims and the nose, thus maximising the area of the bearing surface.

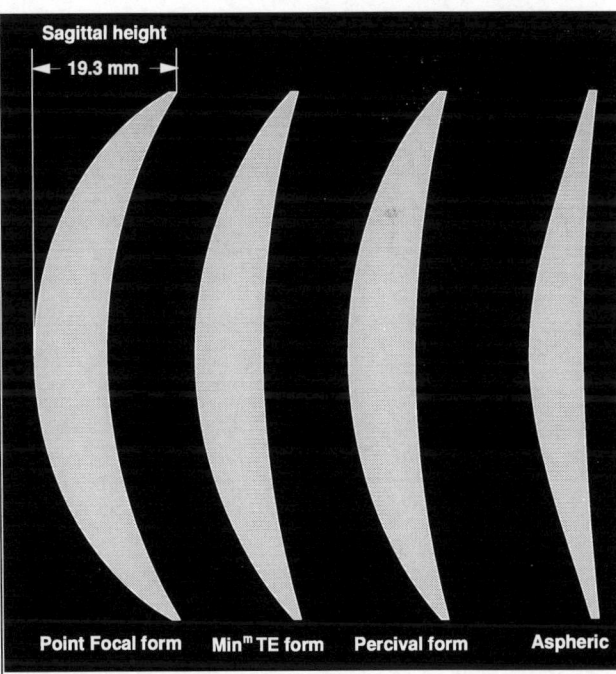

Fig. 19 Full scale sections through three best form spherics and an aspheric lens. Powers +6.00D, diameters 70 mm, material CR 39. The sagittal heights and centre thicknesses are as follows:

Lens	Sagittal height (mm)	Centre thickness (mm)
Point focal	19.3	10.5
Minimum TE	14.4	9.2
Percival	13.2	9.0
Aspheric (CR 39)	9.1	7.1

† From A G Bennett's 1965 analysis of Ministry of Health figures.

4.2 Uncut sizes, finished lenses, and lens thickness

Unlike minus lenses, where if we order an uncut size too large[‡] the excess material is cut away in the glazing process, this does not happen with plus lenses. Consider figure 20 which illustrates the problem with plus lenses. These diagrams illustrate the minimisation of lens thickness achieved with an uncut of just the right diameter. *It is absolutely essential for the dispenser to order the minimum sized uncut from which the lens can be cut.* This ensures the lightest and thinnest version of the chosen lens type and, since bigger uncuts are more expensive, it also guarantees the least expensive uncut of this type from which the job can be glazed.

Because aspheric lenses are flatter than spherics, there is less need to curve the upper and lower rims of the frame to match the lens. This is apparent by implication in figure 20 where the temple side of the rim is seen to be lower (bent further backwards) from the position of the nasal rim. This makes aspherics easier to glaze in thick metal rims.

4.3 Plus aspherics have a shallow back curve

On the whole, plus aspherics have about a 2 dioptre flatter back surface than a similarly powered Percival form spheric lens. In an uncoated aspheric this produces a large reflected image which is especially noticeable by an observer when the wearer is facing a window. Such reflections prevent the observer seeing the wearer's eyes, so eye contact is lost and the observer finds this disturbing. It follows that *a multi-AR coating should be advised with all aspherics*, and this is no doubt why a lot of these lenses come with an antireflection coating as standard.

There are certain *precautions one must take when heating frames with AR coated plastic lenses*. Because of the difference between the thermal coefficient of expansion of the lens material and the coating, it is necessary to take special care to avoid coating cracks and lens deformation when putting plastic lenses into frames, or when adjusting the glazed frame with heat.

- ❑ Do not expose lenses to high temperatures when fitting and adjusting with the frame heater. If it is likely to require a lot of heat to adjust the frame, remove the lens on the side being adjusted.
- ❑ Do not heat the first lens when fitting the second one.
- ❑ Adjust the frame curve as much as possible before fitting the lens.
- ❑ Use accurate formers and check for excessive strain.
- ❑ Check the surface curves of glazed plastic lenses for warping caused by glazing strain. Warping will cause irregular refraction and blur.
- ❑ Advise patients not to leave the lenses in direct sunlight, such as on a dashboard.
- ❑ Advise patients not to wear the lenses in a sauna.

4.4 Centration of single vision lenses

Statements about centration, the placement of the optical centre, relate to both plus and minus lenses. The requirement for good optical performance is that the vertex distance must be correct to provide the necessary vergence at the eye when it looks along the optical axis of the lens, and the optical axis should pass through the eye's centre of rotation to ensure that the lens performs to its design specifications in oblique gaze. Figure 21 shows the correct and incorrect optical axis and optical centre settings, as described in the diagram and the legend.

Horizontal centration of the optical centre should therefore match the monoPD for distance vision, and vertical centration depends on the pantoscopic tilt according to the

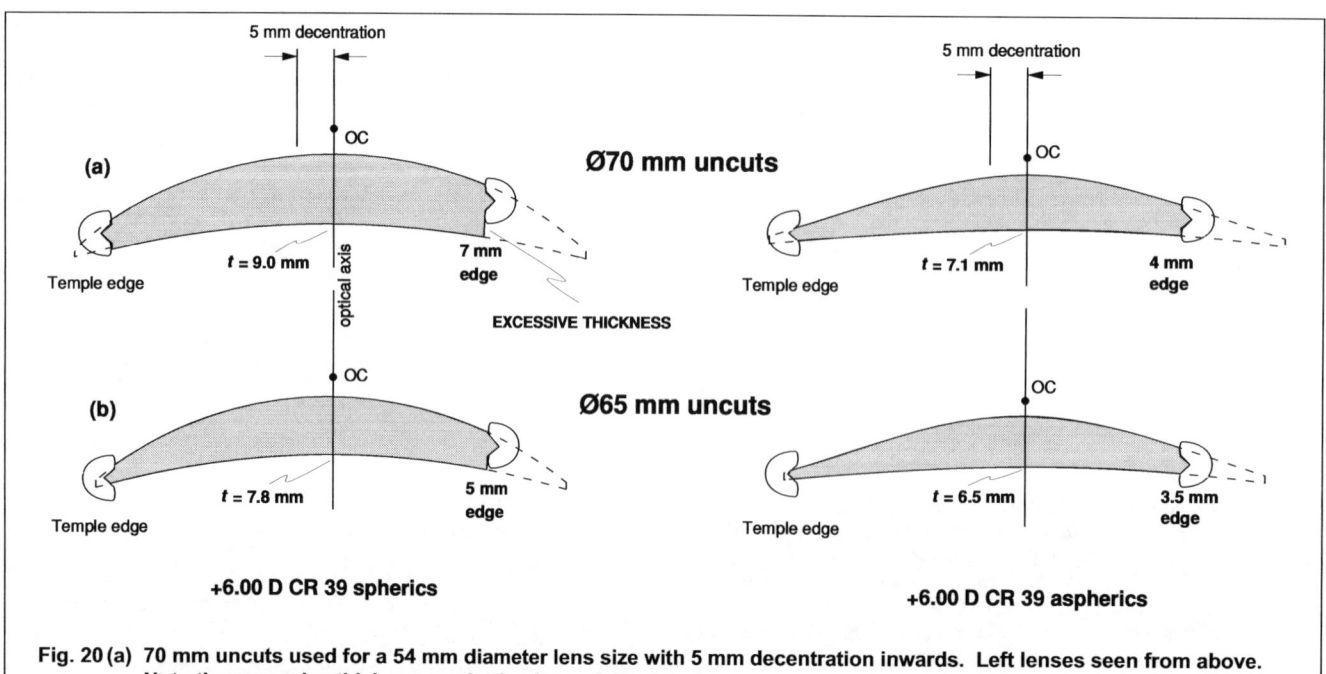

Fig. 20 (a) 70 mm uncuts used for a 54 mm diameter lens size with 5 mm decentration inwards. Left lenses seen from above. Note the excessive thickness on both edges of the spheric.
(b) In the case of the spheric, note the reduction in thicknesses with a 65 mm uncut diameter. The saving in edge thickness in the case of the 65 mm aspheric uncut is less dramatic, but the lens is nonetheless thinner overall.

[‡] Although the extra material is removed in glazing, the oversized uncut will have cost more than one of the optimum size, so the dispenser should still endeavour to determine the correct size.

rule on page 9, repeated here for convenience:

For each degree of pantoscopic tilt the optical centre should be moved 0.5 mm downwards from the pupil centre position in the primary position of gaze.

For spherics and aspherics alike it is important to place the optical centre so that the optical axis of the lens agrees with the pantoscopic tilt. However, aspherics are more sensitive to tilt and decentration errors than spherics, as can be seen from the results below for a +6.00 BVP measured in the +30° zone (ocular rotation upwards). +10° tilt is too large a pantoscopic angle by this amount, and +5 mm decentration is 5 mm too much decentration downwards. The results give the Mean Oblique Error (MOE), which is how much the mean power departs from +6.00 DS, and the Oblique Astigmatic Error (OAE) which ideally should be zero.

	Aspheric		Spheric	
	MOE	OAE	MOE	OAE
normal	+0.03	+0.28	−0.01	+0.34
+10° tilt	−0.07	+0.59	+0.20	+0.83
−10° tilt	−0.15	−0.01	−0.07	+0.12
+5 mm dec	−0.99	−1.19	−0.12	+0.26
−5 mm dec	+0.52	+0.86	+0.25	+0.58

In this example, except for the +10° tilt, the aspheric's errors are greater than the spheric's. These are large tilt and decentration errors and, hopefully, would not occur in practice, but they do illustrate the need for careful centration, more especially with aspherics. The effects increase with lens power so, as always high powered lenses are likely to cause more problems unless care is taken with centration and pantoscopic tilt.

4.5 Prescribed prism

Whenever possible with spheric lenses we obtain prescribed prism by decentration. This gives the same optical performance as having the prism worked. In both cases, it is assumed that the extra thickness is glazed to the back of the frame which is the same as saying the back surface has been tilted; see figure 22. If we were to decentre aspheric lenses to obtain prescribed prism, the vertex of the aspherical surface would no longer occupy the position assumed when designing the lens. During the design the optical axis of the lens is assumed to pass through the eye's centre of rotation. This obviously places the vertex of the aspherical surface such that the optical axis of this surface passes also passes through the centre of rotation. However, if we were to decentre the lens for prismatic effect, the vertex of the aspherical surface would no longer occupy a position in which symmetry occurs for ocular rotations on opposite sides its optical axis. To illustrate the effect of decentring an aspheric lens, compared with having prism worked, let us look at 3 D base down obtained by both methods. The

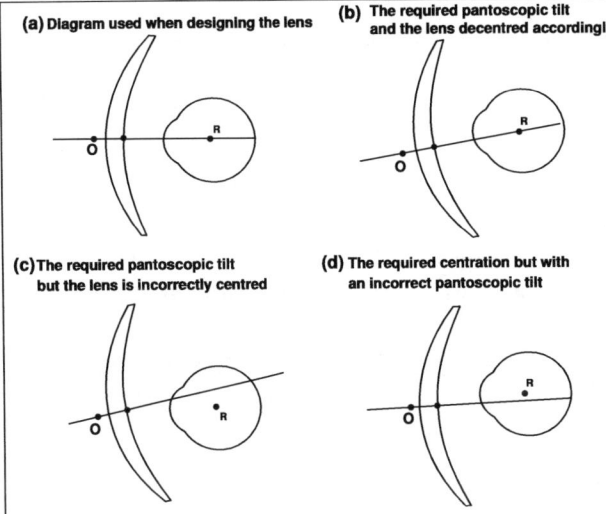

Fig.21 (a) The lens position when lens design is being considered. O is the optical centre. R is the eye's centre of rotation.
(b) The optical axis position when a pantoscopic tilt has been applied.
(c) The required pantoscopic tilt but the optical centre is incorrectly positioned.
(d) The required optical centre position but the pantoscopic tilt is incorrect.

results are shown for a +6.00 lens in the following listing.

Vertical Ocular Rotation	No prism sph / cyl	Decentred for 3^Δ sph / cyl	Worked for 3^Δ sph / cyl
+30°	+5.77 / +0.21	+6.04 / +0.74	+5.83 / +0.09
+20°	+5.91 / +0.10	+6.09 / +0.44	+5.94 / +0.02
+10°	+5.98 / +0.03	+6.07 / +0.18	+5.98 / +0.01
0°	+6.00 / 0.00	+5.97 / +0.02	+6.00 / +0.01
−10°	+5.98 / +0.03	+5.72 / +0.15	+5.96 / +0.09
−20°	+5.91 / +0.10	+5.50 / +0.22	+5.87 / +0.22
−30°	+5.77 / +0.21	+5.33 / +0.28	+5.71 / +0.37

It is apparent from the above results that on looking away

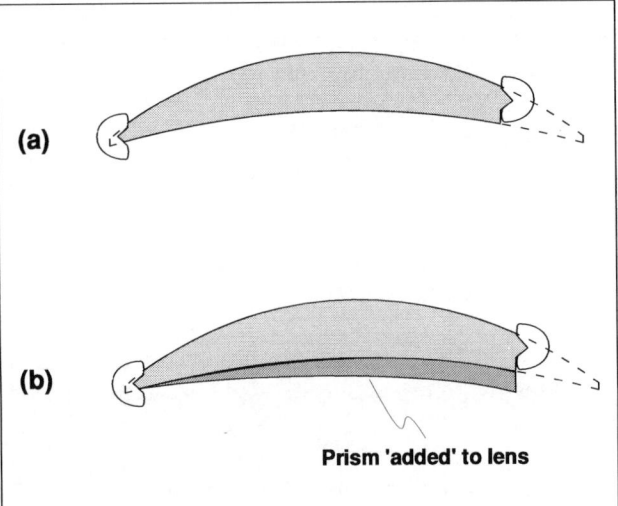

Fig. 22 (a) A decentred lens without prescribed prism.
(b) The lens with prescribed prism, shown in darker shading to illustrate the manner in which it is glazed. In effect, the back surface is tilted.

from the base direction (positive ocular rotations), the oblique astigmatic error is worse in the decentred lens, whereas on looking towards the base direction the sphere power is mostly in error. These deductions can be seen more easily if we subtract the 'no prism' performance from the two cases producing the prism. For example, in the first row (+6.04 / +0.74) − (+5.77 / +0.21) gives an error of +0.27/+0.53 for the lens with 3^Δ produced by decentration. These deductions are shown in the following table.

Vertical Ocular Rotation	No prism sph / cyl	Difference between prism and no prism	
		Decentred for 3^Δ sph / cyl	Worked for 3^Δ sph / cyl
+30°	+5.77 / +0.21	+0.27 / +0.53	+0.06 / −0.12
+20°	+5.91 / +0.10	+0.18 / +0.34	+0.03 / −0.08
+10°	+5.98 / +0.03	+0.09 / +0.15	0.00 / −0.02
0°	+6.00 / 0.00	−0.03 / +0.02	0.00 / −0.02
−10°	+5.98 / +0.03	−0.26 / +0.12	−0.02 / +0.06
−20°	+5.91 / +0.10	−0.41 / +0.12	−0.04 / +0.02
−30°	+5.77 / +0.21	−0.44 / +0.07	−0.06 / +0.16

It is now quite evident from these results that the lens with the worked prism has a better performance than the decentred one: the errors or departures from the no prism case are more nearly zero for the worked prism. We can therefore conclude:

Prescribed prism in aspherics must be worked for optimum performance of the lens.

The differences between the two cases are less with lower amounts of prisms, but we should nevertheless strive to achieve the best performance by having prism worked on aspheric lenses.

4.6 Single vision lenses solely for near vision

There is a difference of opinion between manufacturers about inward decentration of aspheric lenses for near vision. With spheric lenses we normally decentre the optical centres inwards to account for the right and left visual axes converging to fixate an object for near vision; see figure 23. In practice, one either measures the Near Centration Distance (NCD) directly, or one can determine it from a table of interpupillary distances (PDs) and working distances. From figure 23, it is evident that the NCD is dependent on PD, working distance w, and the fitting distance s, as shown in the formula which is simply derived from similar triangles in the figure.

Table 15 lists NCDs for working distances from 25 cm to 50 cm for PDs in two millimetre steps from 54 to 76 mm.

As an example, a patient with a PD of 64 mm, and a working distance of 35 cm, has an NCD of 59 mm, so each lens for near vision would be decentred inwards
$$(64-59)/2 = 2\tfrac{1}{2}\ \text{mm}^\dagger.$$

† Note, in passing, it is conventional in practice to write half millimetres and half prism dioptres as proper fractions.

Table 15 Near Centration Distance (NCD) as a function of interpupillary distance (PD) and working distance. Results to the nearest millimetre.

	Working distance (cm)						
PD	20	25	30	35	40	45	50
54	48	49	50	50	51	51	51
56	49	51	51	52	52	53	53
58	51	52	53	54	54	55	55
60	53	54	55	56	56	57	57
62	55	56	57	58	58	58	59
64	56	58	59	59	60	60	61
66	58	60	61	61	62	62	66
68	60	61	62	63	64	64	65
70	62	63	64	65	66	66	66
72	63	65	66	67	67	68	68
74	65	67	68	69	69	70	70
76	67	69	70	71	71	72	72

Decentration for near vision lenses is designed to allow the eyes to look through the optical centres at the fixation point, as shown in figure 24, and assuming equal powered right and left lenses, to experience zero horizontal differential prism when looking at other object positions. However, such decentration means that the optical axes do not pass through the centres of rotation (R), and one needs to ask whether this upsets the lens performance for near vision.

Plus lenses will incorporate some base out prism effect if near vision lenses are centred for distance rather than near vision, and this may or may not be acceptable by the patient. One must not forget that patients under 45 years of age use lenses for near vision which are centred for distance vision, anyway! But, disregarding this last point, how do the oblique performances of near vision aspherics compare in lenses centred for distance with similar lenses centred for near vision? In the results below, ΔA_{vs} is the difference between the accommodation required in oblique gaze and paraxial gaze. OAE is the Oblique Astigmatic Error.

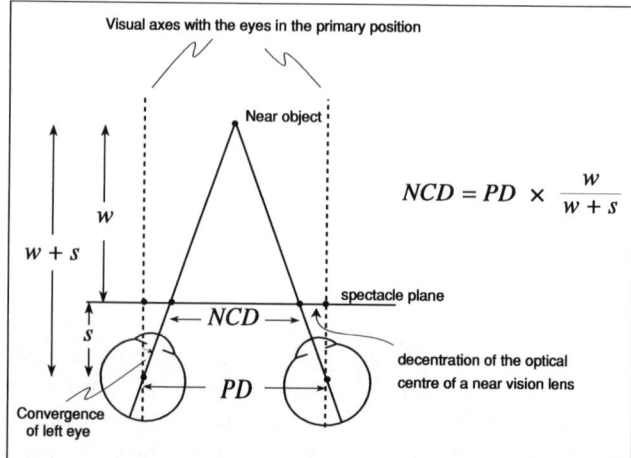

Fig. 23 The Near Centration Distance (*NCD*) as a function of the working distance (*w*), the fitting distance (*s*), and the interpupillary distance (*PD*).

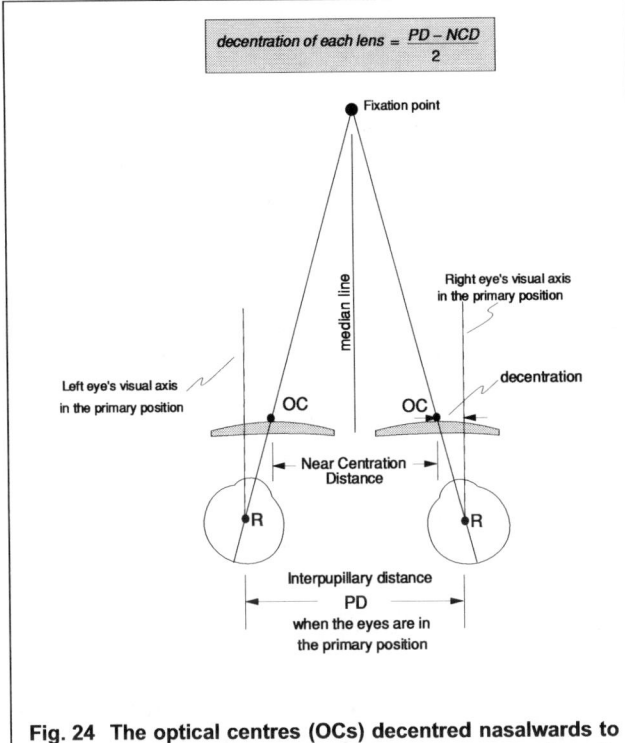

Fig. 24 The optical centres (OCs) decentred nasalwards to allow the visual axes to experience zero prismatic effect for the fixation point on the median line.

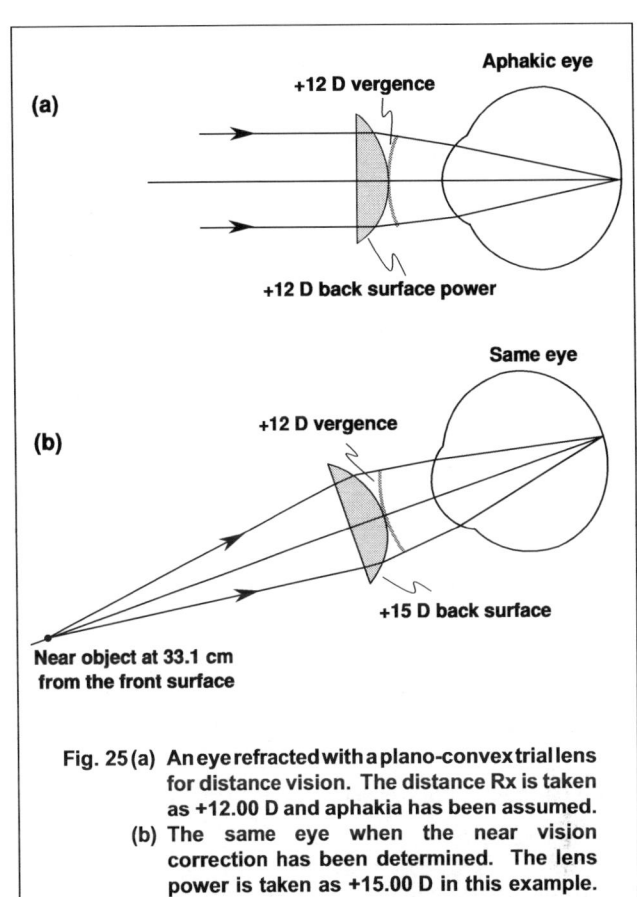

Fig. 25 (a) An eye refracted with a plano-convex trial lens for distance vision. The distance Rx is taken as +12.00 D and aphakia has been assumed.
(b) The same eye when the near vision correction has been determined. The lens power is taken as +15.00 D in this example.

Comparison of the effect of distance centred versus near centred plus aspheric lenses for near vision. The eye is rotated 20° nasalwards and the object is 37 cm from the front surface of the lens, measured along the chief ray. ΔA_{vs} is the difference between the accommodation looking along the axis and accommodation with 20° ocular rotation. Ideally, ΔA_{vs} and the Oblique Astigmatic Error (OAE) should be zero.

	Centred for distance		Centred for near	
BVP	ΔA_{vs}	OAE	ΔA_{vs}	OAE
+3.00	+0.05	−0.02	−0.01	+0.05
+6.00	+0.15	−0.05	+0.02	+0.09
+9.00	+0.17	−0.03	+0.04	+0.11
+12.00	+0.15	+0.09	+0.07	+0.14

Inspection of the table above shows very little difference between the two sets of results. Each of the Oblique Astigmatic Errors (OAE) is negligible and the decentred lens requires very slightly less accommodation than the lens centred for distance. Therefore, the rule is the same as for spherics:

Decentre to match the near centration distance.

4.7 High plus lenses in near vision

A problem of effectivity arises with high powered plus lenses for near vision. During the refraction a thin, probably plano-convex lens will be used in the trial frame for near vision. Consider a case of an aphakic patient for whom a +15.00 D power is obtained with such a trial lens. The convex surface of the trial lens faces the eye and its centre thickness is 4 mm. Assuming the distance Rx is +12.00 D at a vertex distance of 10 mm, then the near point object will be held 33.1 cm from the front surface of the +15.00 D reading lens to obtain a clear retinal image; see figure 25.

Now suppose the reading lens dispensed is a +15.00 D spheric lenticular with a back surface power of −3.00. Putting the object point at 33.1 cm from the front surface of the lens, measured along the chief ray at 10° to the principal axis, the Mean Oblique Image Vergence (MOIV) is +11.51 D instead of +12.00 D, with an OAE of +0.17 D. This means the lens is undercorrected by 0.49 D. That is, a Near Vision Effectivity Error (NVEE) exists. Ordering a +15.50 D lens with the same back surface power gives a MOIV = +11.99 D, near enough to the +12.00 D required for a clear retinal image with the object at the patient's preferred distance of 33.1 cm from the front surface. This near vision effectivity error, resulting in the need for additional plus power in the dispensed lens, is entirely due to the difference between the lens forms used for the test and the finished spectacles. The problem is only significant with reading lens powers of +8.00 D and over. In these cases we must therefore adjust the power obtained using the trial lens and it is for the dispenser to ensure that the optometrist has already done this, or to apply the correction himself after ensuring that it has not already been done by the prescriber.

Table 16 allows us to obtain the correction value without too much effort.

Dispensing Single Vision Lenses

Table 16 Near vision effectivity compensation:

order value = trial lens near Rx + correction value.

Trial lens Rx for near	Correction value for the stated Add		
	Add 2.00	Add 2.50	Add 3.00
+8.00			
+8.50			
+9.00			+0.25
+9.50			
+10.00		+0.25	
+10.50	+0.25		
+11.00			
+11.50			
+12.00			
+12.50			
+13.00			+0.50
+13.50			
+14.00		+0.50	
+14.50			
+15.00			
+15.50	+0.50		
+16.00			+0.75

The values in Table 16 relate to a fitting distance of 28.5 mm for Rodenstock Perfastar aspheric lenses and convexo-plane trial lenses, but are applicable to a spheric lens as well.

Rodenstock data.

What happens if the correction for NVEE is not made?

In the above example, if the lens is ordered as a +15.00 instead of the corrected lens +15.50, then the patient must move the object further away to obtain a clear image. Again, calculation shows that the object would have to be moved about 7 cm further away. If this is inconvenient for the patient, who may have a particular visual task which is more comfortably executed at the preferred distance of about 33 cm, then not compensating the dispensed lens for the NVEE would probably produce a complaint. On the other hand, many such patients have 6/6 acuity or better, and would still be able to read N5 at 40 cm working distance, the distance at which clear vision would be obtained in an uncompensated lens. So, unless there is a particular task distance involved, a patient is likely to accept an uncompensated lens without complaint. Nevertheless, the dispenser should compensate all reading lenses with powers over +8 D.

4.8 Field of view in high plus single vision lenses

The field of view with high plus lenses is markedly reduced because of the large prismatic effect at the margin of the seeing area. For example, consider a plus lenticular as shown in figure 26. Notice how in (a) the ray through the centre of rotation makes a relatively large angle of 35.5° when it enters at the margin of the optic zone. In object space, however, the fixation field of view on one side of the axis is reduced to 23.4° and there is a region in which objects cannot be seen by fixation. This region is called a ring scotoma because it is ring shaped. This is not to say that objects are not visible in this region, because if we consider the field of half illuminance it extends to about 41°, although objects from about 23° to 35° cannot be fixated. This is often quoted as a problem with high plus lenses, although patients seem not to complain about it. Evidently, they have to turn their heads more than usual, and this is how they cope with it. When aphakia was the optical approach of dealing with cataract, before the intraocular lens became the standard procedure, then there was a significant proportion of first time high plus lens wearers, and explaining about ring scotoma might have been important to help the patient adapt to the lenses. Aphakia is now rare and first time high plus lens wearers are consequently rare too. Nevertheless, the dispenser should be aware of ring scotoma with plus lenses. The effect is likely to be less noticeable anyway nowadays because we would dispense aspherics and these lenses have a reduced ring scotoma; see figure 27.

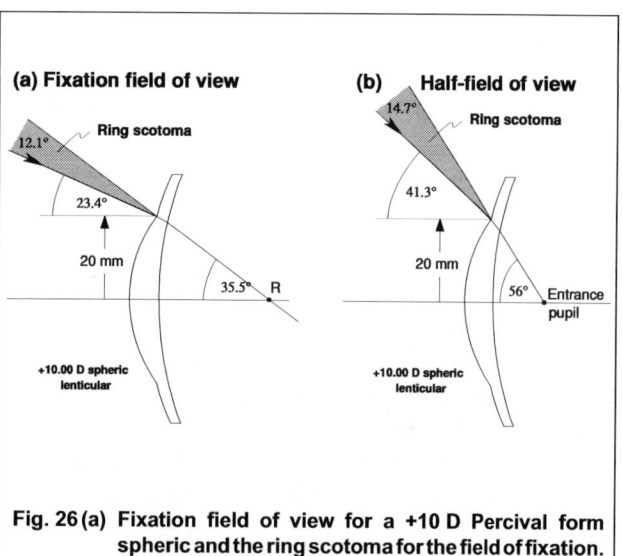

Fig. 26 (a) Fixation field of view for a +10 D Percival form spheric and the ring scotoma for the field of fixation.
(b) The ring scotoma for the field of half illuminance.

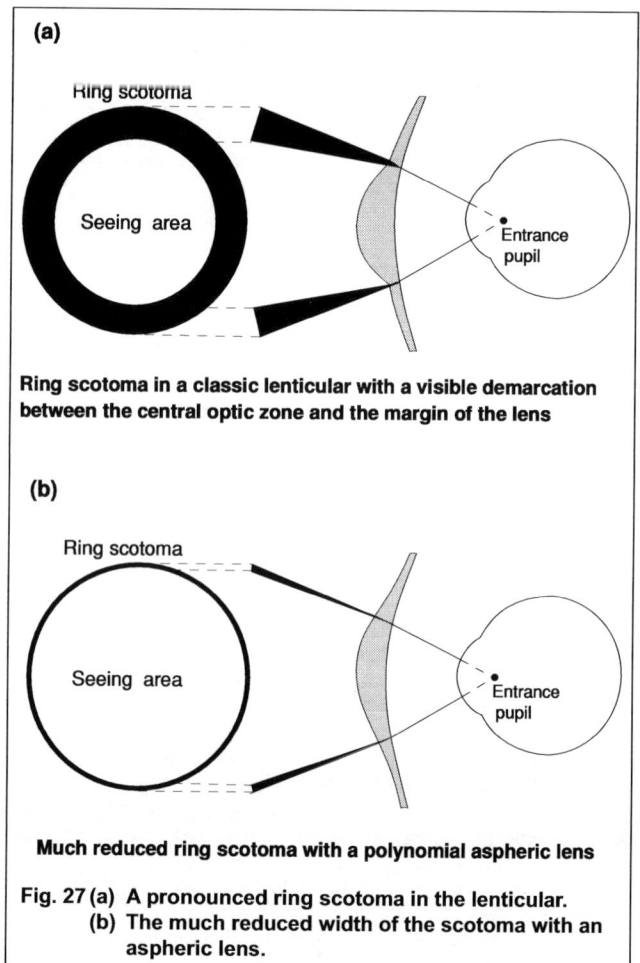

Fig. 27 (a) A pronounced ring scotoma in the lenticular.
(b) The much reduced width of the scotoma with an aspheric lens.

Vertex distance consequences

Dispensing high powered lenses always requires the utmost care on the part of the practitioner. Most errors in the performance of lenses, whether inherent in the compromises of lens design or due to inaccuracies on the part of the dispenser, are likely to have bigger adverse effects on the patient's vision than would be the case with low power lenses. Vertex distance must be considered with lenses over about 5 dioptres power, since dispensing at a different vertex distance from that used to determine the prescription can introduce defocus blur due to effectivity changes. Figure 28 illustrates this effect schematically. The higher the lens power and the greater the difference between the vertex distance used for the test and that occurring in the dispensed spectacles, then the greater will be the effectivity power change. When this change is significant, meaning 0.25 dioptre or more, then the dispenser must adjust the power of the dispensed lenses accordingly. An elementary calculation soon shows the following results:

Lens	Vertex distance	Power change required
Minus	increased	stronger
Minus	reduced	weaker
Plus	increased	weaker
Plus	reduced	stronger

In practice, the simplest way of determining any necessary power change with a vertex distance change is to consult a table. Table 17, on page 28, gives the compensated power change concomitant with a range of vertex distance changes from 2 to 8 mm. Vertex distance changes in between these values can be found from interpolation of the results in the table. In Table 17, those few results shown in light grey print can be ignored since they do not affect the power of the lens when we round the value to the nearest 0.25 D.

Other vertex distance effects

Several small advantages are to be gained by keeping the vertex distance as small as possible. The field of view is larger with a small vertex distance. This comes about in a manner similar to the practical analogy of walking closer to a window and finding one's field of view through the window is greater. Both distortion and Transverse Chromatic Aberration (TCA) increase with the distance of the chief ray from the optical axis. So, with a small vertex distance distortion and Transverse Chromatic Aberration are marginally less because the chief ray meets the lens closer to the optical axis for a given eye rotation. These effects are very small. For example, a Percival +6.00 spheric worn at a vertex distance of 16 mm, assuming the fitting distance is 30 mm, has a distortion of 9.46% and a TCA of 0.26^Δ. Fitted 6 mm nearer, and adjusting the power to +6.25 from Table 17, the respective values are 9.35% and 0.24^Δ. These are exceedingly small differences, but nonetheless, they are improvements with a smaller vertex distance. The differences are greater with a −6.00 lens. Fitting at 10 mm, with a −5.75 determined from the table, assuming −6.00 is correct at 16 mm vertex distance, the reduction in TCA is 0.05^Δ and in distortion 2.00%.

When a smaller vertex distance is used, spectacle magnification moves in the direction of unity, so that there is less change of retinal image size. High powered lenses also alter the apparent size of the wearer's eye to an observer. With minus lenses the eye appears smaller, whilst it appears larger with plus lenses; both these magnifications tend to unity with a smaller vertex distance.

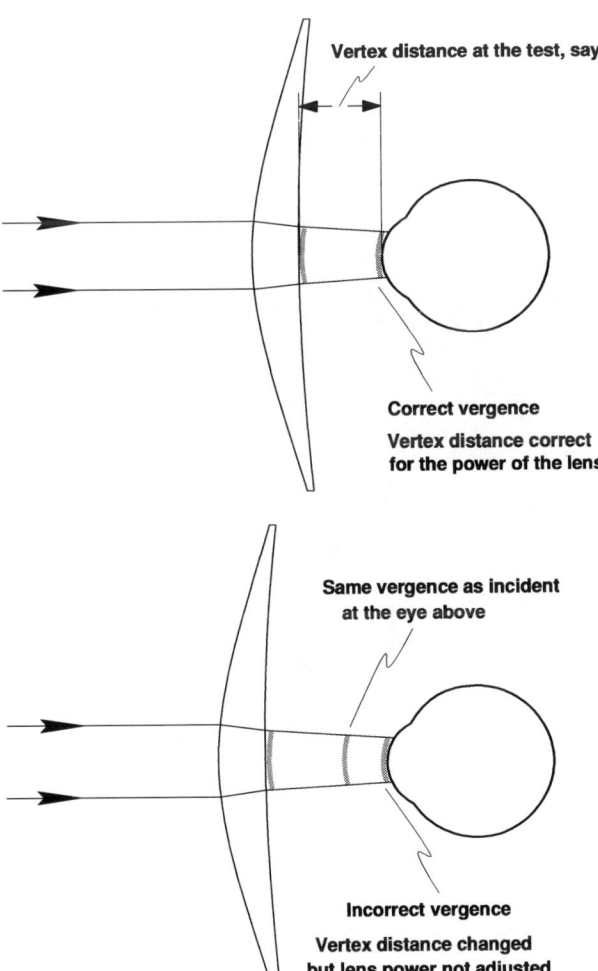

Fig. 28 (a) Correct vergence at the eye since the vertex distance is correct for the lens power.

(b) Effectivity error by failure to adjust the lens power when altering the vertex distance. Lens power is too great in this position.

Summary of effects of keeping the vertex distance small

* Field of view is maximised.

* Less change in retinal image size.

* Less change in the apparent size of the eye.

* Reduction in TCA and distortion.

Table 17 Compensated power for lenses when the vertex distance is changed

Plus lenses: increase in vertex distance (mm) Minus lenses: decrease in vertex distance (mm)				Original Power	Plus lenses: decrease in vertex distance (mm) Minus lenses: increase in vertex distance (mm)			
8	6	4	2		8	6	4	2
4.34	4.38	4.42	4.46	**4.50**	4.54	4.58	4.62	4.67
4.81	4.85	4.90	4.95	**5.00**	5.05	5.10	5.15	5.21
4.27	5.32	5.38	5.44	**5.50**	5.56	5.62	5.69	5.75
5.73	5.79	5.86	5.93	**6.00**	6.07	6.15	6.22	6.30
6.18	6.26	6.34	6.42	**6.50**	6.59	6.67	6.76	6.86
6.63	6.72	6.81	6.90	**7.00**	7.10	7.20	7.31	7.42
7.08	7.18	7.28	7.39	**7.50**	7.61	7.73	7.85	7.98
7.52	7.63	7.75	7.87	**8.00**	8.13	8.26	8.40	8.55
7.96	8.09	8.22	8.36	**8.50**	8.65	8.80	8.96	9.12
8.40	8.54	8.69	8.84	**9.00**	9.17	9.34	9.51	9.70
8.83	8.99	9.15	9.32	**9.50**	9.68	9.88	10.07	10.28
9.26	9.43	9.62	9.80	**10.00**	10.20	10.42	10.64	10.87
9.69	9.88	10.08	10.28	**10.50**	10.73	10.96	11.21	11.46
10.11	10.32	10.54	10.76	**11.00**	11.25	11.51	11.78	12.06
10.53	10.76	10.99	11.24	**11.50**	11.77	12.05	12.35	12.67
10.95	11.19	11.45	11.72	**12.00**	12.30	12.61	12.93	13.27
11.36	11.63	11.90	12.20	**12.50**	12.82	13.16	13.51	13.89
11.78	12.06	12.36	12.67	**13.00**	13.35	13.71	14.10	14.51
12.18	12.49	12.81	13.15	**13.50**	13.87	14.27	14.69	15.13
12.59	12.92	13.26	13.62	**14.00**	14.40	14.83	15.28	15.77
12.99	13.34	13.71	14.09	**14.50**	14.93	15.39	15.88	16.40
13.39	13.76	14.15	14.56	**15.00**	15.46	15.96	16.48	17.05
13.79	14.18	14.60	15.03	**15.50**	16.00	16.52	17.09	17.69
14.18	14.60	15.04	15.50	**16.00**	16.53	17.09	17.70	18.35
14.58	15.01	15.48	15.97	**16.50**	17.06	17.67	18.31	19.01
14.96	15.43	15.92	16.44	**17.00**	17.60	18.24	18.93	19.68
15.35	15.84	16.36	16.91	**17.50**	18.13	18.82	19.55	20.35
15.73	16.25	16.79	17.37	**18.00**	18.67	19.40	20.18	21.03
16.11	16.65	17.23	17.84	**18.50**	19.21	19.98	20.81	21.71
16.49	17.06	17.66	18.30	**19.00**	19.75	20.56	21.44	22.41
16.87	17.46	18.09	18.77	**19.50**	20.29	21.15	22.08	23.10
17.24	17.86	18.52	19.23	**20.00**	20.83	21.74	22.73	23.81

Other powers and vertex distance changes (Δd) can be evaluated by interpolation for values within the table or by using the well-known expression

$$F_{new} = \frac{F_{old}}{1 + \Delta d \cdot F_{old}}$$

where Δd is positive for an increase and negative for a decrease in vertex distance.

Note that Δd is entered in metres.

An approximate expression for finding the change in power is $\Delta F = - \Delta d \times F^2$. The same conventions apply to Δd.

Vertex distance measurement

The vertex distance is the measurement from the back vertex of the lens to the anterior corneal vertex, with the eye looking along the optical axis of the lens. The prescriber has very little difficulty measuring this to the nearest millimetre, either with a millimetre rule or with a manufacturer's gauge designed for the purpose, because he/she can see both the back vertex of the trial lens and the corneal vertex when using a trial frame. The dispenser, however, is faced with some difficulty. How does he/she determine the vertex distance in finished spectacles? There are two cases to deal with: unglazed frames and glazed frames. The latter is the easier to deal with and is indicated in the legend of figure 29.

The problem really is with unglazed spectacles and since this includes new frames it is the majority of cases. There are two solutions to obtaining the vertex distance, one for minus and one for plus lenses.

Empty frame and minus lens Rx – the vertex distance

From figure 30, we see that we can measure the distance a from the front rim to the cornea. Then we need to estimate the sag s of the expected front surface power. This power is obtained from Table 6 on page 8, then the sag s can be obtained from Table 18. Assuming minus lenses are glazed with no bevel showing, as in figure 30, and further assuming minus lenses have a 1 mm centre thickness t, then from the diagram we see that the estimated vertex distance is

$$vertex\ distance\ =\ a + s - t.$$

We need the sags for an appropriate range of vertical lens diameters, refractive indices, and surface powers. With minus lenses there is a limited number of front surface powers required, as Table 6 will confirm. Now let us look at an example. Note that with all tables, in-between values are found by interpolation, and this is the case with the +2.50 DS front surface power in the example below.

Example

Prescription lens power −8.00.
Refractive index 1.523
Front surface power of lens from Table 6   +2.50
Vertical lens diameter 48 mm
Sag of +2.50 front surface from Table 18   1 mm
Measured distance a (as in figure 30)   14 mm

Hence, $vertex\ distance\ =\ a + s - t = 14 + 1 - 1 = 14$ mm. Note that this is equal to the measurement a.

If we peruse Table 6, looking at the range of powers and the refractive indices we would use for them, plus the fact that vertex distance errors are unimportant below lens powers of 5 dioptres, the sag of the front surface is going to be about 1 mm. So s and t cancel and for practical purposes we can conclude that:

For minus lenses, the distance from the front rim to the cornea is a good value for the expected vertex distance.

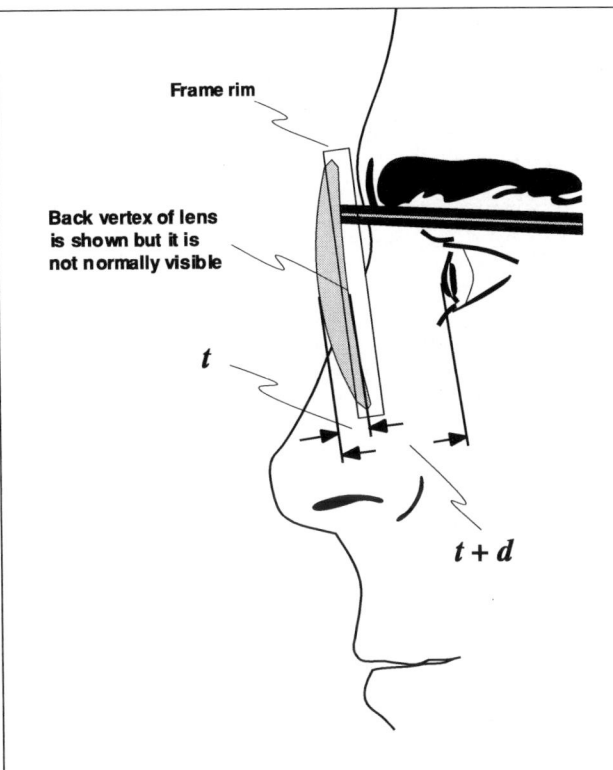

Fig. 29 Measuring the vertex distance in a glazed frame. Both the front vertex of the lens and the cornea are visible, so one can measure this distance $t + d$. Then measure the lens thickness t with calipers and deduct this to give the vertex distance d.

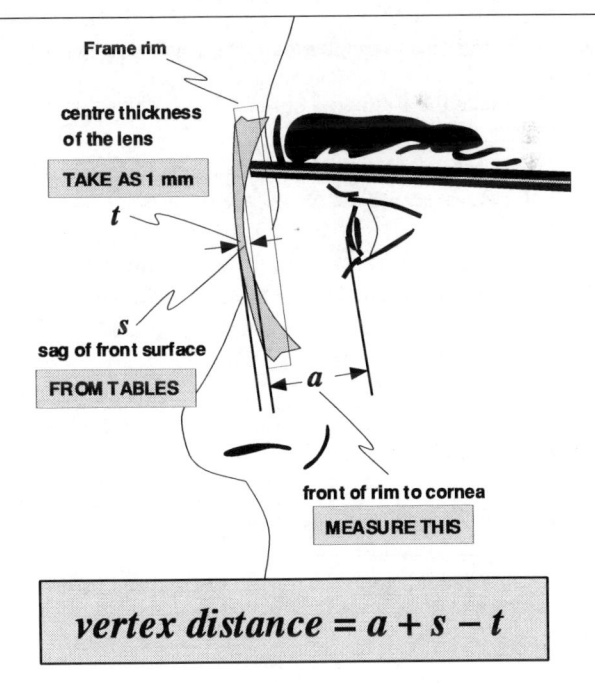

Fig. 30 Estimating the vertex distance for an empty frame which is to take minus lenses.
Measure the distance a. Find the expected front surface power from Table 6 and determine the sag from Table 18. Take minus lenses to have a centre thickness of 1mm, then the expected vertex distance is $a + s - t$, which is $a + s - 1$, with $t = 1$ mm.

Dispensing Single Vision Lenses

Table 18 Sags, to the nearest mm, used in estimating the vertex distance in unglazed frames

Surface power	36	38	40	42	44	Vertical lens size 46	48	50	52	54	56	58	60
						Sag (to nearest mm)							
1.523 index													
1.00	0	0	0	0	0	1	1	1	1	1	1	1	1
2.00	1	1	1	1	1	1	1	1	1	1	2	2	2
3.00	1	1	1	1	1	2	2	2	2	2	2	2	3
4.00	1	1	2	2	2	2	2	2	3	3	3	3	3
5.00	2	2	2	2	2	3	3	3	3	4	4	4	4
1.6 index													
1.00	0	0	0	0	0	0	0	1	1	1	1	1	1
2.00	1	1	1	1	1	1	1	1	1	1	1	1	2
3.00	1	1	1	1	1	1	1	2	2	2	2	2	2
4.00	1	1	1	1	2	2	2	2	2	2	3	3	3
5.00	1	2	2	2	2	2	2	3	3	3	3	4	4
1.7 index													
1.00	0	0	0	0	0	0	0	0	0	1	1	1	1
2.00	0	1	1	1	1	1	1	1	1	1	1	1	1
3.00	1	1	1	1	1	1	1	1	1	2	2	2	2
4.00	1	1	1	1	1	2	2	2	2	2	2	2	3
5.00	1	1	1	2	2	2	2	2	2	3	3	3	3

Empty frame and plus lens Rx – the vertex distance

We shall make the following simplifying assumptions:

1. For plus spherics the back surface is –4.00 D.
2. For aspherics, the back surface is –2.00

These assumptions lead to the following further simplification. By inspection of Table 18, near enough, 2.00 dioptre surfaces have a sag of about 1 mm, and 4 dioptre surfaces a sag of about 2 mm.

Figure 31 will be used to indicate the method. The procedure is:

1. Measure the distance a from the back of the rim to the cornea.
2. Measure the distance b from the back of the groove to the back of the rim.
3. Then the vertex distance is

$$vertex\ distance = a + b + s.$$

Using this method, with glazed frames so that the lenses can be removed for the measurements and then replaced to check the predicted vertex distance against the measurement obtained by the method shown in figure 29, gave an accuracy of about 1 mm, and the error never exceeded 2 mm.

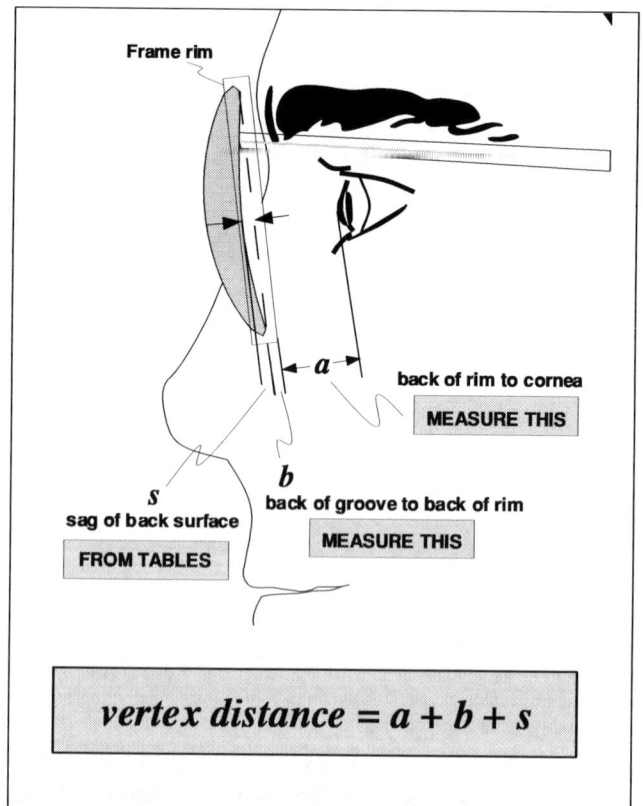

Fig. 31 Estimating the vertex distance for an empty frame which is to be glazed with plus lenses.
Measure the distance a. Measure the distance b from the groove to the back of the rim. Then the expected vertex distance is $a + b + s$.
s is taken as 2 mm for spherics, and 1 mm for aspherics.

Ordering single vision spectacles

It is essential to ensure that the order for spectacles sent to the laboratory contains all the essential data to specify the spectacles. Prescription laboratories, not unjustifiably, have been known to complain about the time and expense involved in querying incomplete orders, so it is incumbent on the dispenser to provide all the necessary information for the efficient execution of the order. The following list is a guide to ordering and includes factors such as tints and toughened lenses which we have not mentioned in this article. Also, although it is not uncommon practice to order the horizontal centration by quoting the PD or the NCD, with high powered lenses one should quote the right and left mono-measurements to avoid centration error effects and ensure the optimum performance of the lenses.

- Lens material: glass or plastic type.
- Tint, AR coating, Hard Coat, UV blocker — specify type.
- Lens type: meniscus, toric, flat, aspheric, lenticular. If lenticular, state type and optic zone aperture where there is a choice.
- Base or sphere curve, where necessary to match a previous lens or to ensure best form.
- Special processes: toughening, thickness control.
- Rx details: sphere and cylinder powers
  cylinder axes
  prism.
- Horizontal centration, quoting right and left decentrations for aspheric lenses where the mono-PDs differ.
- Vertical centration for lenticulars, snooker spectacles, asphericss, and where a vertical PD exists.
- If a balance lens is required, specify.
- Type of edge finish, where special.
- Frame style, colour, and size, with any special instructions regarding alterations made to an enclosed frame, especially alterations to the lens shape and/or bridge.

The dispensing optician's rôle

Twenty years ago when there were few lens designs to choose from and when there were even fewer lens materials, the dispensing optician's function was concerned with little more than frame selection, lens selection from a very limited range, ordering, checking, and fitting. Generally, a well trained receptionist was able to do this work almost as well. Now, with the multiplicity of materials, the advent of computer designed lenses, and the optometrist's tendency not to dispense, the dispensing optician's rôle has changed almost out of recognition. He/she is expected to advise the patient on the use of spectacles in any number of vocational and occupational situations and on the effects of lenses on perception, to undertake supervised auxiliary optometric functions and, naturally, to be au fait with the huge range of single vision, bifocal, and multifocal lenses available. The following list suggests the sort of initial procedure which a dispensing optician would be expected to undertake when presented with a patient and his/her prescription record card. The order of the listing is not sacrosanct, but is a most probable scenario.

1. Peruse the history and symptoms and the past records. Looking at the current symptoms indicates why the patient is attending for a consultation. One needs to note the change in the prescription and consider whether the new prescription solves the problems associated with any visual symptoms reported. As a simple example, suppose the patient has reported "blurring with small print", and the only change is an increase of 0.50 D on the Add, then the dispenser would be happy that new spectacles would solve the problem. Of course, the dispenser would have to advise on the new restrictions on the range of clear vision with a higher Add.

2. One should look through past records to determine any non-tolerance problems that might have occurred in the past, such as lens type, form or material difficulties. In the absence of a series of past records, the patient should be questioned about his/her spectacle wearing history, and his/her current spectacles should be thoroughly measured and the details recorded. Changes in cylinder axes, and meridional power changes, may induce perceived distortion of stereoscopic space so the patient should be advised in these cases.

3. Centration and prescribed prism in the patient's current spectacles should be compared with the new prescription. The dispenser needs to check the muscle balance and fixation disparity results to ensure that prism has not been omitted, and to confirm the base direction and amount of any prescribed prism; we do not want base out prisms to relieve exophoria, or a badly written numeral to be misinterpreted, and such like. Even simple things like the sphere, cylinder, and axis should be scrutinised for fidelity. It is not unknown for a cylinder to be written in one form (plus or minus) and then to be written in the alternative form but without the 90° axis change!

4. Unaided vision and acuities should be checked against previous records, noting in particular any age related worsening of acuity which may affect the patient's visual routines and, unless discussed may lead to dissatisfaction with the spectacles later.

5. In presbyopic cases, the dispensing optician should check the validity of the Add. The working distance will be needed for this and although the optometrist should record the working distance at which the Add was prescribed, not all do this. The dispensing optician should measure this distance and record it if the optometrist has not done so. Any discrepancy between the dispenser's estimated Add and the Add written on the Rx card should be queried: mistakes are expensive!

After this preliminary procedure, the new dispensing can begin . . .

Availability of Full Aperture Single Vision White Lenses

Glass Lenses

SPHERICS   **Maker / Supplier**

Spectacle crown   White   All laboratories

UV   Hoya

Slab-off process on glass single vision   Norville

1.6 index
- Altoglass 1.6 — Shamir
- Punktal 1.6 — Zeiss

1.7 index
- LHI — Hoya
- 1.7 index glass lens ($V = 35$) — Jai Kudo
- Rodalent 1.7 ($V_e = 39.3$) — Rodenstock
- Altoglass 1.7 — Shamir
- Tital ($V_e = 39.3$) — Zeiss

1.8 index
- THI - II — Hoya
- 1.8 index glass lens ($V = 35.0$) — Jai Kudo
- Nikon Pointal ($n = 1.807$, $V = 34.4$) — Nikon
- 1.8 Index MAR coated ($V = 35$) — Norville
- Rodalent 1.8 ($V_e = 35.4$) — Rodenstock
- Altoglass 1.8 — Shamir
- Lantal 1.8 ($V_e = 35.4$) — Zeiss

1.9 index
- 1.9 index glass lens ($V = 30.6$) — Jai Kudo
- 1.9 Index MAR Coated Glass 65 mm — Norville
- Rodalent 1.9 ($V_e = 30.4$) — Rodenstock
- Altoglass 1.9 — Shamir
- 1.9 MAR — SOLA
- Lantal 1.9 ($V_e = 30.3$) — Zeiss

ASPHERICS

1.6 index   Cosmolux (plus and minus)   Rodenstock

Plastic Lenses are on the next page

Plastic Lenses

FULL APERTURE SPHERICS
                                                                      Maker / Supplier

Lens	Maker / Supplier
CR 39, CR 39 Hardcoated and CR 39 MAR coated	All labs
RLX Plus, in-the-mould hard coat single vision	Signet Armorlite
Small diameter (Ø60), shallow curve stock lenses	SOLA & WLC
Dip coatings - Tints, Hydrophobic and Anti-scratch	BPI
Tintable Hardcoated CR 39 Hilux Hard Easy Tint	Hoya
Slab-off CR 39	Norville

Mid index plastics (refractive index and *V*-value in brackets)

Lens	(index, V)	Maker / Supplier
Polycarbonate	(1.586, 30)	All labs
Unor 1.6	(1.61, 42)	BBGR
Myoperal (See AS Ormex)	(1.561, 37)	Essilor
Hilux Eyas Spheric	(1.60, 41)	Hoya
1.61 Spheric HMAR	(1.61, 42)	Jai Kudo
Ultra Clear 1.6	(1.6, 42)	Pentax
1.60 Super 16 Plus	(1.6, 42)	Seiko
Altolite 1.56 Spheric	(1.56, 37)	Shamir
Altolite 1.6 Spheric	(1.6, 41)	Shamir
SA 1.56 SV HC	(1.56, 36)	Signet Armorlite
SA 1.6 SV HC	(1.60, 42)	Signet Armorlite
TX (SG = 1.16)	(1.557, 43)	Taylor Optical
Multiplus Xtra Lite Spheric	(1.59, 36)	WLC
Multiplus 1.61	(1.61, 42)	WLC

High index plastics

Lens	(index, V)	Maker / Supplier
Stylis Spheric	(1.67, 32)	Essilor
Hilux Eynoa Spheric	(1.67, 31)	Hoya
Cosmolit 1.67 hardMAR	(1.67, 31.4)	Rodenstock
SV 1.67	(1.67, 32)	Seiko

FULL APERTURE ASPHERICS (including bi-aspherics)

CR 39

Lens	Maker / Supplier
Aspherlite	American Optical
Hyperal	Essilor
Nulux	Hoya
Norlite Aspheric	Norville
SolAspheric	SOLA
Cosmolit 1.5	Rodenstock
Altolite 1.5 Aspheric	Shamir
Kodak 1.498 SV HC Aspheric	Signet Armorlite
Clarlet 1.5 AS and Hypal	Zeiss

Trivex

Lens	Maker / Supplier
PNX (n = 1.53, V = 45, SG = 1.11)	Hoya
Trilogy Aspheric (n = 1.53, V = 45, SG = 1.11)	Norville
Altolite Trivex Aspheric	Shamir

Spectralite

Lens	(index, V)	Maker / Supplier
Spectralite Aspheric	(1.54, 47)	SOLA

Mid index

Lens	(index, V)	Maker / Supplier
AO 55	(1.54, 47)	American Optical
Hyperal Ormex	(1.56, 37)	Essilor
Altolite 1.56 Aspheric	(1.56, 37)	Shamir
Kodak 1.56 SV HC Aspheric	(1.56, 38)	Signet Armorlite

Full aperture mid-index Aspherics cont.

Polycarbonate	AO Rugged (plus powers)	(1.59, 30)	American Optical
	Multiplus Xtra Lite 15 AS	(1.59, 30)	WLC
	Tilium AS Polycarbonate	(1.59, 31)	BBGR
	Cosmolit Polycarbonate	(1.59, 31)	Rodenstock
	Altolite Polycarbonate	(1.59, 31)	Shamir
1.6	AOXT16	(1.60, 42)	American Optical
	Asphor 1.6	(1.61, 42)	BBGR
	Ormix 1.6 Aspheric	(1.60, 42)	Essilor
	AS Ormil	(1.60, 34)	Essilor
	Nulux Eyas Aspheric	(1.60, 41)	Hoya
Bi-Aspheric	Nulux EP **Bi-Aspheric**	(1.60, 41)	Hoya
	1.61 Aspheric	(1.61, 42)	Jai Kudo
	Nikon Lite III AS	(1.60, 42)	Nikon
Bi-Aspheric	Norlite 1.6 Bi-Aspheric		Norville
	Ultra Clear 1.60 AS	(1.60, 42)	Pentax
Atoroidal back surface	Impression Mono 1.6	(1.60, 41)	Rodenstock
	Cosmolit 1.6	(1.60, 41)	Rodenstock
Bi-Aspheric	SLU AZ 1.6 Bi-Aspheric	(1.60, 42)	Seiko
	SLU 1.6 Aspheric	(1.60, 42)	Seiko
	Altolite Aspheric 1.6	(1.60, 42)	Shamir
	Kodak 1.6 SV HC Aspheri	(1.60, 37)	Signet Armorlite
	1.6 Aspheric Teflon coated	(1.60, 42)	SOLA
	Multiplus Xtra Lite Aspheric	(1.59, 36)	WLC
	Multiplus 1.61 AS	(1.61, 42)	WLC
	Clarlet 1.6 AS	(1.60, 36)	Zeiss
High Index	Asphor 1.67	(1.67, 32)	BBGR
	AS Stylis	(1.67, 32)	Essilor
	Nulux Aspheric	(1.67 and 1.70)	Hoya
Bi-Aspheric	Nulux EP **Bi-Aspheric**	(1.67 and 1.70)	Hoya
	1.67 Aspheric	(1.67, 32)	Jai Kudo
	Nikon Lite IV-AS	(1.67, 32)	Nikon
Customised Bi-Aspheric	Seemax 1.67	(1.67, 32)	Nikon
Biconcave Aspheric	Norlite 1.67 Bi-concave aspheric	(1.67, 32)	Norville
	Ultra Clear 1.67	(1.67, 32)	Pentax
	Super Atoric 1.67	(1.67, 32)	Pentax
	Cosmolit 1.67 aspheric	(1.67, 32)	Rodenstock
	Impression Mono 1.67	(1.67, 31)	Rodenstock
Bi-Aspheric	SSV AZ Bi-Aspheric	(1.67, 32)	Seiko
	Super SV 1.67 Aspheric	(1.67, 32)	Seiko
	Altolite 1.67 Aspheric	(1.67, 32)	Shamir
	Kodak 1.67 SV HC Aspheric	(1.67, 32)	Signet Armorlite
	Kodak 1.67 Bi-concave Aspheric	(1.67, 32)	Signet Armorlite
	1.67 Aspheric Teflon coated	(1.67, 32)	SOLA
	Multiplus 1.67 AS	(1.67, 32)	WLC
	Clarlet 1.66 AS	(1.66, 32)	Zeiss
Very High Index	AS Fusio 1.74 (aspheric)	(1.74, 33)	Essilor
	1.74 Aspheric	(1.74, 33)	Jai Kudo
	NLV-AS	(1.74, 33)	Nikon
	Norlite 1.74 Spheric and Aspheric	(1.74, 33)	Norville
Biconcave Aspheric	Norlite 1.74 Bi-concave Aspheric	(1.74, 33)	Norville
	Ultra Clear 1.74 AS	(1.74, 33)	Pentax
	Cosmolit 1.74	(1.74, 33)	Rodenstock
	SPG 1.74 Aspheric	(1.74, 33)	Seiko
Bi-Aspheric	SSV AZ Bi-Aspheric	(1.74, 33)	Seiko
	Altolite 1.74 Aspheric	(1.74, 33)	Shamir
	Kodak 1.74 SV HC Aspheric	(1.74, 33)	Signet Armorlite
	Multiplus 1.74 AS HMAR	(1.74, 33)	WLC
	Clarlet 1.74 AS (aspheric)	(1.74, 33)	Zeiss

Dispensing Progressive Addition Lenses

After the age of 45, most people experience difficulty with reading, the eye's ability to alter focus having reduced to the extent where 3 dioptres of accommodation requires 100% ciliary muscle contraction compared with only 5% contraction to do the same focusing task at 20 years of age[1]. After 50 years of age, the ability to accommodate has reduced to such an extent that bifocal wearers have difficulty with objects just beyond the artificial far point through the reading segment, to the extent that they cannot focus those objects at 'intermediate' distances properly neither through the distance portion nor through the segment. They either tolerate this problem or seek help in the form of trifocals or progressive addition lenses (PALs). Trifocals have never been popular, most practitioners barely dispensing one pair per year. However, progressive addition lenses have grown in popularity in the last decade, so much so that practitioners feel relatively confident in dispensing them nowadays. New designs have improved patient adaptation. This confidence is in stark contradiction to the situation two decades ago when, for whatever reasons, the success rate for adaptation to progressive lenses was very poor, to say the least. Even so, there is still a proportion of patients who fail to adapt to PALs and this must be borne in mind by practitioners when considering this type of correction.

The first commercially available progressive lens, no longer available and now referred to as the Varilux 1, was a glass lens introduced in France in 1959 by the company Essel (now called Essilor). This had a spherical front surface form in the distance portion with the progressive surface confined to the region below this; see figure 1. Progressive power increase follows the continuous shortening of the radius of curvature of the front surface over the progressive zone. In the case of the Varilux 1 lens, this was over a depth of 12 mm, with a spherical distance portion and a 22 mm wide reading zone of constant power.

Good visual acuity in the progression zone is confined to a region known as the progression corridor which may be less than 4 mm wide at its narrowest and about 12 to 20 mm long, depending on the design. The progression corridor is bounded on the nasal and temple sides by areas of surface aberrational astigmatism, a defect which is inherent in the design; see figure 2. The process which provides the increasing power, the progressive increase in curvature of the front surface from the distance to near power, also

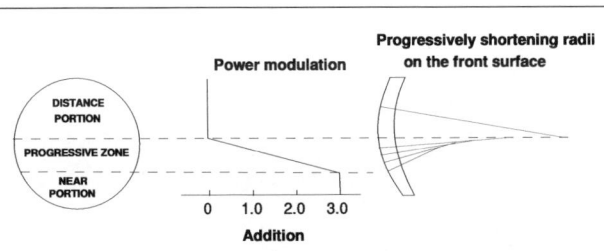

Fig. 1 Schematic diagram of the power progression in the original Varilux I lens. The progressive power is on the front surface which, in this lens, was spherical in the distance portion.

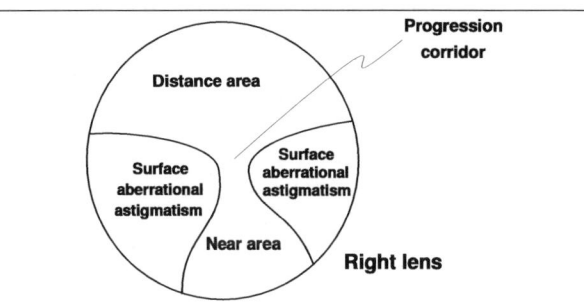

Fig. 2 Schematic representation of the distance, progression corridor and near vision regions on a progressive addition lens (PAL). The progression surface is referred to as non-spherical

produces increasing amounts of surface astigmatism away from the progression corridor. Despite this imperfection in the optical performance of PALs, these lenses have some clear advantages over other forms of presbyopic correction, as well as disadvantages. Both should be explained to the prospective wearer.

Advantages of Progressive Addition Lenses

- No visible segment top.
- The appearance of a single vision lens, thereby improving cosmesis over a bifocal or trifocal lens.
- No image jump, because there is no sudden introduction of a change in prismatic effect.
- The gradual change in power provides distance and near foci and a range of intermediate foci.

Disadvantages of Progressive Addition Lenses

- Areas of surface astigmatism and consequent blur.
- During adaptation, apparent 'rocking' of objects in the lower visual field as the eye scans across those regions of the lens with surface aberrational astigmatism.
- The period of adaptation is less predictable than with other lens types.
- Narrow reading area compared with bifocals.
- Narrow intermediate area compared with trifocals.

This brief review of Progressive Addition Lenses will consider the following themes:

(A) The specification of progressive lenses.
(B) Features of PAL design.
(C) Dispensing PALs.
(D) Patient acceptance of PALs.

Before proceeding with the above sections, it is worth looking at the huge variety of lenses now available. Where, in the very early days, only spectacle crown lenses were available, we now have both white glass and plastics, and photochromic glass and plastics, the latter being a very recent addition to the armoury. Tables 1 and 2 list all the white progressive addition lenses available in the UK at the present time.

Table 1 Availability of White Glass Progressive Addition Lenses

			Maker / Supplier
WHITE	**Spectacle crown**		
	Hard	Truvision	American Optical
		Graduate	Sola
	Soft	AO PRO 15	American Optical
		VariVue	Lentoid
		Navigator	Signet Armorlite
		Insight	Taylor
	Ultrasoft	Gradal 3	Zeiss
1.6 index			
	Hard	Contour H	Crossbows
	Soft	AO PRO 16	American Optical
		Contour S	Crossbows
		Varilux Comfort and Varilux Expert	Essilor
		Progressiv Life 2 and Multigressiv 2	Rodenstock
		Progressiv AT	Rodenstock
		Kodak Progressive	Signet Armorlite
		XL	Sola
		Insight	Taylor
		Gradal HS 1.6 index	Zeiss
	Ultrasoft	Varilux Panamic Clear Glass 1.6	Essilor
		Summit Pro (n=1.6, V=41)	Hoya
		Percepta	Sola
		Genesis	Taylor
		Gradal Individual	Zeiss
		Gradal Top	Zeiss
		Gradal RD (OPAL for int./near use)	Zeiss
1.7 index			
	Hard	Contour H	Crossbows
		Graduate (1.7 index, V = 42)	Sola
	Soft	Varilux Comfort	Essilor
	Ultrasoft	Genesis (V = 42)	Taylor
		Tital Gradal 3	Zeiss
1.8 index			
	Soft	AO PRO 18	American Optical & Lentoid
		Varilux Comfort Clear Glass 1.8	Essilor
		Progressiv Life 2 and Multigressiv 2	Rodenstock
		Lantal Gradal Top	Zeiss
	Ultrasoft	Panamic Clear Glass 1.8	Essilor

For near and intermediate use only (OPALs)

	Office (1.523)	Taylor
	Gradal RD (1.6 index)	Zeiss

Excerpt from *Ophthalmic Lens Availability*.
Compiled by Dr A H Tunnacliffe and published by the Association of British Dispensing Opticians.

Table 2 Availability of White Plastic Progressive Addition Lenses

WHITE				Maker / Supplier
CR 39	**Hard**		Truvision	American Optical
			Contour H	Crossbows
			NSP Progressive	Norvilles
			Graduate	Sola
	Soft		AO PRO 15	American Optical
			Contours S	Crossbows
			Varilux Comfort, Varilux Expert	Essilor
			Varilux Omega (high plus)	Essilor
			Concord and Outlook	Lentoid
			New Image	Norville
			Essilor Natural	Norville
			Progressiv SI	Rodenstock
			Progressiv Start 2	Rodenstock
			Progressiv Life 2 and Multigressiv 2	Rodenstock
			Kodak Progressive and Navigator Precision	Signet Armorlite
			SolaMax and XL	Sola
			Insight	Taylor
			Vartek	WLC
			Gradal HS	Zeiss
	Ultrasoft		AO b'Active	American Optical
			Omni	American Optical
			Varilux Panamic Orma	Essilor
			Hoyalux GP, Hoyalux GP Wide and Summit Pro	Hoya
			Protek 1.5	Jai Kudo
			Presio CX-16	and Ci-15 Nikon
			NCF5 Aspheric Progressive	Norville
			AF 1.50	Pentax
			Progressive AT	Rodenstock
	Back surface progressive		Impression	Rodenstock
			Kodak Precise	Signet Armorlite
			Percepta	Sola
			Genesis	Taylor
			Gradal 3, Gradal Top and Gradal Individual	Zeiss
			Clarlet PAL 1.5 (Gradal 3 based budget lens)	Zeiss
Trivex	**Soft**		Trilogy Image (n = 1.53, V = 45, SG = 1.11)	Taylor (Younger lens)
Spectralite	**Soft**		AO Compact 55 (n = 1.537, V = 47)	American Optical
			Graduate Gold (n = 1.537, V = 47)	Sola
			SolaMax (n = 1.537, V = 47)	Sola
	Ultrasoft		XL Gold and Percepta (n = 1.537, V = 47)	Sola

Short corridor progressives — collected here for convenient reference

			AO Compact (CR 39 and 1.6)	American Optical
			Petite	Crossbows
			Summit CD (n =1.60, V = 41)	Hoya
			Protek 1.5 and 1.56	Jai Kudo
			Outlook	Lentoid
			Presio 14 and Presio *i* 13 series	Nikon
			Mini AF 1.50 (also 1.60 and 1.67)	Pentax
			Super Atoric 1.67 (10, 12 & 14 mm corridors)	Pentax
			Progressiv Life XS (CR39 and 1.6 index)	Rodenstock
			Kodak Concise (CR 39, 1.56, 1.6 and 1.67)	Signet Armorlite
			Piccolo	Taylor and Lentoid
			Gradal Short I	Zeiss

PLASTIC PROGRESSIVE ADDITION LENSES – WHITE (cont.)

Mid index Plastic Progressives   Maker / Supplier

Hard   Graduate Polycarbonate   Sola

Soft   AO Compact 16 & AO PRO 16 ($n = 1.6$, $V = 42$)   American Optical
            AO PRO 55 ($n = 1.55$, $V = 36$)   American Optical
            Varilux Comfort Ormex and Ormil   Essilor
            Varilux Expert Ormex   Essilor
            Concord ($n = 1.57$)   Lentoid
            Tegra Outlook (Polycarbonate)   Lentoid
            Natural ($n = 1.60$, $V = 36$)   Norville
            Multigressiv 2 and Progressiv Life 2 ($n = 1.6$)   Rodenstock
            Progressiv SI ($n = 1.6$)   Rodenstock
            Kodak Progressive 1.56, 1.60 & Polycarbonate   Signet Armorlite
            Navigator ($n = 1.56$ and $n = 1.60$)   Signet Armorlite
            Insight ($n = 1.56$)   Taylor
            Clarlet 1.6 Gradal HS   Zeiss

Ultrasoft   Omni (Polycarbonate)   American Optical
                 Panamic Ormil 1.6 and Polycarbonate   Essilor
                 Hoyalux EX and EX Wide ($n = 1.60$, $V = 41$)   Hoya
                 Hoyalux Summit Pro ($n = 1.60$, $V = 41$)   Hoya
                 Protek 1.56 ($n = 1.56$, $V = 38$)   Jai Kudo
                 Presio DX-16 and Presio *i* Ei-15   Nikon
                 Seiko Genius ($n = 1.60$, $V = 42$)   Norville

Back surface progressive   Seiko Synergy ($n = 1.60$, $V = 42$)   Norville
                              NCF6 Aspheric Progressive ($n = 1.6$, $V = 36$)   Norville
                              AF 1.60 ($n = 1.60$, $V = 40$)   Pentax

Back surface progressive   Impression ($n = 1.6$, $V = 40.5$)   Rodenstock
                              Progressiv AT (through the lens ray trace design)   Rodenstock
                              Kodak Precise ($n = 1.56$, $V = 36$ & $n = 1.60$, $V = 32$)   Signet Armolite
                              Percepta (Polycarbonate and $n = 1.6$, $V = 42$)   Sola
                              Clarlet 1.6 Gradal Top and Gradal Individual   Zeiss

High Index Plastic Progressives

Soft   Presio Presio FX-14 and Fi-13 ($n = 1.67$, $V = 32$)   Nikon
            Kodak Progressive ($n = 1.66$, $V = 32$)   Signet Armorlite

Ultrasoft   Panamic 1.67 ($n = 1.67$, $V = 32$)   Essilor
                 Protek 1.67 ($n = 1.67$, $V = 32$)   Jai Kudo
                 Hoyalux LX and LX Wide ($n = 1.71$, $V = 36$)   Hoya
                 Summit Pro ($n = 1.70$, $V = 36$)   Hoya
                 Presio FX-16 and Fi-15 ($n = 1.67$, $V = 32$)   Nikon
                 Seiko Genius Wing ($n = 1.67$, $V = 32$)   Norville

Back surface progressive   Seiko Synergy ($n = 1.67$, $V = 32$)   Norville
                              AF 1.67 and Super Atoric 1.67   Pentax
                              Percepta 1.67 ($n = 1.67$, $V = 32$)   Sola
                              Clarlet 1.67 Gradal Top   Zeiss

Very High Index Plastic Progressives

Ultrasoft   Protek 1.74   Jai Kudo
                 Presio Gi-15 and Gi-13 ($n = 1.74$, $V = 33$)   Nikon
                 Seiko Synergy ($n = 1.74$, $V = 33$)   Norville

For near and intermediate use only (OPALs – Occupational Progressive Addition Lenses)

Technica   American Optical
Interview   Essilor
Continuum   Norville
Office Perfalit 1.5   Rodenstock
Access Enhanced Near Vision Lens   Sola
Office   Taylor and Lentoid
Clarlet Business and Gradal RD   Zeiss

(A) Specifying progressive addition lenses

There is no easy way of comparing the optical properties of PALs although, if a manufacturer is prepared to go to the expense, there is a method available which employs a 'scanning focimeter' interfaced with a computer. This instrument can take up to 1000 readings across the lens and plot a number of important parameters. In 1982, the American Optometric Association Commission on Ophthalmic Standards recommended that diagrams should be used to display isocylinder lines, the orientations of the aberrational astigmatism, and isospherical power lines. Some manufacturers present isocylinder line diagrams, but to the author's knowledge, only Sola will allow the practitioner access to the whole lot. In fact, Sola go even further: they also plot the power profile of the Addition along the umbilical line.

These technical terms are best understood by referring to a diagram. Figure 3 shows (a) isocylinder lines, (b) a vector plot of the amount and orientation of the aberrational astigmatism, (c) the Add power lines, and (d) the Add profile down the umbilical line for the Sola Graduate lens.

Isocylinder lines

These are also known as isoastigmatic lines. A scanning focimeter can usually take up to as many as 1000 readings at a matrix of points across the PAL uncut's progression surface. In measuring lenses, it is usual for the manufacturer to specify the base curve and the Addition, the distance portion normally being taken as plano for comparison

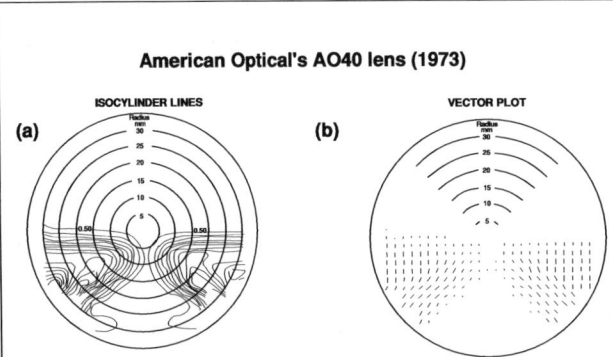

Fig. 4 Closely spaced isocylinder lines indicate a relatively large rate of change of astigmatism in the aberration zones. This is an early progressive lens with a *hard design*. Hard designs typically have surface aberrational astigmatism and distortion concentrated in the lower nasal and temple areas.

purposes (note, though, that the isocylinder line distribution is affected by the distance power and will vary from minus to plus powers). Figure 3(a) shows lines joining those points where the surface aberrational astigmatism is 0.50, 1.00, 1.50 dioptres, and so on. The width of the distance portion is usually specified by the distance between 0.50 D isocylinder lines at some specified height on the lens, whilst the reading width is measured between the 050 or 1.00 D lines* at the centre of the near checking circle. The lens diameter here is 60 mm, so the width of the progression corridor between the 0.50 D isocylinder lines can be seen to be very narrow. A relatively narrow progression corridor occurs on all PALs, although there is a difference between three basic types known as *hard, soft* and *ultrasoft* designs;

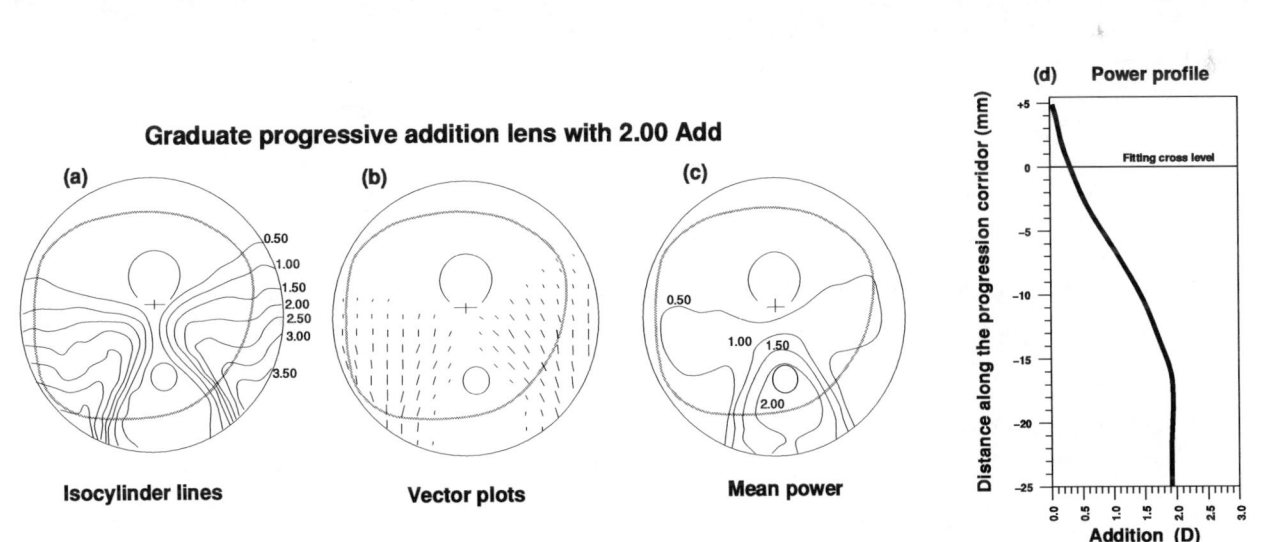

Fig. 3 (a) Isocylinder lines join points on the progression surface where the surface aberrational astigmatism is of the same magnitude. Such plots are usually made on a plano distance portion lens with a specified base curve and Add.
(b) A vector plot, by the length and orientation of each line, indicates the relative amounts of surface aberrational astigmatism and the direction of the cylinder power. Vertical lines are desirable because the patient will not experience apparent rotation of horizontal and vertical object lines through such regions. There will be less apparent 'rock or sway' of objects, making such lenses easier for adaptation by the patient.
(c) The mean power plot indicates the distribution of the progressive addition, the lines joining points of equal Add (isopower lines).
(d) The power profile indicates the start and the progression of the Add along the umbilical line in the progression corridor. The umbilical line down the centre of the progression corridor joins those points with zero surface aberrational astigmatism. The fitting cross is also indicated in figures (a) through (c), together with the distance checking area (upper horse-shoe shaped ring), and the near checking area (the lower circle).

(Adapted from Sola's diagrams).

---

* Experiment shows that the width of the distance and intermediate portions measured between the 0.50 D isocylinder lines is in good agreement with practical measurements. Because the pupil is smaller in near vision, more blur can be tolerated and measurement between the 1.00 D isocylinder lines agrees well with practical measurement for the reading width.

the softer the lens design, the wider the progression corridor and the easier is the adaptation by the patient. Improved 'softness' is achieved in the design by allowing some surface aberrational astigmatism to appear in the upper nasal and temple peripheral areas.

Hard, soft and ultrasoft design PALs

Depending on the distribution and the amount of surface aberrational astigmatism, progressive addition lenses were first classified as either *soft* or *hard* in design (Woodcock, 1985)[2]. With further design developments from 1994 onwards, the surface aberrational astigmatism was either reduced or moved lower down the lens, relative to the fitting cross. This has lead to what the author describes as *ultrasoft designs* which present the patient with much the easiest adaptation.

The early *hard design* lenses had a very narrow progression corridor and a relatively wide reading area, with a full-width spherical distance portion. All early PALs were of a *hard design*. Closely spaced isocylinder lines, as seen in figure 4, indicate a relatively rapid rate of change of the surface aberrational astigmatism over the progression surface. The name 'hard design' is used to indicate this relatively large rate of change of surface aberrational astigmatism. These early *hard designs* concentrated the surface aberrational astigmatism and distortion in the lower nasal and temple areas of the lens, areas which are considered to be used least in a spectacle lens.

Hard design lenses are typically described as having a relatively wide reading area. However, note the word 'relatively'. This is relative to *soft design* PALs and not to bifocals. In all modern PALs the reading area is narrow when compared with even 25 mm diameter bifocal segments!

Soft design PALs came later in the evolution of progressive lenses. In the *soft design* PALs, the surface astigmatism extends into the marginal parts of the distance portion in some designs, thus allowing a reduction in its amount and producing a wider progression corridor, but at the same time introducing some astigmatic blur into the periphery of the distance portion. Early *soft designs*, some of which are still available, have a relatively narrow width of the reading portion. Generally speaking, *soft designs* offer easier adaptation[3] for the patient and for general use the distance and reading portion widths are found adequate. Because of their wider intermediate portion, they are also more suited to prolonged intermediate use. Figure 5 illustrates these properties with the Sola XL lens. Note the width of the reading area compared with the Graduate in figure 3.

Most *ultrasoft design* lenses have less surface aberrational astigmatism so the rate of change of this aberration is less, even compared with *soft design* lenses. At the same time, designers have been able to increase the reading area, compared with early soft design lenses, thus making *ultrasoft* PALs arguably the only progressive lens type to consider, with the exception of occupational PALs which are best where prolonged intermediate visual tasks are undertaken, as when viewing a computer monitor for lengthy periods.

Vector plots

Figure 3(b) and 5(b) show the surface aberrational astigmatism indicated by vectors. The length of the lines indicates the magnitude of the astigmatism and the orientation of each line is along the power meridian. Each vector is drawn centred on that point where the astigmatism was measured on the lens. This diagram is a good indicator as to how easy or difficult it will be for a patient to adapt to the lens. Vertical vectors indicate that horizontal and vertical lines on objects will be seen as such. However, where the vectors are oblique the

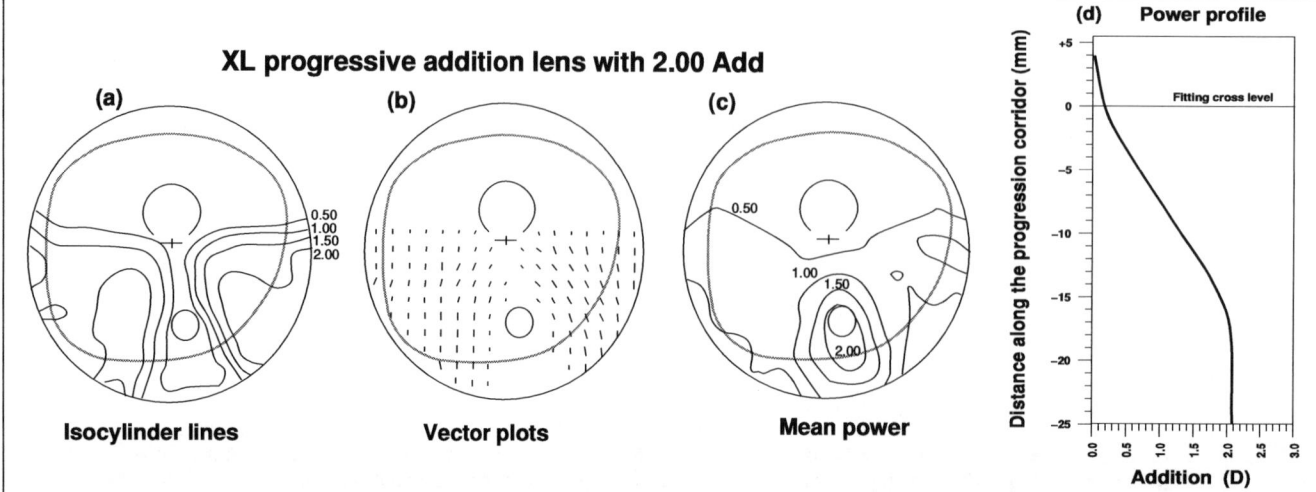

Fig. 5   A soft design lens. Notice that there is less aberrational astigmatism than in the hard design Graduate in figure 3. This has been achieved by reducing the width of the reading area, although the progression corridor is a little wider. From the practical point of view, the author finds this lens suitable for general use and at a Visual Display Unit (VDU). Distortion of vertical lines barely exists. Compared with hard designs, the narrower reading area means that more head turning is necessary when reading a newspaper. Notice there are more oblique vectors in the less important nasal area.

patient will experience a rotation of horizontal and vertical object lines (as well as others not parallel or perpendicular to the vector). When looking across the lens from side to side where the vectors are not vertical, the patient's eyes meet varying amounts and obliquities of astigmatism which cause a disconcerting apparent rocking or swaying movement of perceived objects. Compare the vector lines in figures 3 or 5 with those of an older, discontinued lens in figure 4. Small wonder that adaptation to progressives is now easier than it was in the nineteen-seventies. The AO 40 lens in figure 4 had a 25 mm wide reading area, but today's hard designs have a narrower reading area, not more than 17 mm (measured with a 2.00 Add), with a consequent reduction in the astigmatism which produces easier adaptation.

Isopower lines

Figures 3(c) and 5(c) show how the Add is distributed over the lens. Evidently, the region of the full Add is limited compared with bifocals. With a *soft design* Sola XL and a +2.00 Add, the author finds he can read about 2 newspaper column-widths (8 to 9 cm) without turning the head. This almost doubles with the hard design Graduate but I cannot use this latter design for very long on the VDU (computer Visual Display Unit or monitor screen). However, with the introduction of the *ultrasoft design* Sola XL Gold in 1994, the author found his reading area increased significantly, besides having a wider intermediate zone.

Distance and reading widths

Table 3, below, indicates the widths of some PAL reading areas, measured at the level of the centre of the near checking area between the 1.00 D isocylinder lines. Also indicated in this table are the progression corridor lengths, measured from the fitting cross to the centre of the near checking area, and the width of the distance portion between the 0.50 D isocylinder lines 5 mm above the fitting cross. Note that many modern *soft* and *ultrasoft designs* have reading widths similar to the current *hard designs* and also combine wide distance areas. As mentioned earlier, this suggests that *ultrasoft designs* ought to be the first choice for general use because they are easier for patient adaptation.

Most *soft* and *ultrasoft* design PALs have a narrower distance area at the level of the fitting cross than the widths quoted in Table 3 where the measurements were taken 5 mm above the fitting cross. In terms of ocular rotation or head tilt, 5 mm on the lens represents a 10° head tilt or rotation of the eyes to look through the quoted width of distance portion; see figure 6. Someone might do this when working at a desk, say, or might develop the habit of tilting the head forwards slightly when looking left and right at a road junction whilst driving. This is of little practical hindrance since it soon becomes habitual.

The power profile

Figures 3(d) and 5(d) indicate how the Addition increases along the umbilical line in the Graduate and XL lenses. Notice that both of these lenses commence the progression about 4 mm above the fitting cross, which is normally placed at the centre of the pupil with the eyes in the primary position. However, in both cases the power at the pupil centre does not exceed 0.2 D and this seems to be acceptable

Table 3	Measurements (mm) for some CR 39 +2.00 Add on plano distance portion Progressive Addition Lenses			
Lens	Maker	Distance width	Length of corridor	Reading width
Hard designs				
Graduate	Sola	33	16	16
Truvision	AO	45	18	17
Soft designs				
AO PRO	AO	39	20	16
Gradal HS	Zeiss	47	18	15
Image	Younger	46	18	15
Kodak PAL	Signet Armorlite	50	17	14
Progressive Life 2	Rodenstock	44	18	17
Varilux Comfort	Essilor	47	18	15
XL	Sola	46	17	14
Ultrasoft designs				
AO b'Active	AO	47	17	11
GP Wide	Hoya	full	18	14
Percepta	Sola	full	18	13
Summit Pro	Hoya	full	18	13
Varilux Panamic	Essilor	26	18	17
XL Gold	Sola	full	15	15

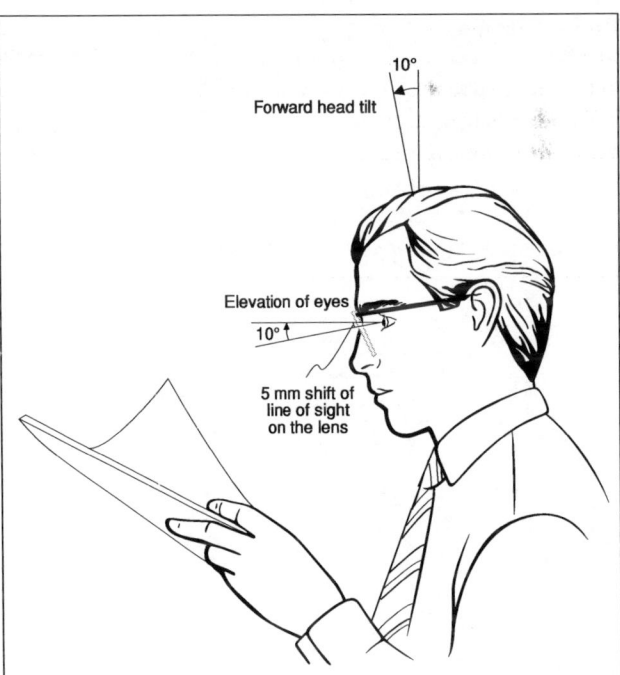

Fig. 6 The widths of the distance portions quoted in Table 3 are measured 5 mm above the fitting cross. To use this part of the lens requires a 10° forwards head tilt since each 1 mm on the lens is corresponds to about 2° head tilt or eye rotation. This fact can also be used to realise the importance of ensuring the head is erect during the measurement of the fitting cross height. A forwards or backwards head tilt of just 2° during this measurement results in a 1 mm too high or 1 mm too low fitting, respectively!

in practice. Starting the progression a little above the fitting cross allows a slower rate of change of the power with a consequent reduction in the aberrational astigmatism. The majority of manufacturers seem to adopt this strategy, especially with softer designs.

(B) Features of PAL design

In the early days of progressive lens design, in the 1970s, the principal ideas were to achieve a full aberration-free distance portion and a reading portion about 25 mm or so in width. This necessitated a very narrow progression corridor and a large amount of surface aberrational astigmatism. The AO 40 lens in figure 4 is a good example of this design philosophy.

The AO 40 lens was superseded by the AO Truvision; see figure 7. In this case, in order to reduce the rate of change of surface astigmatism, the astigmatism was allowed to spread upwards on the nasal side of the lens, and the width of the reading area was reduced a little. Both the amount (fewer lines) and the rate of change (wider line spacings) of the surface astigmatism were lessened in this design. These observations are apparent from the isocylinder plots in figures 3(a) and 5(a). Allowing the surface astigmatism to spread into the upper part of the nasal area of the lens seems a reasonable philosophy since this part of the lens is less likely to be used when compared with the upper temple region. In any case, the nose intrudes into the nasal visual field to some extent.

Second generation PALs

In 1973, the Varilux 2, now known simply as the Varilux*, appeared on the scene to introduce what has subsequently been referred to as 'second generation PALs'. The philosophy here was to spread the astigmatism into the distance portion, thus making the upper half of the lens non-spherical too. The upshot of this design manoeuvre is to further spread out the isocylinder lines reducing both the amount and rate of change of surface astigmatism. This can also be appreciated from figure 4. Spreading the surface astigmatism into the distance area assumes there is a tolerance on the blur which will be experienced. Maintenaz, the designer of the Varilux 2, assumed 0.3 D to be the tolerable limit of surface aberrational astigmatism[4], although others are quoted as having found 1.00 D is acceptable.

Asymmetric and symmetric designs

First generation PALs had optical properties which were

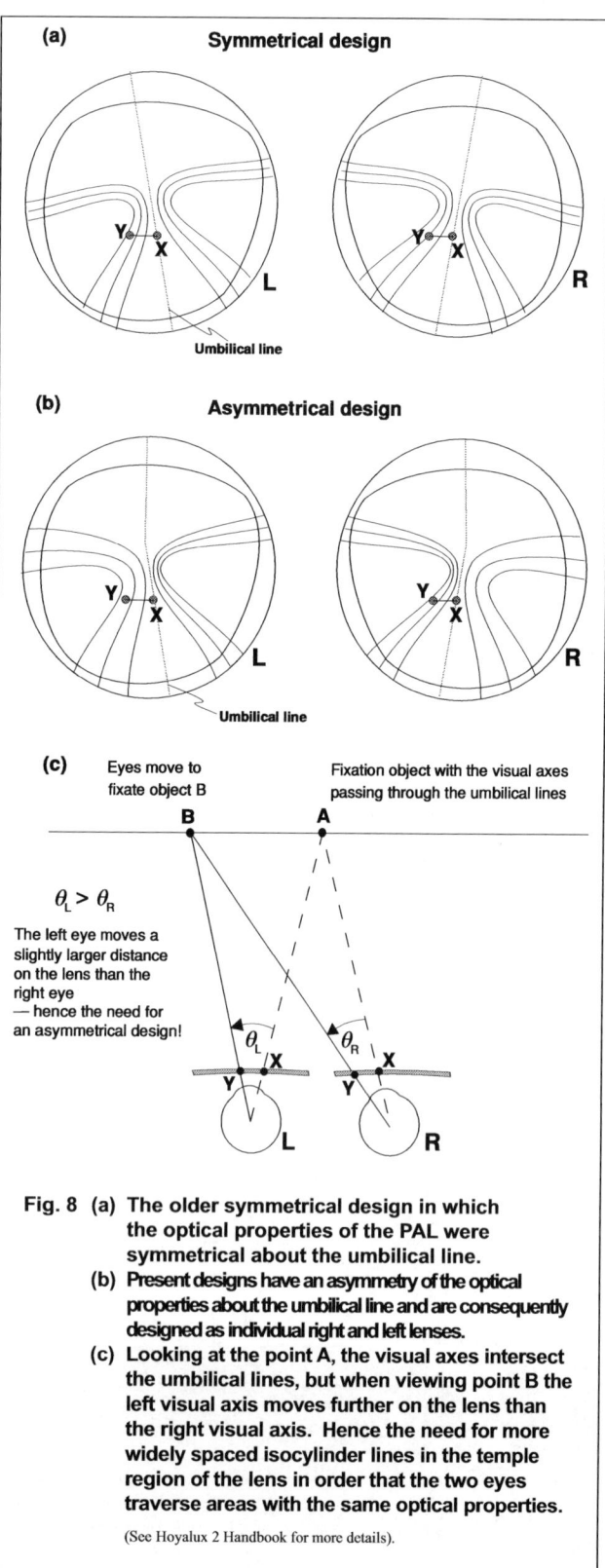

Fig. 7 The Truvision superseded the AO 40 lens. Note that compared with figure 4, the isocylinder lines spread a little upwards in the nasal area, where they are considered to be least troublesome since this area of the lens is probably the least used. The reading portion is only two-thirds the width of that in the older, harder AO 40 lens. Notice that many of the vectors on the temple side are more nearly vertical too.

Fig. 8 (a) The older symmetrical design in which the optical properties of the PAL were symmetrical about the umbilical line.
(b) Present designs have an asymmetry of the optical properties about the umbilical line and are consequently designed as individual right and left lenses.
(c) Looking at the point A, the visual axes intersect the umbilical lines, but when viewing point B the left visual axis moves further on the lens than the right visual axis. Hence the need for more widely spaced isocylinder lines in the temple region of the lens in order that the two eyes traverse areas with the same optical properties.
(See Hoyalux 2 Handbook for more details).

* Withdrawn in 2003.

symmetrical about the umbilical line; see figure 8(a). This enabled the manufacturer to produce a lens which could be used for either right or left eyes, the near inset being achieved by setting the lens with a 10° tilt inwards at the bottom. From the point of view of stocking and production, this method had an appealing simplicity, but it failed to take account of the fact that the two eyes make slightly different traverses across the lens in lateral movements from a fixation position in which the two visual axes intersect the umbilical lines; see figure 8(c). In consequence, a better design for binocular vision is an asymmetrical design, as in figure 8(b), in which the surface aberrational astigmatism changes more gradually in the temple region of the lens. This takes account of the fact that the left eye moves a little further on the lens than the right in changing fixation from object A to object B.

Manufacturers of asymmetrical designs have to stock double the number of lenses but patients have the benefit of more comfortable binocular vision, which no doubt accounts for some of the increased acceptance of PALs in recent years.

Mono and multi-designs

First and second generation designs did not take account of the differing needs of patients in different stages of presbyopia. Under the age of 50, the amplitude of accommodation is sufficient to make focusing adjustments either through the distance or reading portions. For example, a 45 year old patient with a 1.00 Add has an artificial far point of 100 cm through the reading power and can focus to 33 cm through the distance portion, although this would not be comfortable for very long. Nevertheless, there is an overlap of these focused regions indicating that for general use, at least, the intermediate portion of a PAL is not so important in early presbyopia. On the other hand, a 70 year old patient with a 3.00 Add can only see clearly to 33 cm through the reading power and cannot focus down to 100 cm through the distance Rx. There is therefore an important range of intermediate distances which need to be considered in the design of PALs for patients with higher Adds. The early designs did not do this and Essilor has coined the phrase mono-design for those types[5].

Essilor introduced the Varilux Multi Design (VMD) to address this problem, using 12 different progressive surfaces, a different one for each Add from 0.75 to 3.50. As shown in figure 9, Essilor's VMD design has a slower rate of change in power from the distance to the intermediate region. Concomitant with the more gentle progression is a wider progression corridor, better distribution of the surface aberrational astigmatism and improved binocular vision.

Perhaps we should refer to this multi-design concept as the **third generation** of PALs since other manufacturers have adopted a multi-design concept to some extent. American Optical Company introduced the Prima lens* for early presbyopes, having Adds of 0.50, 0.75 and 1.00. When the need for a higher Add arises the patient is then transferred to the Omni. In early 1993, American Optical extended

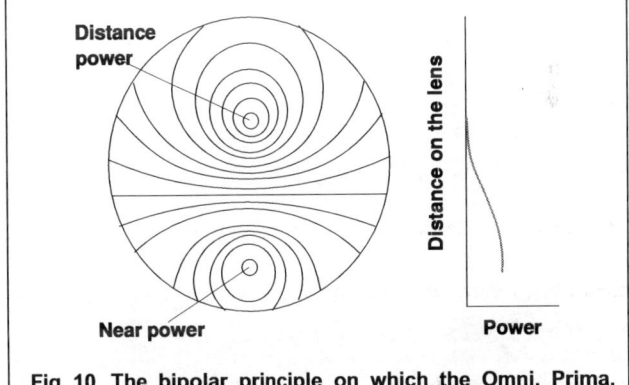

Fig. 10 The bipolar principle on which the Omni, Prima, Technica and AO PRO progressive lenses are based. The principle produces lenses with less aberrational astigmatism than other designs, although its intrusion into the distance portion is somewhat greater.

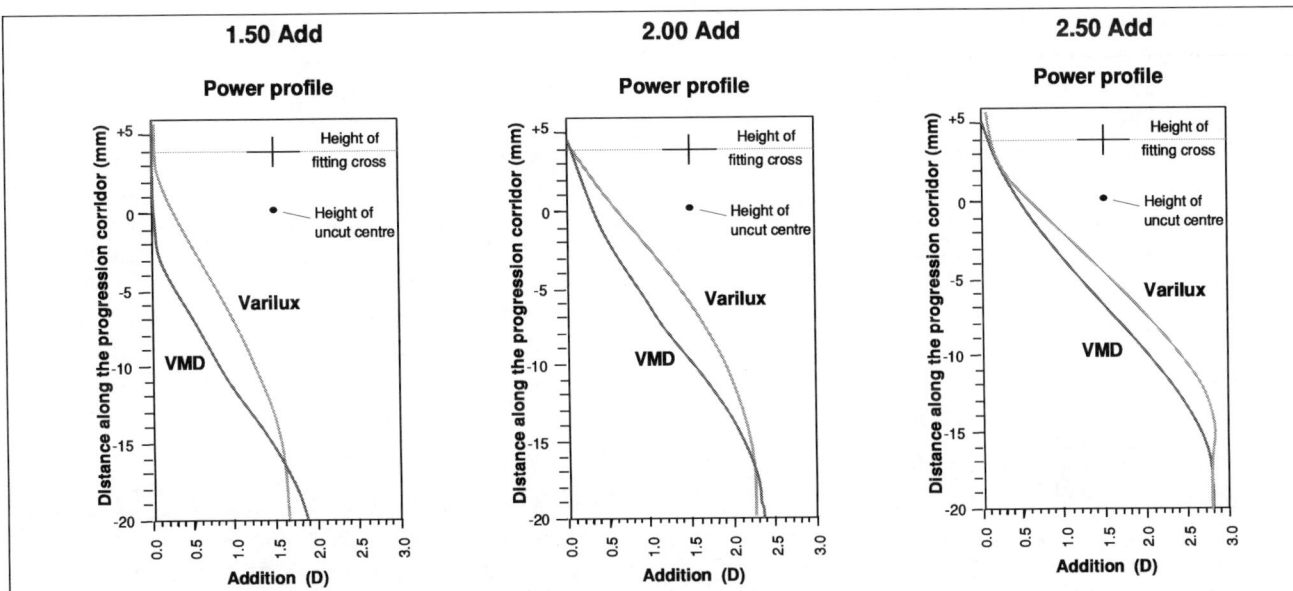

Fig. 9 Power profile illustrating a fundamental difference in the rate of change of power between the Varilux monodesign type and the more recent Varilux Multi Design. The more gentle change in power of the VMD produces a wider intermediate zone and allows a better distribution of the aberrational astigmatism, the latter improving the performance in binocular vision. Also notice there is less emphasis on the intermediate power in the lowest Add.

* Withdrawn in 2003.

Omni progressive addition lens — 2.00 Add

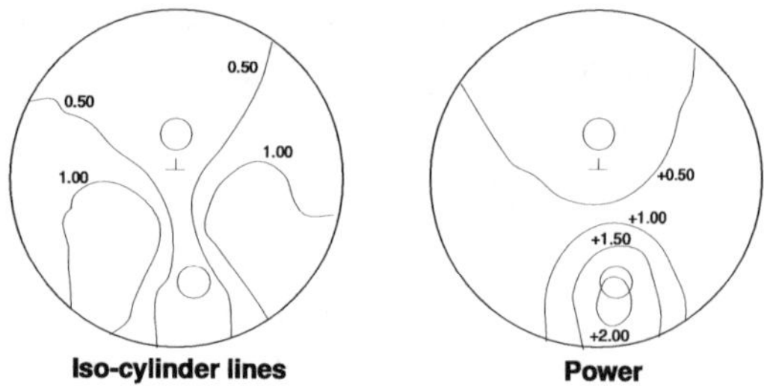

Fig. 11 Isocylinder lines and power lines on a 2.00D Add Omni progressive addition lens. This lens has the softest design of any general purpose PAL, but as with all designs, there is a compromise between the width of the distance and reading portions and the spread of the aberration over a larger part of the lens. The AO PRO design, using the same bipolar principle, is a little less soft, having slightly more astigmatism and a rather wider distance portion.

this multi-design concept in the UK with the introduction of the AO PRO lens. Using the same bipolar principle of design employed in the Omni and Prima, in which the power increases from the distance to the near power in the manner shown in the bipolar layout diagram of figure 10, they "created stable distance and near viewing zones for all Add powers and also introduced a specific corridor length for each Add".

The very soft nature of the Omni can be seen from the isocylinder lines in figure 11. The AO PRO diagrams are somewhat similar to figure 11, but the design is a little less soft; see figure 12.

Aspherisation and PALs – the Fourth Generation

Aspheric design principles, used in single vision lenses since the launch of Rodenstock's Cosmolit lens in 1986, have become a main feature in PAL design. The AO PRO uses this approach, and several soft lens designs before this have used the principle, but without making particular mention of it. Perhaps the most striking advance using aspherisation came with the launch of the Sola XL Gold in early 1994.

AO PRO isocylinder lines

Add 2.00

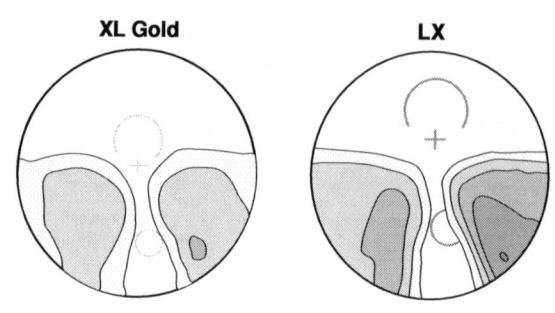

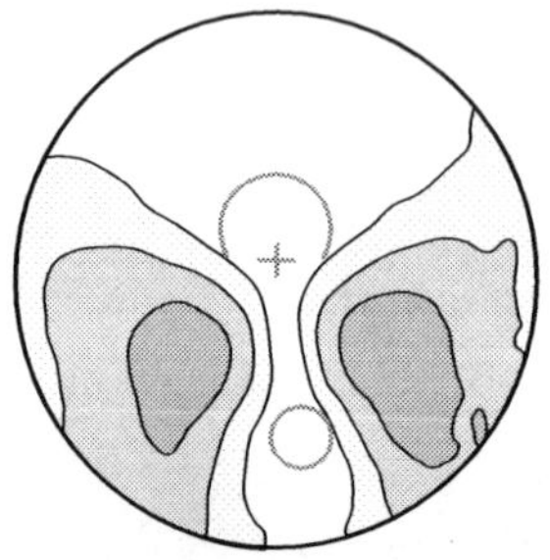

Fig. 12 AO PRO: a third generation design which "creates stable distance and near viewing zones" for all Adds.

Isocylinder lines on plano distance portion with a 2.00 D Add

Fig. 13 Comparison of the isocylinder lines in the XL Gold and XL progressive addition lenses. Note the wider progression corridor in the XL Gold version, a fact which makes reasonably well suited to applications where intermediate vision is important, such as the ubiquitous problem of the Visual Display Unit.

The XL Gold was preceded by the XL which was available in CR 39 plastic, but the XL Gold comes in Sola's mid-index plastic Spectralite ($n_d = 1.537$, $V_d = 47$, $SG = 1.21$). The XL Gold lens owes something to the XL in its design, but more aspherisation has been employed. Just as single vision aspherics can be made flatter than their spheric counterparts, aspherisation in the progressive lens design allows a flatter and therefore thinner lens to be produced with less surface aberrational astigmatism; see figure 13. The progression corridor has been made about 1½ mm longer in the 2.00 Add XL Gold than in the XL, and this also enables a reduction in surface aberrational astigmatism to be made.

Through the lens design – the Fifth Generation

In the latter part of the 1990s, computer ray tracing, long applied to single vision design, was adopted for the much more difficult analysis of progressive surfaces. Hot on the heels of this major advance, computer ray tracing was used to incorporate the progression and the prescription cylinder correction into the back surface. Computer ray tracing, using the lens in conjunction with a mathematical model eye, immediately allowed these designers to determine the nature of the retinal image of point objects in different parts of and at different distances in object space. Analysis of the retinal image is used to optimise the design of the progressive surface. Design by computer ray tracing also allows easy determination of the vertex sphere power of the lens in three dimensions. This latter method is used to evaluate the quality of oblique vision in single vision lenses. So, designers can now use this long-established means of inferring the quality of vision which a PAL wearer might expect.

The camera and ophthalmic lens company Pentax call their ray tracing design method *Retina Forward Design*™ which uses computer ray traces through the lens to determine the nature of the retinal images of a range of point objects. Using 5000 ray traces through the lens, spot diagrams on the retina are assessed for the quality of the image. Each spot is an intersection of a ray with the retina, pencils of rays

Dispensing Progressive Addition Lenses

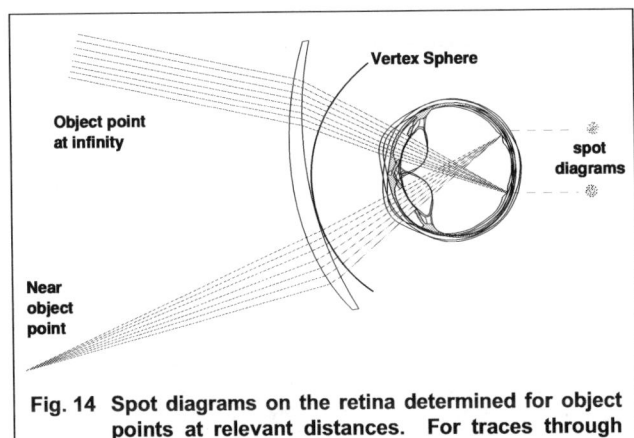

Fig. 14 Spot diagrams on the retina determined for object points at relevant distances. For traces through the progression corridor the object point is set at intermediate positions between distance and near.

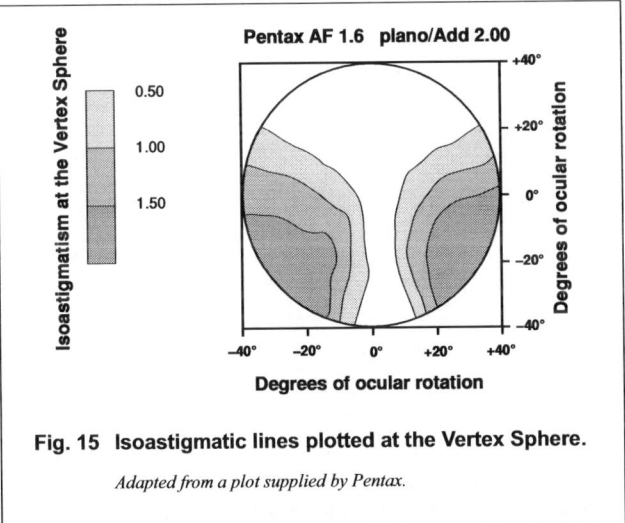

Fig. 15 Isoastigmatic lines plotted at the Vertex Sphere.

Adapted from a plot supplied by Pentax.

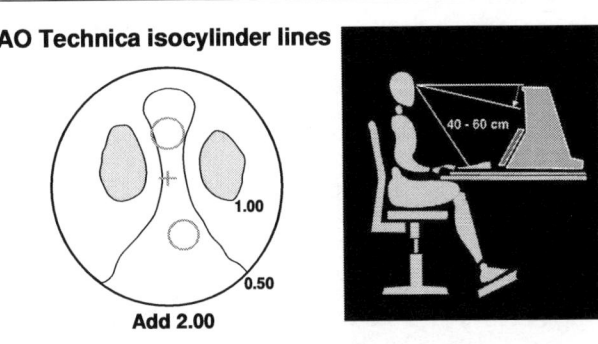

Fig. 16 The Technica progressive addition lens, is designed for continuous intermediate and near work, such as VDU use. 80% of the Add is placed 15° below the primary position of gaze. The distance portion is suitable for occasional use, but the lens should be regarded as an occupational PAL — OPAL. OPALs are not suitable for driving.

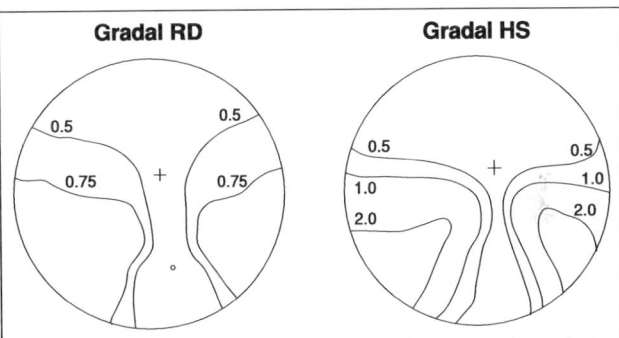

Fig. 17 Isocylinder lines on *Gradal RD* and *Gradal HS* lenses with a 2.00 prescription Add.

being limited by the eye's pupil. Figure 14 illustrates the principle.

Assuming a distance from the lens to the eye's centre of rotation, a 10° pantoscopic tilt and aspheric design principles, spot diagrams are evaluated for different fixation point positions. Each spot diagram is improved to better represent a point retinal image by a computer process which amends the surface parameters until the image is optimised. This gives the lens its name for the UK market: AF, standing for All Focus, although this is something of an exaggeration since there are still aberrations present, as can be seen from figure 15. Because ray traces through the lens are performed, it is possible to specify the mean power and aberrational astigmatism at the Vertex Sphere, something which opticians would appreciate since they are familiar with evaluating best form lenses in this way. The isoastigmatism plot of figure 15 is determined at the Vertex Sphere.

What Pentax has managed to do is to make this ultrasoft design lens perform well across the prescription range. Isoastigmatism (isocylinder) plots look much the same from −4.00 sph to +4.00 sph with a 2.00 Add.

OPALs – lenses for intermediate and close-work*

The Technica, introduced in 1988, is the only lens designed for people who require continuous use of the intermediate and near portions but relatively little use of the distance area. Inspection of the isocylinder lines in figure 16 immediately demonstrates the emphasis on near and intermediate vision. American Optical Company state that the lens is aimed at presbyopic professionals such as surgeons, architects, accountants and engineers, and at hobbyists with near and intermediate visual needs. Nowadays, we would include computer use. The lens is of bipolar design, like the Omni and the AO PRO.

In 1994, Zeiss and Rodenstock each introduced a progressive lens with only intermediate and near portions which might be called *Occupational Progressive Addition Lenses*, or OPALs. Zeiss' lens, the *Gradal RD*, the 'RD' translating loosely as 'Room Distance', indicating it is intended for use in indoor situations, either at work or at home. The lens has been designed with a 30 mm long progression corridor, which should be contrasted with the 18 mm corridor length of the Zeiss Gradal HS general purpose PAL; see the isocylinder plots in figure 17. In the Gradal RD, +0.50 DS is added to the distance Rx, but the Add is reduced accordingly to maintain the correct near vision power.

Rodenstock approached their design by using the idea of a single vision aspheric lens with the near vision power reducing to provide intermediate vision out to about 1 metre. As such, the resulting lens ought to be called a *degressive*, but, for simplicity, the author calls all intermediate/near lenses

* See pages 57 - 61 for more detail on OPALs.

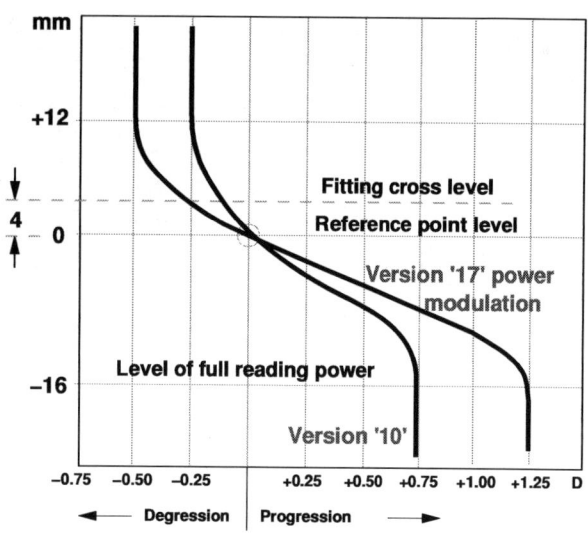
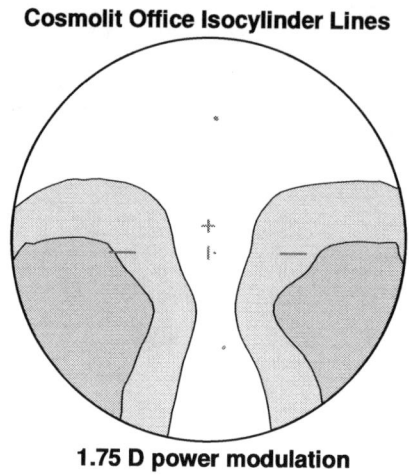

Fig. 18 CR39 near vision aspheric lens with variable power allowing clear vision to about 2 metre. For presbyopes requiring an intermediate focus in the upper portion of the lens – an Occupational Progressive Addition Lens (OPAL). Ideally suited for office workers, VDU users, draughtsmen, architects, surgeons, etc. The isocylinder plots shows 0.50 and 1.00 D isocylinder lines, so these lenses are 'very soft' in design and therefore present extremely easy adaptation. In effect, they are readers with a generous intermediate portion.

OPALs, irrespective of whether they have a progressive or a degressive surface. Rodenstock's original lens was called Cosmolit P, but it has now been replaced by the *Office*; see figure 18. In the second half of 1994, Essilor released a similar lens called Proximal, later replaced by the *Interview*. Both the Cosmolit P and the Proximal had a fairly limited power range, the lenses being intended as alternatives to reading glasses for near-emmetropic presbyopes. On the other hand, the Gradal RD and the Technica both have a more comprehensive power range allowing them to be prescribed for the majority of presbyopes. Rodenstock's new *Office* has a much increased range from −6.00 to +6.00 combined powers. There are now a number of OPALs available; see the bottom of Table 3, page 38.

The intermediate and reading fields of view with OPALs are significantly greater than with even the softest of regular wear PALs. Figure 19 illustrates this for the author's spectacles.

The effect of increasing Addition

It is generally true the width of the intermediate and reading areas narrow as the Add increases on PALs[6]. The corridor length is also increased in the design in order to try and restrict the increase of surface aberrational astigmatism. This is of some significance when dispensing second and subsequent PALs where the Add will probably have increased. A patient with a higher Add will notice a reduced width of the reading portion which, unless forewarned about, might give rise to complaint. In the author's personal experience, this narrowing of the reading area is apparent with as little as 0.25 D increase in the Add. Figure 20 shows this narrowing of the reading area with 1.50, 2.00 and 2.50 D Adds on a typical modern PAL. Also, note the increased surface aberrational astigmatism and the closer line spacing of the isocylinder lines, all of which suggests PAL wearing patients must be advised of the possibility of adaptation problems when a larger Add is dispensed.

One of the problems older presbyopes can find with PALs is the limited reading area with a high Add PAL being compounded by the presence of an age-related drop in the visual acuity. Slataper (1950)[7] published results on age norms for visual acuity, showing it begins to reduce after 50 years of age. In 50% of the population over 70 years old the acuity was less than 6/6, the norm being about 6/7.5, whilst at 80 years of age the norm is 6/12 with only 15% retaining

Fig. 19 Sola XL Gold PAL and Zeiss Gradal RD OPAL fields of view. The author's binocular reading fields were measured using an A3 landscape page printed with continuous rows of figure 8s.

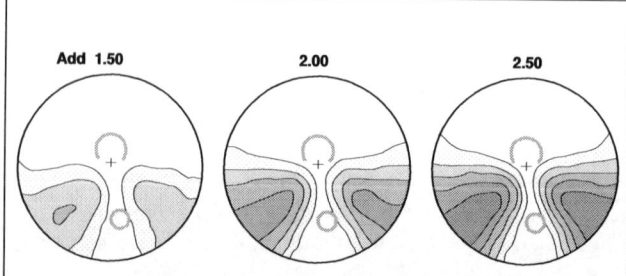

Fig. 20 Isocylinder lines on plano distance portion lenses with three different Additions. Note the increase in surface aberrational astigmatism with consequent narrowing of the reading and progression areas as the Add increases. Evidently, patients with lower Adds have wider fields of view.

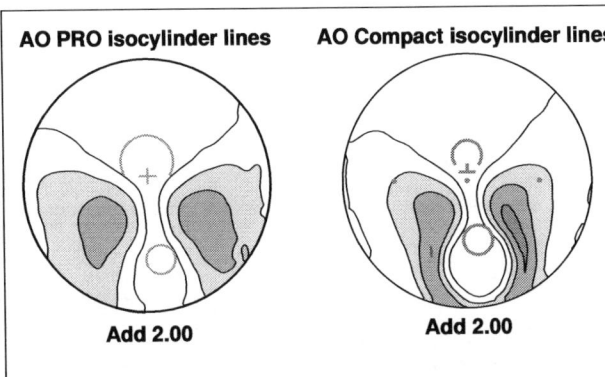

Fig. 21 The AO PRO here has a 19 mm corridor length whilst the AO Compact's is only 13 mm. Note the harder nature of the Compact design, something which must not be forgotten when considering Short Corridor Length PALs.

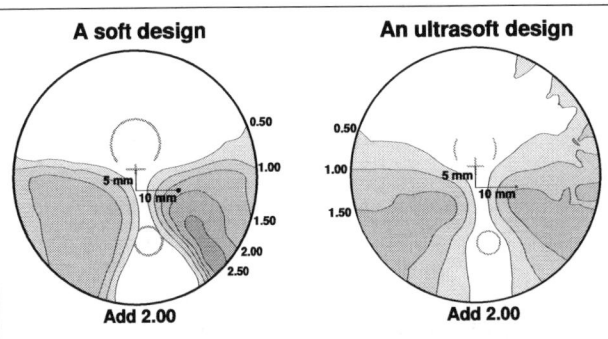

Fig. 22 Using the author's empirical criterion, a soft design PAL has surface aberrational astigmatism (SAA) in the range 1.50 D to less than 2.00 D on a lens with a 2.00 Add. The reading area is a little reduced in width compared with a hard design but there is less overall SAA. Ultrasoft PALs have less than 1.50 D SAA at the author's critical point.

6/6 or better. The norms here exclude subjects with any pathological conditions such as incipient cataract.

Especially where the Add has increased, the dispenser should be concerned when dispensing a new pair of PALs to an elderly patient with less than 6/6 acuity. Where the patient has worn PALs for some time, he/she may find that the reading vision is unsatisfactory because the field of view is too small for reading. Lenses which perform well with high Adds should obviously be considered, but sometimes the only solution is single vision readers to be worn when any 'serious' close-work is to be undertaken. Alternatively, for indoor use something like the AO Technica could be considered since it has a narrow distance portion with relatively wide reading and intermediate zones. The problem here is that there is no guarantee that any PAL will be acceptable.

Short corridor PALs

In the late 1990s, a fashion change in spectacle frames saw shallow lens shapes ('eyesizes') becoming the rule rather than the exception. PAL manufacturers rushed to address the problem of long corridor lengths not being suitable for such shallow lens shapes. In the process of reducing the corridor length comes a hardening of the PAL design; see figure 21. Consequently, we should expect the reading and intermediate fields of view to be less than with longer corridor lengths. Cautions concerning more limited fields of view when the surface aberrational astigmatism increases, mentioned on the previous page when associated with a stronger Add, will also need to be borne in mind by the dispenser when dealing with *Short Corridor Lenses*.

There are about a dozen *Short Corridor PALs* now available and they are listed in Table 3 on page 37.

A simple method of classifying PALs

We have used isocylinder line distribution to classify PALs as hard, soft or ultrasoft in design. Providing one has access to isocylinder plots*, it is possible to use a simple method of classifying progressive lenses, as follows. The method is empirical, but it works well.

The author's empirical method of classifying a *hard design* PAL is to choose a point 5 mm below and 10 mm in from the fitting cross on a lens with a 2.00 Add; if the surface aberrational astigmatism (SAA) at this point is 2.00 or more dioptres the lens is a hard design.

Lenses are classed as *soft design* if $1.50 \leq SAA < 2.00$ dioptres at the point 5 mm down and 10 mm in from the fitting cross; see Figure 22.

Progressive lenses with less than 1.50 D of SAA at the author's critical point have been called *ultrasoft* by the author.

Limit of isocylinder plot usefulness

The advent of computer ray tracing design means that isocylinder plots of the *progressive surface* are not going to be quite so useful for a PAL comparison tool, since the aberrational astigmatism can now be expressed at the vertex sphere. Once all PALs are designed by computer ray tracing, then isocylinder and mean power plots at the vertex sphere will probably become the standard for comparison.

(C) Dispensing progressive lenses

When dispensing progressive addition lenses, two thoughts should be uppermost in the practitioner's mind:

(1) Choosing the patient and (2) choosing the lens.

One thing is certain about dispensing PALs, and that is the uncertainty that the patient and/or the lens has been selected with 100% certainty of success. There is no infallible way of doing this. Given this scenario, the best the practitioner can do is to follow the guidelines derived from experience.

---

* You will find many of the isocylinder plots in *Ophthalmic Lens Availability* which can be purchased from the Association of British Dispensing Opticians. It is compiled by Dr A H Tunnacliffe and is updated at least once per year.

Choosing the patient

Presbyopic patients who may be considered for PALs can be classified into one or more groups:

- Current PAL wearers who are satisfied with them.
- Young presbyopes requiring their first Addition.
- Those who require an intermediate focus in addition to distance and near vision areas on the lens.
- Those desiring the appearance of a single vision lens.
- Those whose lifestyle, work or hobbies do not require wide reading or intermediate areas on the lenses.
- Those who would benefit from the no-jump performance of PALs.
- First-time potential PAL wearers who are prepared to 'gamble' on the chance that they can adapt to PALs.

Patients who are unlikely to succeed with PALs include:

- Previously failed PAL wearers.
- Patients who require a wide reading area and cannot or are not prepared to turn the head more for lateral viewing.
- Patients who are happy with single vision lenses, bifocals or trifocals. This includes those who are not disturbed by or conscious of the segment top in bifocals.
- Patients who are not prepared to 'gamble' on the chance of adapting to PALs, or are not prepared to wait an indeterminate time for adaptation to occur.

Choice of progressive lens

As already mentioned, there is no method by which a lens can be selected with certainty to match the patient's needs. The very fact that all the lenses in tables 1 and 2 are worn successfully by particular patients and, presumably, they have all been rejected by a small proportion of patients, indicates the problem facing the dispenser. Will one type be best for one particular patient? You are never going to know the answer to this question. So how does the practitioner decide on which lens to recommend?

The first thing to do is to question the patient about the points listed earlier when determining whether a patient is likely to be a potential PAL wearer. Perhaps the most important generalisation is the dichotomy of PALs into hard and soft/ultrasoft designs. The author can speak from considerable experience of the success of this subdivision of PALs. I spend a lot of time at a VDU where I need to focus between 40 and 70 cm from the keyboard to the screen, and anywhere between about 35 cm and 70 cm to one side at an angle of about 45° to the front-facing body position. This I can do with any of the soft designs I have tried, but with the three hard designs I have tried I find that I get asthenopia within 15 minutes. On the other hand, I can wear the hard designs for general use where there is no sustained intermediate vision, the wider reading and distance areas being readily appreciated. With harder designs, more head movement is required when scanning a newspaper compared with reading spectacles because the intermediate portion is so narrow, but the extra head movements, although still necessary are much reduced with softer design PALs. With OPALs, head and eye movements are much the same as with reading lenses with the added advantage of intermediate vision, of course.

From my personal experience adaptation is easier with softer designs, an observation which has been made before[3] and simply confirms the raison d'être of their design philosophy. As mentioned several times already, adaptation is by far the easiest with *ultrasoft designs*. Whereas, in the early nineties, I would have recommended a hard design for someone seeking a replacement for bifocals or needing a relatively wide distance portion, such as professional drivers, nowadays I would always recommend an ultrasoft design. For professional drivers just be sure to choose one with a wide field of view. In this respect Sola's Percepta has perhaps to widest distance field of view, the softness being achieved by ensuring the isocylinder lines appear in the lower half of the lens.

Always, the patient must be warned of the relatively narrow reading area, even with hard design lenses, when compared with even the smallest bifocal segment. As the PAL wearer ages and requires an increased Add, it is important to notify them of the reduced reading and intermediate field of view expected with a higher Add. Depending on which lens such a patient is wearing, it may be necessary to change the lens design to one where the reading area is a little wider. For this reason if for no other, it is wise for the practitioner to keep sufficient data to compare lenses.

Whatever the trend, all practitioners are aware of patients who accept hard design lenses for their first pair of progressives, and even those who prefer a hard design after subsequently trying a soft one. This only confirms the fact that there can be no absolute rules, only guide lines. However, with the new generation of aspherised PALs in the 1990s, it is probably true to say that hard design lenses have had their time. We may also witness the 'jelly mould' computer design phenomenon, as we did with cars, in which aspherised PAL isocylinder line plots all 'look the same'!

Other considerations in PAL selection

Tables 1 and 2, on pages 36 and 37, show that there are further considerations we can make when deciding on a progressive lens. As with other types of lens, we would wish to choose a medium or high refractive index in order to control lens thickness. This is now possible with lenses ranging through 1.5, 1.6, 1.7 and 1.8 index for PALs in glass. Powers up to −20.00 are available in glass, depending on the index, and up to +15.00 in CR 39, so power availability is rarely a problem except that there is a more limited choice of design.

Numerous photochromic PALs of hard, soft and ultrasoft designs are available in spectacle crown and 1.6 index glass, and the range in plastics is from 1.5 to 1.67. The power range for these plastic lenses varies between manufacturers but combined powers from −16.00 to +8.00 are available.

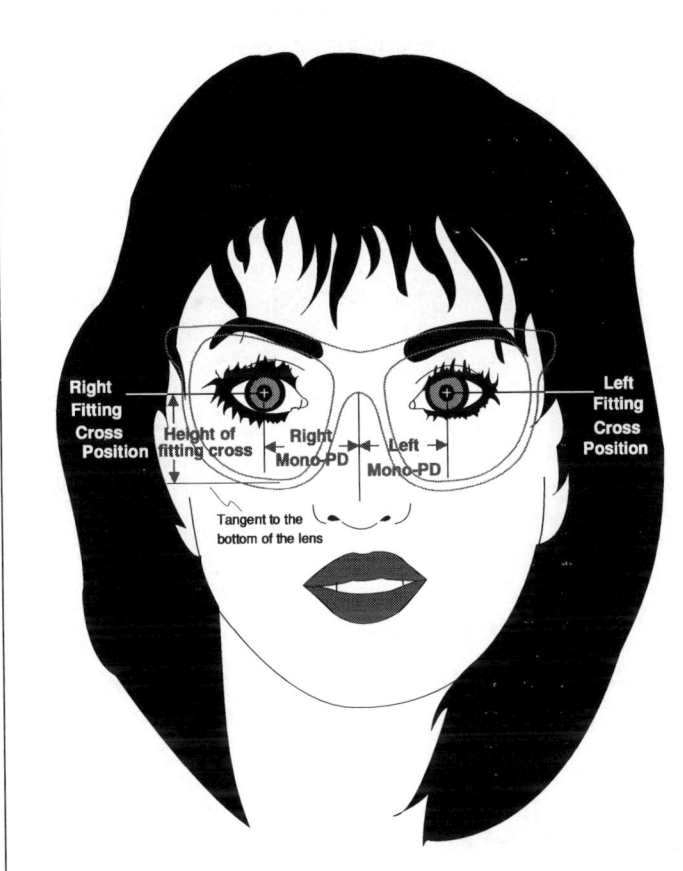

Fig. 23

Essential measurements when ordering progressive addition lenses. The head should be erect and the eyes in the primary position of gaze.

Because the upper part of the progression corridor may be as narrow as 2mm, it is essential to state the right and left mono-PDs in order that each eye centres on the umbilical line of the corridor. This ensures the best possible visual acuity when viewing a near object in the median plane. Mono-PDs quite often differ by 2 mm, and occasionally by as much as 5 mm.

Right and left fitting cross heights should both be measured since they can differ significantly. Once the fitting cross height has been measured, the fitting cross position should be stated with reference to the horizontal centre line of the frame (datum line), rather than stating a height above the lower rim or below the upper rim of the frame. The reason for this is that some practitioners fail to use the correct definition of 'height', a problem which also applies to bifocal ordering. The height of the fitting cross is from the centre of the pupil to the horizontal tangent at the bottom of the lens shape. Measuring from the pupil centre to the nearest point on the lens shape below the pupil is NOT the defined height, and is confusing and often expensive for the laboratory!

However, as with glass PALs, the range of designs is not as wide as in white plastics. A patient already wearing a white PAL successfully may find a photochromic version of the same lens is not available. Also, the photochromic PAL version, if it does exist, does not necessarily have quite the same range of power availability.

High prescription cylinders do not appear to be a contra-indication of successful wear. Indeed, it has been found that such patients had the highest probability of being successful PAL wearers. A possible reason for this is that wearers of high cylinder prescriptions have already experienced some variability of focus over their lenses. For example, a prescription −2.00 DS / −5.00 DC made in 1.523 material with a −5.25 D barrel toroidal base curve would be regarded as a best form lens. However, the performance can be seen to differ for vision at a 30° eye rotation along the base and cross curve meridians in Table 4.

Table 4 Power/vergences experienced with a −2.00 / −5.00 toric lens. Base curve −5.25, n = 1.523. 30° eye rotation. Values at the vertex sphere. Near vision at 35 cm.

	Base curve meridian	Cross curve meridian
Distance vision	Oblique Power	Oblique Power
	−2.18 DS / −5.03 DC	−1.75 DS / −5.03 DC
Near vision	Vergences	Vergences
	−4.86 / −9.94	−4.59 / −9.18

Fitting progressive addition lenses

The essential measurements are well-known (see figure 23):

1 Mono-PDs   and   2 Fitting cross heights.

It is essential that the patient and practitioner are seated on the same level and, most importantly, the patient's head must be erect. As indicated in figure 6, on page 42, a 2° forwards or backwards tilt of the head will result in a 1 mm high or low measurement for the fitting cross position, respectively. Since we measure to the nearest ½ mm, such an error is significant. Similarly, a sideways rotation of the head by 2° will introduce a 1 mm error increase in one mono-PD and a similar reduction in the other.

Mono-PDs are essential because of the narrow entry to the progression corridor which may be as little as 2 mm on a high Addition hard design. Even on a soft design, with a high Add it is unlikely to exceed 4 mm. Accurate centering is not only important for optimum performance of each lens, but comfortable binocular vision is also designed into modern PALs and depends on accurate and precise fitting. The mono-PDs are evidently essential in order to have the patient follow the umbilical line down the lens to the near vision area. Since the right and left mono-PDs can infrequently be as much as 5 mm different, and not unusually as much as 2 mm different, this measurement must be a routine part of the fitting.

Mono-PDs can be measured in one of several ways:

- by use of a PD gauge (also called a pupillometer).
- by use of a face rule, a method which is just as accurate as the PD gauge in experienced hands.
- by placing a strip of cellophane tape vertically across the frame lens shape, or using a dummy lens which might already be in the frame, and marking the pupil centre.
- by using a proprietary measuring aid supplied by a manufacturer, nowadays often consisting of a digital camera and Visual Display Unit system.

The right and left fitting cross heights should both be taken because they are not necessarily going to be the same; facial asymmetry is almost the rule rather than the exception! In figure 23, the height of the fitting cross is indicated as the distance from the horizontal tangent to the bottom of the lens to the pupil centre. Some practitioners quite wrongly state the height to be from the point on the rim immediately below the pupil centre, thus confusing the laboratory and compelling them to operate a second standard. Yet others measure the fitting cross position from the upper rim! These problems are all solved if the position of the fitting cross is stated relative to the horizontal centre line of the frame (datum line). Typically, stating the fitting cross position in this way will result in measurements within the range 3 to 7 mm (for 'long corridor' or standard PALs) although the occasional measurement outside this range will occur.

Marking the pupil centre position within the lens shape on the frame, or indicating it with a proprietary marking aid, has the advantage that both mono-PD and the height of the fitting cross can be determined by taking the frame off the patient's face and determining the measurements in a more controlled situation on a desk top.

Some writers on the subject of PAL fitting state that there are occasions when it might be advantageous to put the fitting cross a millimetre or two below the pupil centre[10]. They cite early presbyopes, the idea being that adaptation will be easier if the progression starts lower down, relative to the eye. Others state that a patient requiring a lot of use of the intermediate portion may prefer to have the fitting 1 to 2 mm higher than the manufacturer's recommended position[11]. My experience has always been that low fitting PALs are more likely to be rejected than high fitting ones. This clinical and anecdotal observation has been borne out by some Danish research[12]. Forty patients were each fitted with 5 pairs of Varilux lenses, one pair with the fitting crosses at the pupil centres and the others 1 and 2 millimetres above and below the recommended position, otherwise the spectacles were identical. They found a range of fitting heights of this lens were acceptable, to a certain degree. They found that complaints of asthenopia appeared more frequently with low fitting lenses. Incidentally, they also concluded that neither the distance nor the reading part of the prescription should be altered from that which would be prescribed normally for other forms of presbyopic correction. However, given the softer nature of PALs nowadays, there should be no reason to place the fitting cross other than in front of the centre of the pupil with the eye in the primary (zero) position of gaze. Remember this position of gaze implies the head is erect, see figure 24.

Customised progressive lenses

The new millennium saw two customised PALs enter the scene. These lenses, the *Gradal Individual* from Zeiss and the *Impression* from Rodenstock, include extra measurements to tailor the lens to the patient's needs. As indicated below, both lenses require additional measurements on the order form for which each company provides the necessary measuring tools.

Each *Gradal Individual* PAL is prepared to the patient's Rx, monocular PDs, boxed lens measurements, DBL, pantoscopic tilt, near working distance and vertex distance and requires a minimum fitting cross height 20 mm. A short corridor version, the *Gradal Short I*, with an 11 mm corridor length and 16 mm minimum fitting height, became available very soon after the initial launch.

Rodenstock's *Impression*[ILT] (ILT = Individual Lens Technology) was released about the same time. It has the progression and cylinder correction combined on the back surface. The ILT version is designed for the individual and requires the following measurements: mono-PDs, fitting cross positions, pantoscopic tilt, dihedral angle (frontal curve or bow of the front – average 4°) and the vertex distance.

Customised designs remove much of the problem of PAL choice since bespoke lenses should provide the very best solution. They come at a premium, of course. They are likely to be the most expensive and a high cost may be prohibitive in many cases. However, given time, this is probably the way PAL dispensing will go. Nevertheless, for some considerable time the majority of lens choices will depend on the practitioner's judgement because many of the current non-customised designs are going to be with us for a long time yet.

Frame selection

In common with all spectacle lenses, PALs should be fitted as close as possible to the eyes. This maximises the field of view, which is especially important in the relatively narrow

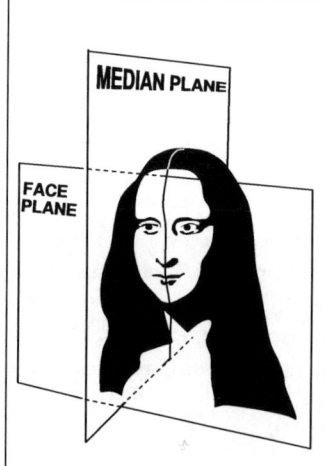

Fig. 24

Two important reference planes which determine the erect head position. The median plane divides the head into two halves through the centre of the nose. The face plane is perpendicular to the median plane and tangential to the eyebrow ridges and the chin. The head is erect when the two planes

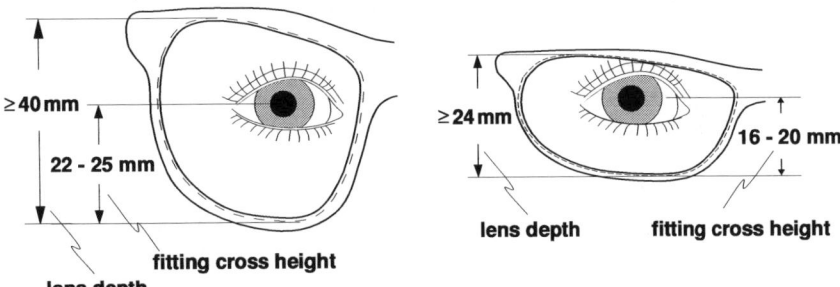

Range of lens depths and fitting cross heights for (a) standard and (b) short corridor progressive lenses

Fig. 25 (a) For Standard 'long corridor' PALs, the depth of the frame below the pupil centre, with the eye in the primary position, should be between 22 and 25 mm, depending on the particular progressive lens. Since, with almost all modern PALs, the full Add is reached between 14 and 18 mm below the fitting cross, this leaves about 8 mm of full reading depth, or a vertical field of about 15 cm at a working distance of 40 cm. Typical positions of the fitting cross will lie between 3 and 7 mm above datum line* in the frame, although 1 or 2 mm outside this range is not impossible; this means the depth of the lens shape between the upper and lower horizontal tangents should be at least 40 mm.

* Corresponds with the Horizontal Centre Line in BS 3521 : Part 1 :1991.

(b) Short corridor progressive lens range of lens depths and fitting cross heights.

progression corridor and reading area, and also minimises distortion[13]. The pantoscopic tilt should be about 10-15°, bringing the lower part of the lens as close as possible to the eyes and increasing the field of view in this area of the lens. (The conventional theory of pantoscopic tilt associated with having the optical axis pass through the eye's centre of rotation, does not strictly apply here since there is effectively an infinite sequence of optical axes in the progression zone.)

For standard PALs, all manufacturers recommend that the depth of the frame should be somewhere in the range 20 to 25 mm below the pupil centre with the eye in the primary position. The reason for this can be appreciated from figure 25 and its legend. In order not to cut into the reading portion, frames should not be used where the lower nasal rim cuts away from the nose, as with 'aviator' or oval shapes for example. However, short progression corridor PALs are designed to cope with the shallow eyesizes which fashion has dictated in the late 1990s. Short corridor PALs, such as Rodenstock's 12 mm corridor length *Progressiv Life XS* allow fitting cross heights as small as 16 mm, and with a minimum of 8 mm above the fitting cross this means that lens depths can be as low as 24 mm. But, remember, such lenses are harder in design than their standard counterparts and therefore patients are likely to have a more difficult adaptation.

Once the frame has been selected, *it should be fitted to the patient before the fitting cross height measurement is taken.* Adjustable pads allow some movement of the frame both at the time of the dispensing and at the collection. Strictly, one should not need to adjust the fitting at collection, but the patient might return and express the desire to have the lenses higher or lower, something which is possible with an adjustable pad frame, to about a 1 mm change of height. With a fixed pad frame, raising or lowering the lenses would involve narrowing or widening the bridge, which in turn would adversely alter the lateral position of the progression corridor. Having taken great care to match it to the mono-PDs, this is clearly undesirable. Ideally, the adjusted frame should be included with the order, which means stocking all measurement combinations of each frame.

Checking glazed PALs

All PALs should arrive at the dispenser's checking desk with two sets of marks: one set of temporary painted

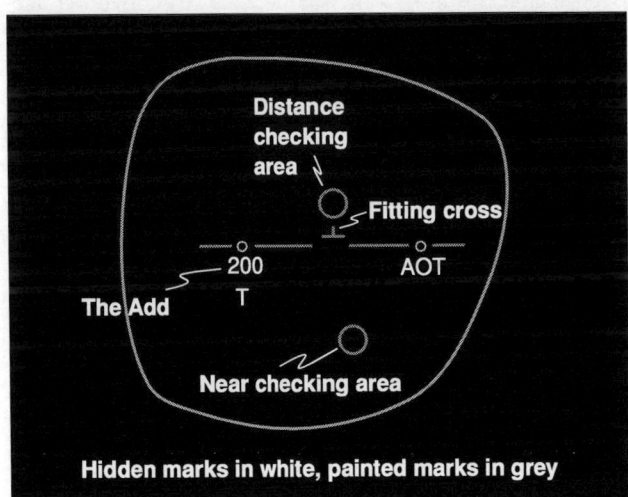

Hidden marks in white, painted marks in grey

Fig. 26 Painted and hidden marks on a right Technica progressive addition lens (American Optical Co.). The upper painted circle is the distance checking area where the distance power should be measured with the focimeter. The lower painted circle is the near checking area. Not all manufactures have 'hidden' circles to determine the horizontal setting of the lens, some use crosses or triangles, the AO PRO has marks which look like a letter 'p', and Zeiss uses a tiny stylised letter Z. These marks are always 34 mm apart. At collection, the fitting cross should be directly in front of the pupil centre with the eyes in the primary position. Prescribed prism should be checked on the horizontal line below the fitting cross, midway between the two horizontal locators.

marks and a permanent set of engraved or cast, 'hidden or semi-visible' marks. Figure 26 illustrates these marks on a Technica occupational progressive addition lens (American Optical). The painted marks are used for checking the distance power (upper circle), the reading power (lower circle), and the horizontal setting of the lens (the horizontal dashed line). For the majority of PALs, when *checking the Add*, remember to measure the difference between the front vertex powers in the near and distance checking areas; this is because the front surface has the additional power on it.

Alternatively, check the *micro-engraved Add* which appears under the temple horizontal locator (hidden circle or other symbol).

There are exceptions to determining the Add by the difference between front vertex powers for near and distance. One obvious case is where the progression surface is the back surface, as in Rodenstock's *Progressiv Life XS* and *Impression* or Seiko's *Synergy*. Another exception is where the lens powers are determined at the vertex sphere, as in the case of Pentax's *AF* and *AF Mini* series. In that case, the manufacturer states the expected focimeter reading for the near vision power with each completed order. Zeiss state on each lens packet the measured power expected in the reading area on the focimeter. It is generally true that where there is a special means of measuring the Add, other than the difference between near and distance area front vertex powers, the manufacturer will specify the method in each case.

Prescribed prism should be checked at the prism checking point which is mid-way between the hidden horizontal line marks (circles, crosses, etc.).

The *fitting cross painted mark* is used to check the fitting at the time of collection. It should appear in front of the pupil centre with the eyes in the primary position of gaze (looking straight ahead with the head erect). After checking the fit and position of the lenses, the painted marks can be removed with acetone.

The *hidden circles*, or other horizontal locator symbols such as crosses, triangles or stylised marks such as ⌐ on most Zeiss progressive lenses, are used if the lenses ever need to be remarked, such as when checking the lenses in cases where the patient returns with some complaint. The hidden marks, which include the Add on the temple side and usually an identification on the nasal side, such as T for Technica in figure 26, can best be seen by holding the lens up to and very slightly to one side of a light source. The marks should be seen against the somewhat darker background immediately at the boundary of the light source and its surround. This is effectively a dark viewing technique where light scatters from the hidden marks, thus increasing their contrast against a dark background. Note that these hidden marks can still be located with coated lenses. Hoya have marketed a dark-ground viewing system which enables hidden markings to be seen with relative ease.

The *identifying mark* can be used to determine the type of progressive lens which a new patient is currently wearing.

There is a complete listing of the identification marks in the Tables section at the back of this book and it is updated annually in the *Ophthalmic Lens Availability* file, marketed by ABDO. The fitting cross is not shown as an engraving or cast mark because this would be directly in front of the pupil in the primary position of gaze. However, its position is needed when checking a complaint of poor lens performance by a patient. The table in the *Ophthalmic Lens Availability* file or at the back of this book also gives the position of the fitting cross above and mid-way between the centres of the circles or other similar hidden marks.

Prism thinning

Because the front progressive surface has gradually reducing radii of curvature towards the bottom of the lens, the lower edge thickness would normally be noticeably less than the thickness of the upper edge; see figure 27. Nowadays, manufacturers remove this excess thickness by what is known as 'prism thinning'. About 0.6^Δ base up prism is removed per dioptre of Add, effectively adding base down prism equally before each eye so that binocular vision is not affected. In order to match right and left lenses when ordering just one lens, it is advisable to inform the laboratory of the prescription in the other eye.

Fowler (1993)[10] has pointed out that prism thinning can sometimes lead to the bottom edge of the lens being thicker than the top edge in medium to high minus lenses. However, if the dispenser forwards the lens shape and size to the surfacing laboratory they should be able to avoid this problem, especially with sophisticated computer software increasingly being able to calculate the precise amount of thinning required.

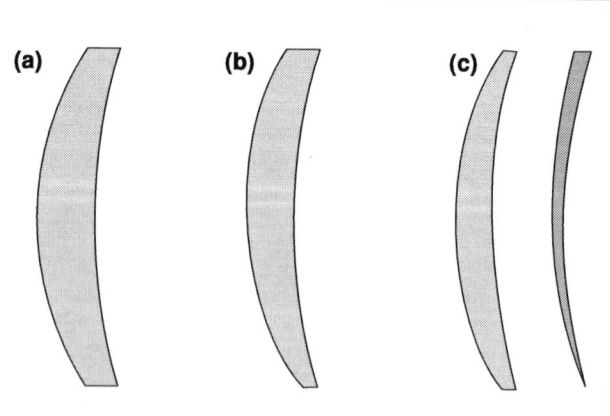

Fig. 27   Prism thinning for reduced weight and improved cosmesis.
(a) An imaginary single vision lens before the front surface is aspherised to produce a progressive addition lens.
(b) The progressive addition lens with continuous shortening of the front surface radius to produce the lower reading portion.
(c) 'Removed' prism (on the right) from the progressive lens to equalize the upper and lower edge thicknesses.

Prescribed Prisms

When a prism is included in a progressive lens, one must realise that the eye will turn towards the apex of the prism and will therefore view through a slightly different position on the lens. In the case of PALs this necessitates altering the fitting cross position on the order. For example, since 1^Δ is about $0.57°$, and from the rule that $1°$ of ocular rotation corresponds to about 0.5 mm displacement of the intersection of the visual axis on the lens, we deduce that a 1^Δ ocular rotation corresponds to $0.57 \times 0.5 \approx 0.3$ mm displacement on the lens. Hence, for example, suppose that the Rx has R. 1^Δ base down and L. 1^Δ base up. This will require the fitting crosses to be ordered 0.3 mm higher in the RE and 0.3 mm lower in the LE (the displacements are towards the prism apices). Horizontal displacements will be necessary with horizontal prisms, too. These fitting adjustments are critical with PALs since the position of the eyes with respect to the progression of the addition is so important for the lenses to perform properly.

(D) Patient acceptance of PALs

When advising prospective PAL wearers, one should always warn them of the fact that not all patients adapt to these lenses. Various reasons are cited for failure to adapt. Borish (1985)[14] reported the preference of 63 subjects in a trial where they were each given the opportunity to compare a progressive addition lens with their present type of correction (reading single vision, bifocals, or trifocals). 42 of the 63 subjects were current bifocal or trifocal wearers. The reasons cited for not selecting PALs in this study were:

Could not locate reading area readily	(4 patients)
Peripheral distortion too bothersome	(4 patients)
Needed or preferred a wide near area	(4 patients)
Needed or liked a wide intermediate area	(5 patients).

Since 16 patients rejected PALs and one did not complete the study, the acceptance rate of PALs over other forms of near correction in this study was $46/62 = 0.74$, or 74%. However, this somewhat pessimistic figure should be viewed in the light of Borish's analysis when he compared the results of first time PAL wearers with those currently wearing bifocals or trifocals; then he found that the acceptance rate was 88%. This agrees with the author's practical experience and results in his informing prospective first-time PAL wearers that about 90% of such patients adapt to these lenses. In Borish's group, the largest proportion of subjects to reject PALs was the current trifocal wearers.

The patient's visual requirements

From the foregoing, it is clear that a patient's visual requirements must be thoroughly investigated, those requiring wide intermediate and/or near vision areas being advised to have some other form of presbyopic correction than PALs, unless the fairly wide intermediate and near areas of a Technica lens would suffice. On the Technica these areas are about twice the width encountered in the Omni, for example, and the lens can be considered an occupational PAL even though it has a narrow distance portion. The Sola XL Gold and AO PRO lenses have a sufficiently wide intermediate area to allow comfortable viewing of a VDU monitor, so fourth generation PALs may well be the solution for both general wear and vocational use too. However, even when the lenses are simply to be used for general purposes, a prospective PAL wearer must be advised that he/she is taking a gamble that adaptation will occur in some unspecified time. Adaptation times, reported by successful PAL wearers returning after some two years, vary from "no time at all" to six months or more. It may well be that *very critical patients* do not make successful PAL wearers, according to Young (1984)[15], whilst less critical patients are able to adapt to the narrow reading area, the peripheral astigmatic blur and the problem of some distortion of vertical and horizontal lines seen through the lower half of the lens. With the present day *ultrasoft design* PALs distortion is less of a problem than the other two factors, the relatively narrow reading area, compared with bifocals, and surface aberrational astigmatic blur.

Of course, because the reading area reduces in width as the Add increases, all patients continuing with PALs should be warned of this fact, especially where they are to have the same type of lens. If they are changing to a lens design with a wider reading area, then they will probably have a narrower intermediate width and more surface aberrational astigmatism to contend with, and they should be warned of this. Adequate instruction in the use of the lenses should be a priority on collection, especially for new wearers. The need for more head movement when using the reading and intermediate areas, caused by their relative narrowness, should be emphasised, although the softness of *ultrasoft* lenses mitigates the effects of the border between clear vision and aberrational blur, making head movements not too much different from those required with reading spectacles, in the author's personal experience. Bear in mind that before the need for a reading correction, a pre-presbyope will probably move the head laterally on changing horizontally from the left column of this page, say, to the right column; so, this degree of head movement is normal and about the same as that which is required when using *ultrasoft* PALs with Adds up to about 2.25, in the author's experience. Nevertheless, when scanning a newspaper, for example, it is true that more head movement is required and even with *ultrasoft design* PALs it should still be mentioned. When adaptation has occurred patients will not notice the extra head movements.

Sullivan and Fowler (1990)[16] have investigated tolerance and non-tolerance of progressive addition lenses amongst 38 patients aged between 43 and 80 years of age, 20 of whom were successful wearers. They found the cause of a patient's problem might be one or more of:

- An incorrect prescription
- A non-tolerance to a prescription
- Incorrect dispensing
- Incorrectly manufactured PALs
- Adaptational difficulties.

Dispensing Progressive Addition Lenses

Table 5 Procedure for dealing with problems with PALs

1. **Ask the patient if the problem is related to any of:**
   - Distance vision.
   - Intermediate vision.
   - Near vision.
   - Right, or left, or both eyes.

2. **Check the frame fitting**
   - Ensure the pantoscopic tilt is correct.
   - Ensure the frame has been fitted as close to the eyes as possible.
   - Ensure there is no warping of the frame.
   - Raise or lower the frame if this appears to help.
   - Alter the bowing (face forming) if this appears to help.

3. **Check the lenses**
   - Remark the hidden circles (or other appropriate symbols).
   - Mark the position of the fitting cross (see Table 5).
   - Check the distance power and axis, the Add, and any prism for each lens.
   - Check whether both lenses have been prism thinned!
   - Check the position of the fitting cross for height and horizontal setting for both lenses.
   - Check that the hidden marks (circles or other) are level.
   - Check the distance from the fitting cross to the point where the full Add is reached on EACH lens as poorly manufactured lenses can introduce asymmetries.
   - Check the base curves of each lens – it is possible for two similar powered lenses to have been made on different base curves.
   - Check for over-tight fitting of lenses in metal rimmed frames as this can significantly warp the lenses.

4. **Check the marked lenses on the face**
   - Check the position of the marked fitting crosses relative to the pupil centres with the head erect and the eyes in the primary position.
   - Check that the minimum depth of lens below the pupil centre is attained (~ 23 mm).

5. **Evaluate patient's use of PALs**
   - Check the patient's head position in relation to the reading material etc.
   - Check that the patient moves the head sufficiently to view laterally placed objects.

6. **Re-examine the patient**
   - Distance Rx.
   - Amplitude of accommodation.
   - Near working distance and the Add, allowing for Near Vision Effectivity Error.
   - Visual acuity — if less than 6/6, single vision readers or some other form of near correction might be better.

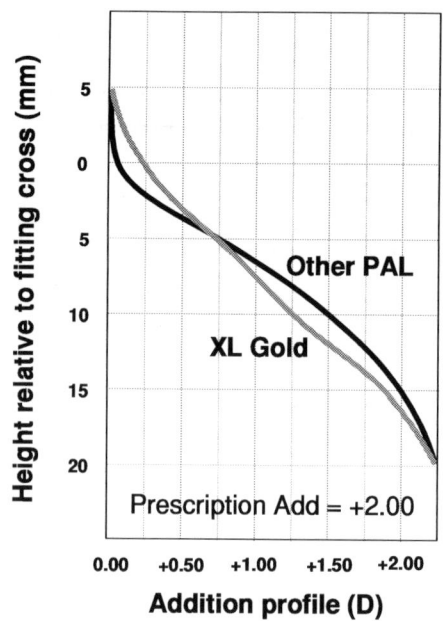

Fig. 28 Plots of the Addition profile along the umbilical line of two lenses. Measurements were made at the six points at 5 mm intervals, the zero on the ordinate indicating the position of the fitting cross. The author found the more linear profile of the XL Gold offered more natural vision when approaching stairs or pavement edges. This is due to a linear profile producing less vergence difference for rays entering the upper and lower margins of the pupil.

The first two potential sources of a wearing difficulty would most likely be checked only after the last three have been investigated.

Incorrect dispensing

This is the first area of difficulty which should be checked when a patient complains of difficulty with new PALs. It is best to have a standard procedure for dealing with complaints, such as the list in Table 6. Perhaps the most common dispensing error is in the determination of vertical positioning of the fitting cross. As noted earlier, the patient and practitioner must be at the same eye-level when this measurement is being determined, and the patient's head must be erect. This review has twice before emphasised the error caused by a forwards or backwards tilt of the patient's head during the fitting cross height measurement. Even when any source of systematic error has been eliminated or minimised, as with all measurements there will be some random error variation, something rarely stressed in dispensing, so it might be a good policy to repeat the measurements three or four times and use the mean value.

Effect of pupil size

It is well known that a small pupil increases the tolerance to blur and this may mean that patients with large pupils have less chance of adapting to PALs than patients with small pupils. In general, pupil diameter reduces with age, being about 3 to 4 mm after 45 years of age on average. However, occasionally one sees presbyopes with pupil diameters of about 6 mm for distance fixation in the light adapted state and this may be a contra-indication for progressive lens wear. However, the author is not aware of any work which has been done on the relationship between pupil size and non-tolerance of PALs.

The author has found that those PALs with a linear Add profile along the umbilical line present more comfortable vision when using the intermediate portion for ascending stairs, for example; see figure 28.

Faulty lenses

Given reasonable accuracy in the measurements, Sullivan and Fowler[16] found that small dispensing errors are insufficient to explain non-tolerance of PALs. In the same investigation, however, they found some cases where the right and left Adds, measured at the near checking centres, varied by more than 0.50 D, so the possibility of manufacturing errors must not be dismissed in 'grief' cases. One measurement which is possible to make on the focimeter is the distance from the fitting cross to the point at which the full Add is found. This should be done in grief cases when all other checks have failed to find the cause of a problem, since asymmetry of this type would indicate a faulty lens.

Summary

Accurate measurement is essential. The position of the fitting cross in PALs should be opposite the centre of the pupil with the eye in the primary position (head erect and looking straight ahead). Considerable care is needed in positioning the patient's head and eyes in both multifocal and bifocal fitting. Fitting the progression too low in PALs causes more difficulty than fitting it too high. Also, since the minimum width in the progression corridor between the 0.50 D isocylinder lines is often no more than 4 mm, one should evidently follow the manufacturer's exhortations to use the mono-PDs for horizontal centration. As with bifocals, vertical height differences are important.

Even with satisfactory dispensing, the success rate with PALs is probably less than with bifocals, although may well change with the fourth generation of aspheric design based lenses and custom designed PALs. Prior to these latest designs, various studies have reported PAL success rates between 73% and 93%. Nevertheless, no matter how good the lens or the fitting, a small percentage of patients are unlikely to adapt to PALs. Potential wearers should be so advised, but with emphasis on the high success rate with PALs.

Whether a patient can or cannot adapt to PALs is unpredictable. Besides accurate fitting and explaining to patients that they will have to move their head more for reading than they would in bifocals, because of the narrow reading area, some precautions might be made in patient selection. In the author's experience, patients with less than 6/6 acuity may be unhappy with PALs, probably because the surface aberrational astigmatism around the narrow reading area reduces the acuity further. If a patient with 6/9 acuities, say, wishes to have PALs, a fourth generation design with its relatively lower amount of surface aberrational astigmatism, or a hard design with its wider reading area might be effective. Patients requiring a wide near field of view should generally be advised not to have PALs, unless one of the OPALs is acceptable.

Patient selection and instruction is important. Wearers who are satisfied with single vision reading spectacles, or with bifocals or trifocals, are probably not good candidates to try PALs. The patient must be prepared to accept some peripheral blur through the lenses and must be made aware that more head turning is required than with bifocals. Patients with occupations demanding a wide field of view for near vision may not be suitable for PALs, even if they are prepared to turn the head a lot, although OPALs are likely to be accepted where distance vision is not a priority. This is especially true where the work has long, straight lines across the field of view; OPALs and the fourth generation PALs present less distortion in the lower half of the lens than earlier design PALs. Instruction in the use of PALs is vital, with some emphasis on moving the head to find the correct region on the lens.

In the final analysis, the PAL patient is taking a gamble with about a 90% probability of successful wear, and this should be explained at the outset. To a lesser extent, there is still a gamble being taken with subsequent stronger Add pairs because the reading and intermediate areas become somewhat narrower as the Add increases. This applies to all progressives.

At the present time, there are some 40 or so manufacturers' versions of PALs available, ranging through 1.523 spectacle crown, CR 39, mid-index plastic, 1.6, 1.7 glass and plastic, 1.8 index glasses, photochromic glass and photochromic plastic.

All PALs fall into one of three basic types – *hard*, *soft* and *ultrasoft* designs. Until fairly recently, practitioners would have been advised to have at least one soft and one hard design in their regular armoury of PALs, but the current fourth generation of PALs has probably changed that situation. Perhaps now only fourth generation lenses are required to suit both first-time and continuing wearers, and those with a high Add. Over time the choice may boil down to customised computer ray trace designed lenses, but these lenses will always have a premium cost. Of course, the practitioner also needs be aware of the special types such as high and very high index lenses, and the vocational lenses such as the Technica OPAL, the Gradal RD, Rodenstock's Office and others.

Patients requiring lengthy periods of intermediate vision should certainly be fitted with an *ultrasoft design*. Those requiring wide aberration-free distance field of view might be fitted with a hard design, which will also tend to have a wider reading area than a soft design, although this is narrower than a bifocal reading area. Sola's Percepta is a modern *ultrasoft design* with a very wide distance field of view, so it isn't necessary to go for a hard design. VDU users will generally find an *ultrasoft design* suitable, subject to exhortations to move the head for laterally placed work, although an OPAL would be better for prolonged use.

One thing is certain, there is no test or measurement that the practitioner can undertake which will allow him to choose the ideal PAL for a patient, although more confidence in a good outcome is now the rule rather than the exception with fourth generation lenses and customised lenses.

Essential fitting measurements

- Each mono-PD should be recorded and indicated on the order.

- Manufacturers specify a fitting cross which should be placed opposite the pupil centre with the eyes in the primary position, account being taken of any difference between the right and left fittings.

- A minimum depth below the pupil centre is required, usually about 23 mm for standard PALs, although this may be as low as 16 mm for the (harder) short corridor lenses.

References

1. Fisher, R.F. (1977) The force of contraction of the human ciliary muscle during accommodation. *J. Physiol.* **270**, 51.
2. Woodcock, F.R. (1985) Varifocal update. *Optician*, **190**, 5025, 15.
3. Wittenberg, S., Richmond, P.N., Cohen-Setton, J. and Winter, R.R. (1989) Clinical comparison of the Truvision Omni and four progressive addition lenses. *J. Am. Optom. Assoc.* **60**, 114.
4. Cited by Sullivan, C.M. and Fowler, C.W. (1988) Progressive and variable focus lenses. *Ophthal. Physiol. Opt.* **8**, 402.
5. W. Koeppen (1990) The New Generation. *Optometry Today*, 15 January, 10.
6. Sullivan, C.M. and Fowler, C. (1991) Reading addition analysis of progressive addition lenses. *Ophthal. Physiol. Opt.* **11**, 147.
7. Slataper, F.J. (1950) Age norms of refraction and vision. *Arch. Ophthal. N.Y.* **43**, 468.
8. Fowler, C. and Sullivan, C. (1990) Variations on a Theme. *Optician*, 23rd March, page 20.
9. Wittenberg, S. (1978) Field study of a new progressive addition lens. *J. Am. Optom. Assoc.* **49**, 1013.
10. Fowler, C. (1993) Current Topics in Progressive Addition Lenses. *Optician*, Sept. 10th.
11. Fannin, T.E. and Grosvenor, T. in *Clinical Optics*, Butterworths 1987, page 286.
12. Kilum, D., Blue, H., Burchardi, P., Praest, B., Rahlff, J. and Trobeck, H. *Essilor's Third International Symposium on Presbyopia*. Haiti, 1985. Vol. 3, page 80.
13. Tunnacliffe, A.H. (1989) Spectacle correction of aphakia. *Optician*, **197**, 5200, 37-40 and 5201, 24-29.
14. Borish, I.M. *Essilor's Third Symposium Internationale de la Presbytie*. Haiti, 1985. Vol. 3, page 72.
15. Young, J.M. (1984) The progress of progressives. *Ophthalmic Optician*, 24, 300.
16. Sullivan, C.M. and Fowler, C.W. (1990) Investigation of Progressive Addition Lens patient tolerance to dispensing anomalies. *Ophthal. Physiol. Opt.* **10**, 16.

Occupational Progressive Addition Lenses

Introduction

Progressive Power Lenses (PPLs) or, as I prefer to call them, Progressive Addition Lenses (PALs), have been with us commercially since the introduction of what was then called the Varilux lens in 1959. The single property which distinguishes these lenses from other ophthalmic lenses is the progression of the *Addition* or the *Power* from the distance prescription in the upper portion to the near prescription in a smaller region of the lower portion. The progression corridor, where intermediate powers are met, is a relatively narrow region of clear vision leading from the distance vision power to the near vision power. This intermediate region is very useful for short term inspection of objects beyond the near portion focus. However, for prolonged intermediate vision tasks, say 30 minutes or more, viewing through this narrow corridor is likely to present asthenopic symptoms. In 1988, the American Optical Company introduced a progressive lens with a very narrow distance portion but with relatively wide intermediate and near vision portions. This was the *Technica*, which is still available today. In keeping with the acronym PAL, we might refer to this lens type as an Occupational Progressive Addition Lens (OPAL). Figure 1 shows isocylinder plots for the *Technica* and the Sola *XL Gold* PAL, indicating the extra width in the intermediate and near vision portions of the *Technica*. It may not be just coincidence that the late eighties saw the advent of the personal and office computer as we now know it with windows and multitasking. Hence, people began to spend long periods of work-time at the Visual Display Unit (VDU), thus placing a large demand on the intermediate vision of presbyopic VDU users. It was not until 1994 that other manufacturers responded to this need with the development of progressive lenses where the power varied from an intermediate vision focus to the near vision focus.

The *Gradal RD* lens from Zeiss has +0.50 DS added to the distance Rx and the reading Rx remains as prescribed. The *Gradal RD* can reasonably be regarded as an OPAL since it is, in effect, a modified PAL in design. However, 1994 also saw the introduction of two other intermediate/near progressive lenses which were, by design, effectively modified near vision lenses. The first of these was the *Cosmolit P* from Rodenstock, followed in the Autumn of 1994 by Essilor's *Proximal* lens. Both of these were superseded by updated designs in late 1998 to early 1999. The *Cosmolit P* was replaced by the *Cosmolit Office*, now referred to as the *Office Perfalit 1.5*, whilst the *Proximal* gave way to the *Interview*. These lenses do not really fall into the classification of 'progressive', being, if anything, 'degressive' from the near vision power. However, for the sake of uniformity in nomenclature, I am going to refer to all of these lenses as OPALs. Figure 2 shows the isocylinder lines of the *Gradal RD* and the power or addition profile. The very small surface aberrational astigmatism means that in practice the patient has a full field of clear vision for intermediate and near vision. I have tried four OPALs and can vouch for their efficacy: reading a newspaper requires no strained head and eye positions. It is possible to see clearly over a relatively wide area on the lens thus giving presbyopes the sense they are using a single vision spectacles. With this property in mind, some manufacturers describe these lenses as *dynamic reading lenses* or **enhanced reading lenses**.

Including the AO *Technica*, with its narrow distance portion, there are currently eight OPALs available, as listed below.

Lens	Manufacturer
Technica	American Optical
Interview	Essilor
Continuum	Norville
Office Perfalit 1.5	Rodenstock
Access	Sola
Office	Taylor
Clarlet Business	Zeiss
Gradal RD	Zeiss

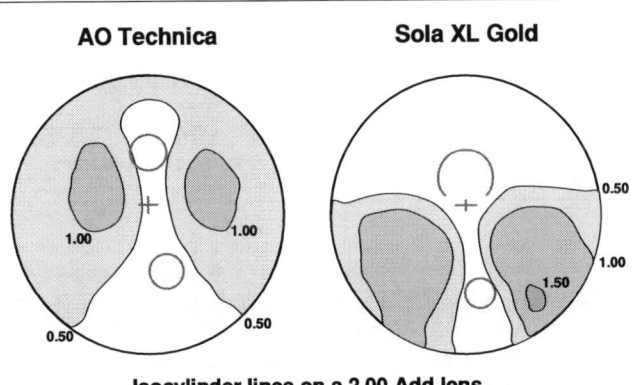

Isocylinder lines on a 2.00 Add lens

Fig. 1 Isocylinder line plots illustrate the extra width of the intermediate and near vision portions on the *Technica* lens compared with the *XL Gold*, the latter having a wide intermediate area for a PAL.

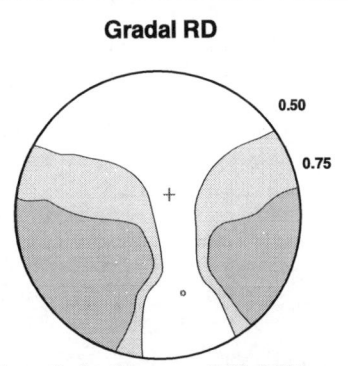

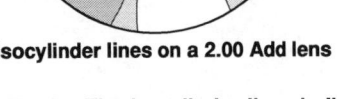

Isocylinder lines on a 2.00 Add lens

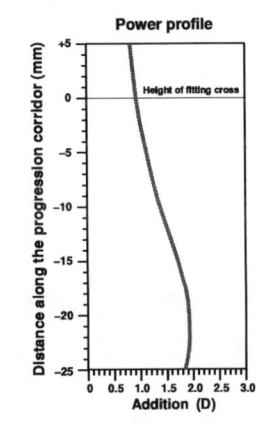

Fig. 2 The isocylinder lines indicate wide intermediate and near vision regions on the Gradal RD whilst the power profile shows how the Addition starts with some plus power, rather from the zero power as in PALs.

Occupational Progressive Addition Lenses

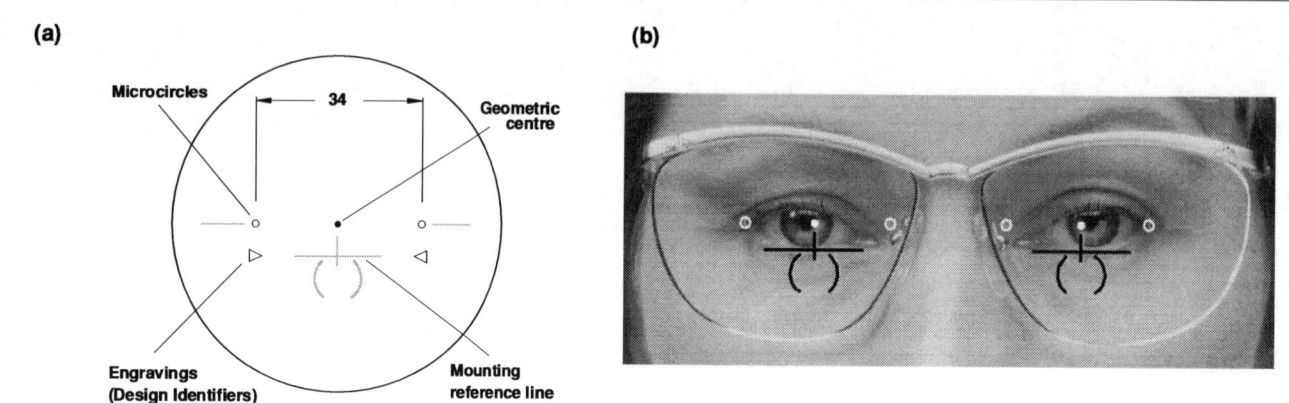

Fig. 3 Essilor's *Interview* lens. (a) The lens markings. (b) The fitting procedure involves placing the Mounting Reference Line on the lower limbus, with the eyes in the primary position, and with the 'crosses' on the right and left mounting reference lines centred for the NCD.

One of the problems faced by the dispenser is that there in no single method of fitting these lenses, so it is necessary to have the fitting details for each lens.

Properties of the lenses

Essilor's *Interview* OPAL

The *Interview* from Essilor was released in the UK in late 1998 and is available in CR 39 material. It can be described as an Enhanced Reading Lens. The full Add is achieved 9 mm below the pupil centre. At the pupil centre the patient has 0.8 D less Add power than the prescribed near vision Add. Figure 3 shows the lens markings in part (a) and the *fitting* is demonstrated in (b) where *the Mounting Reference Line is fitted on the lower limbus and centred for the NCD*.

Range: Ø65, 70 and 75
−4.00 sph to +2.00 maximum
cyl to −2.00.

Care must be taken to determine the artificial far point distance since with highish Adds it may be too close for some intermediate tasks. The distance to the artificial far point is shown for various Adds in the following table; bear in mind that the weakest spherical power is 0.80 D less than the Add!

Add	Artificial Far Point distance
1.00	5.00 m
1.50	1.43 m
2.00	0.83 m
2.50	0.59 m
3.00	0.45 m

Rodenstock's *Office Perfalit 1.5* OPAL

The *Office Perfalit* 1.5*, available in CR 39, was launched in January 1999. It is described by Rodenstock as a near vision aspheric lens with variable power allowing clear vision from the reading distance to about 2 m and being

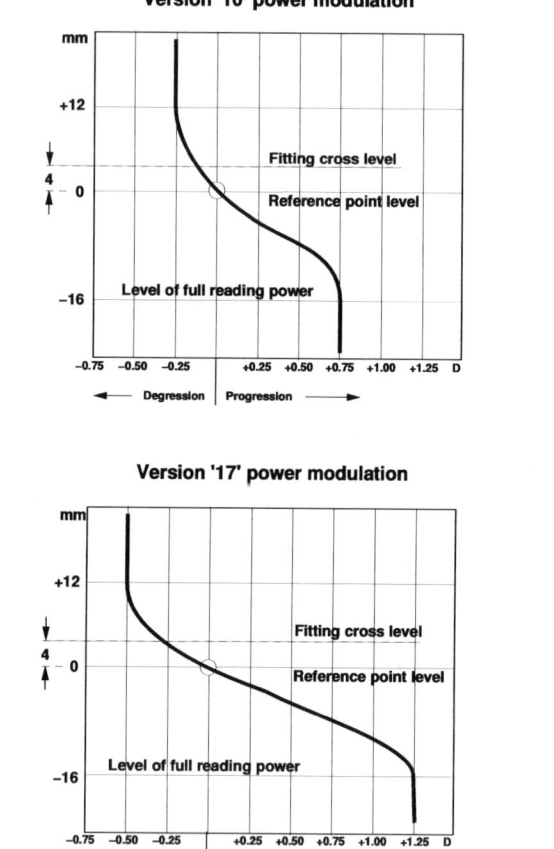

Fig. 4 The power modulation on Rodenstock's *Office Perfalit 1.5* lens. Two versions are available, one with a 1.00 D and the other with a 1.75 D power change. These are designated '10' and '17'.

ideally suited for office workers, VDU users, draughtsmen, architects, surgeons, etc. The horizontal locators are two horizontal ellipses 34 mm apart, thus   o   o , and the lens is engraved with an R, the Rodenstock logo. Either an engraved '10' or '17' appears under the under the ellipse on the temporal side, indicating a power modulation of 1.00 or 1.75 D, respectively; see figure 4. On the nasal side is a two-digit engraving representing the base curve and the refractive index. *The fitting is as for PALs* — place the

* Rodenstock's name for their CR 39 material.

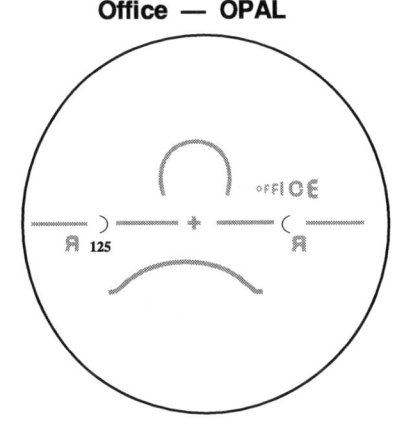

Age	Near Add	Power modulation (Office Dynamic Power)*
Under 50	0.75 to 1.50	0.75
50 & over	1.75 to 2.25	1.25
	2.50 & over	1.75

* Shamir's term for the decrease in power from the Near Addition.

Fig. 5 On the left, the table used to choose the power modulation, or Dynamic Power. On the right are the painted (stamped) markings in yellow and the microengravings black. The power modulation of 1.25D is indicated by 125 under the nasal horizontal indicator ')'. The near vision power should be checked below the yellow curved arc in the lower half of the lens.

fitting cross at the zero pupil point; that is, opposite the centre of the pupil with the eye in the primary position of gaze. The frame must have 22 mm depth below and 14 mm above the zero pupil point. When ordering specify monocular PDs and the heights of each fitting cross relative to Horizontal Centre Line (Datum Line). Determine the power for the normal reading correction at 40 cm. For Adds from 1.25 to 1.75, order *Office 10*, and for Adds 2.00 and higher, order *Office 17*. The *Office Perfalit 1.5* range is:

Ø75 −6.00 sph to +3.25 combined power
       cyl to +4.00

Ø70 plano to +4.75 combined powers
       cyl to +4.00

Ø65 & 60 plano to +6.00 combined powers
       cyl to +4.00

Prism to 2^Δ.

Shamir's *Office* OPAL

The Israeli firm Shamir designed their *Office* lens, figure 5, before Rodenstock confused the issue by using the same name. The Shamir lens is available in the UK via Taylor Optical. It should be ordered by stating the near vision power and the power reduction which is required in the progression: 0.75, 1.25 or 1.75 D. The particular power modulation required can be determined according to the Age and the Near Add in figure 5. Near Rx power range availability is

Ø75/80 −3.00 to +6.00 combined powers.

Shamir advise the optician to ensure that there is a minimum of 13 mm above and 16 mm below the pupil centre to the frame rim when viewed with the patient's eyes in the primary position. The fitting cross is placed at the pupil centre with the eye in the primary position, so that mono-PD measurements are required and **the fitting method is identical with that for PALs**.

Sola's *Access* OPAL

Sola introduced the *Access* lens to the UK scene in 1997. Available in CR 39 material, it is described as an enhanced reading lens, implying that lens has been designed by considering power reduction from the near vision prescription. To simplify dispensing, the right and left lenses are symmetrical and the **fitting point should be placed 3 - 5 mm below the zero pupil point**, the visual point with the eye in the primary position. This is close to the horizontal centre line which Sola has found suitable for the fitting point placement, further simplifying the fitting procedure. The minimum intermediate power can be ordered −0.75 or −1.25 D lower than the near vision Rx and the modulation occurs over a 12 mm depth; see figure 6. In clinical trials Sola found that 80% of wearers preferred Access to conventional single vision readers.

The availability is:

Diameters up to 75 mm
−2.00 DS to +4.00 combined powers
cyl to +4.00.

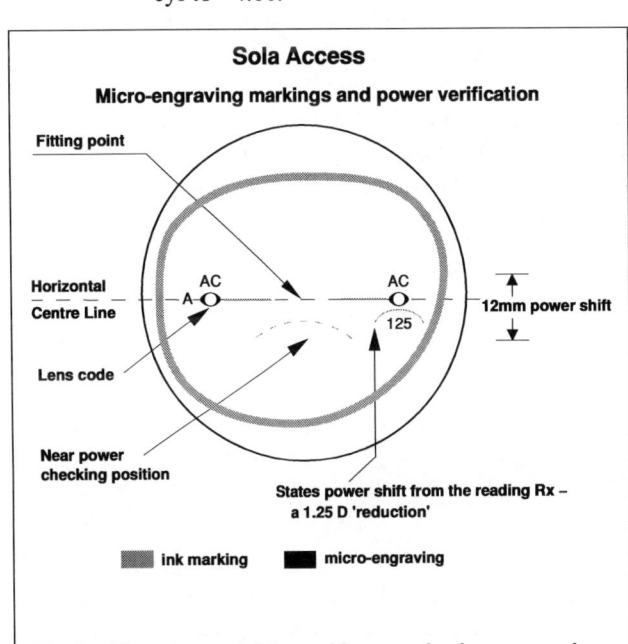

Fig. 6 The stamped ink markings and micro-engravings on Sola's Access occupational progressive lens.

Occupational Progressive Addition Lenses

American Optical's *Technica* OPAL

As mentioned earlier, American Optical Company's **Technica** lens was the first to address the problem of relatively narrow intermediate and reading zones with PALs. Technica is a modified PAL and the only OPAL with a (narrow) distance portion. It is based on AO's bipolar design with 80% of the Add placed 15° below the zero pupil point (7.5 mm below the fitting cross). *Fitting is the same as for a PAL*.

The availability is:
    Ø75/83 −5.00 to +6.00 combined powers
    cyl to 4.00   Adds 1.00 to 3.50.

The micro-engravings are   o   o
                                Add   AOT
                                T

with the fitting cross 2 mm above the level of the hidden circles.

Zeiss' *Gradal RD* OPAL

The Zeiss **Gradal RD** is again a modified PAL available in 1.6 index glass and CR 39. Designed for 'indoor use', the RD translating loosely as 'Room Distance', it has a 25 mm long progression and is *fitted as one would fit a PAL* with the fitting cross at the zero pupil point. The lens is ordered by stating the distance Rx and the near vision Add, whence the laboratory will add +0.50 DS to the distance Rx and deduct the same amount from the Add, leaving the near vision power with the full reading Rx and providing an artificial far point at 2 m. Availability is:

Distance Rx
    Ø70/75 −7.00 to +4.50 combined powers
    Ø65/70 −0.50 to +6.50 combined powers
    Ø60/65 −0.50 to +6.50 combined powers.

Normal prescribed near Adds are available from 1.00 to 3.00, with cyls to 6.00, which gives the *Gradal RD* the widest power range of all the OPALs.

The micro-engravings on the Gradal RD are

           5   □
        Add   RD

where the '5' in the left hidden square indicates the 0.50 DS added to the distance Rx. The fitting cross is 6 mm above the level of the hidden squares which are, as usual 34 mm apart.

Zeiss' *Business* OPAL

In 1998 Zeiss released an OPAL called **Business** which is described as a dynamic reading lens for enhanced near vision. Its design is based on an aspherical front surface resulting in a thin, light lens with a good cosmetic appearance and optical qualities optimised for vision within

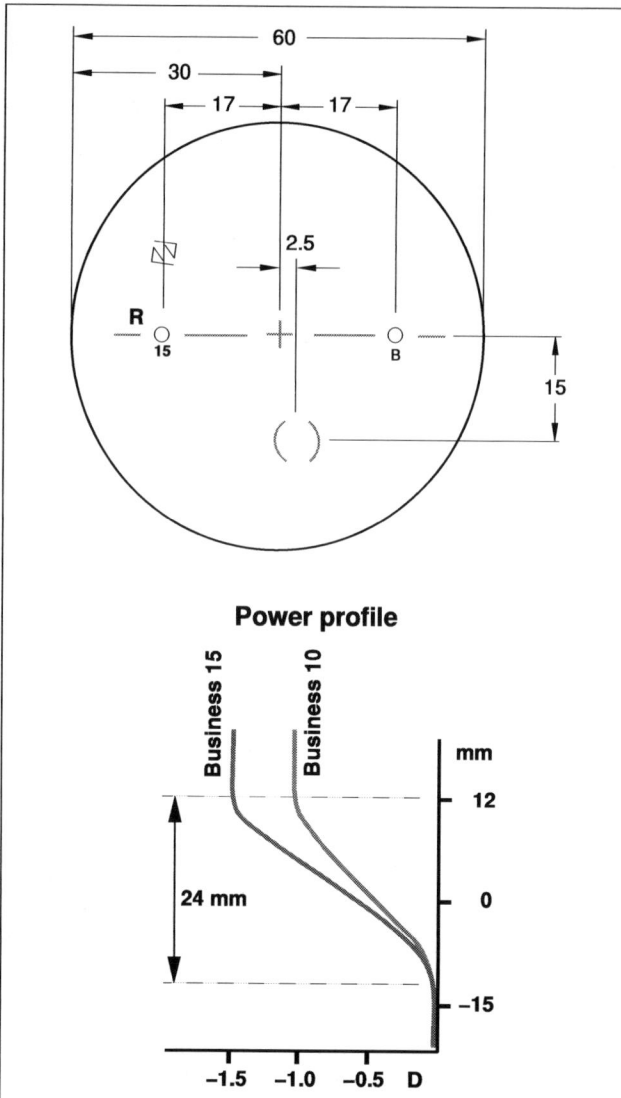

Fig. 7 Ink markings and micro-engravings on the Zeiss Clarlet Business lens (top diagram). At the bottom are the power modulations of 1.00 D and 1.50 D on the Clarlet Business 10 and 15, respectively.

the patient's reach. An asymmetrical design ensures that both eyes experience the same quality of vision during version movements. Available in CR 39 under the Zeiss name Clarlet, it comes in two forms: 1.00 D and 1.50 D reductions from the reading Rx, see figure 7, so that the artificial far point will be 1 m or 0.67 m, respectively. *Clarlet* Business 10* should be chosen for near Adds to and including 1.75 and *Clarlet Business 15* for near Adds of 2.00 and over. The code 15 under the temporal circle indicates *Clarlet Business 15*. This will be 10 when *Clarlet Business 10* is supplied. The B under the nasal circle identifies the lens as *Clarlet Business*.

For *fitting*, apply the centre of rotation rule: for each 1° of pantoscopic tilt decentre the centration cross 0.5 mm down from the pupil centre in the primary position of gaze (the zero or distance visual point). Mono-PDs are required. Prescribed prism is measured at the centration cross.
The power range available is:
    Ø75 and 70   −2.00 to +4.00
    Ø65 and 60   +0.25 to +4.00
    cyl to 4.00   Adds 0.75 to 3.00.

* Zeiss' name for their CR 39 material.

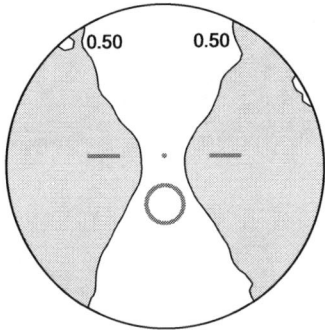

Fig. 8 Sola's Continuum Computer Lens, marketed here by Norville Optical Company.

Continuum Computer Lens from Norville Optical

A lens for intermediate and near vision with a power modulation of 1.00 D; see figure 8. It should be ordered as the reading prescription. The ***fitting height*** is to be measured to 3 mm above the lower limbus with the eye in the primary position. The lenses should then be centred horizontally at this height according to the mono-NCDs. Lens depth should be not less than 30 mm.

Range   Ø75   −2.00 to +4.00 combined powers.

Personal comments on OPALs

I have worn four of the eight OPALs listed here. All of them allow clear vision of an A4 page, and with natural head and eye movements an A3 page is fully clear in either portrait or landscape orientation. In addition, the whole of the computer screen and everything within 1 metre is easily focused with normal head movements. These lenses deserve recognition by dispensers, especially for patients over 50 years of age with regular alternating near and intermediate vision requirements such as office and computer work, bench or deskwork involving measurements and/or inspection over distances up to 1 or 2 metres, and any number of occupational or recreational tasks with similar visual requirements.

Dispensing OPALs

Two OPALs, the AO Technica and the Gradal RD have fixed distance artificial far points; the Technica's is at infinity and the Gradal RD's is at 2 m. However, in all the other OPALs, which can be considered as enhanced readers, the ***distance to the artificial far point*** depends on the near vision Add. For example, with a 1.50 D Add and a power shift of 1.25 D, as in the Access lens, the weakest power will only exceed the distance Rx by +0.25 DS placing the artificial far point at a distance of $1/(1.50 - 1.25) = 4$ m from the lens. However, with a +3.00 Add included in the near vision Rx the artificial far point will be at a distance of $1/(3.00 - 1.25) = 0.57$ m.

This exercise should be considered by the dispenser in all OPAL types which have a fixed power modulation from the reading Rx; that is, with the *Interview*, *Rodenstock's Office*, *Shamir's Office*, *Access* and *Business* lenses. Determining the distance to the artificial far point can be critical in cases with near vision Adds over 2.00 D, since as the case of the 3.00 Add above exemplifies, a far point distance of 57 cm may well be too near for viewing a computer monitor screen.

One unfortunate dispensing factor is that OPALs do not all have the same fitting method and only in the four cases of the *Technica*, *Rodenstock's Office*, the *Shamir Office* and the *Gradal RD* is the method identical with the fitting of PALs.

Full details of markings, prisms, tints and coatings will be found in *Ophthalmic Lens Availability*, a continuously updated manual of ophthalmic lenses marketed in the UK and available from Association of British Dispensing Opticians.

Dispensing Bifocal Lenses

Introduction

The word bifocal means two foci, referring to the lens having two portions each with a different power. The purpose of bifocal lenses is to give patients two different powers within the same lens. Although bifocals are also used to control juvenile stress myopia and to control accommodation in accommodative squint, they are most commonly used for presbyopic patients who cannot accommodate sufficiently for close work and therefore cannot manage with a single vision lens for both distance and near vision.

As shown in figure 1, bifocals are made in several forms:

- *Fused bifocal*, made with two types of glass of different refractive indices.
- *Solid bifocal*, made from a single piece of glass or plastic.
- *Bonded* or *cemented bifocal*, where a segment with the additional power is attached to the main lens.
- *Split bifocal*, where the two powered portions are effectively each a single vision lens, the two being bonded together at the join in modern lenses.

Most bifocals have a segment in the lower half which has additional plus power. This is the *conventional bifocal*. However, there are some bifocals designed for occupational or special uses where there may be more than one segment, or the segment may be positioned elsewhere than in the usual downward gaze position. Most such lenses are manufactured with the segment(s) in fixed positions, but it is possible to bond a segment in any position on a single vision main lens. Figure 1 shows an example of a Double-D segment bifocal where both segments have the same reading Add, the upper one being intended for some specialist use on upwards gaze.

Sola Optical produce an unusual bifocal described as having a progressive power segment. Ostensibly, it has a 30 mm D segment, but the upper half of the segment has a power progression producing an intermediate focus. It is recommended that this segment is fitted with the top about 3 mm below pupil centre with the eyes in the primary position. The initial Addition at the upper margin depends on the reading Add: the details can be seen in figure 2.

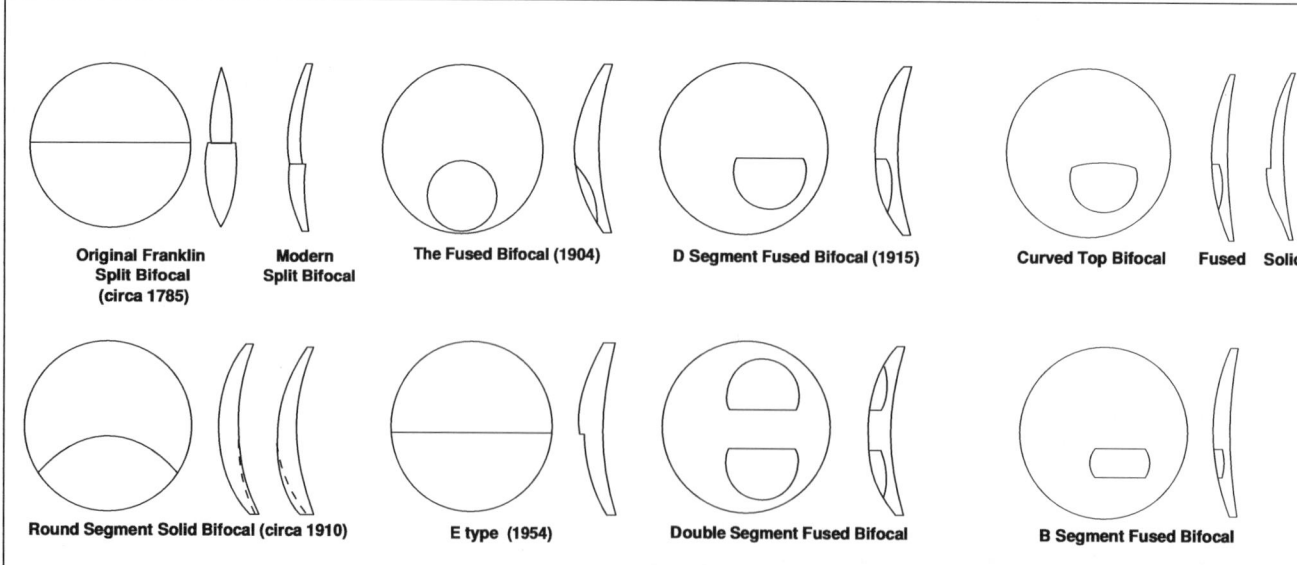

Fig. 1 Illustrating the main types of bifocal. Round, D-segment, and Curved Top bifocals are usually designated with R, D, and C letters. So, in modern nomenclature, we have:
- B = ribbon segment
- C = curved top segment
- D = D-shaped segment
- E = straight top full width segment
- R = round segment.

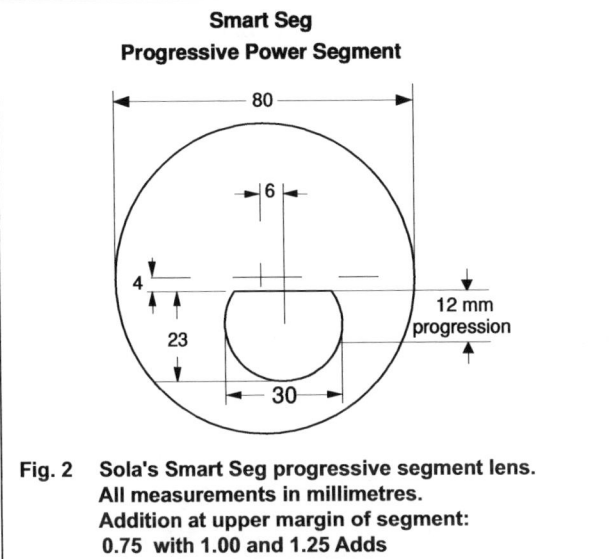

Fig. 2 Sola's Smart Seg progressive segment lens.
All measurements in millimetres.
Addition at upper margin of segment:
0.75 with 1.00 and 1.25 Adds
1.00 with 1.50 to 2.50 Adds
1.25 with 2.75 and 3.00 Adds.

It is worth listing the advantages and disadvantages of bifocals. The following listing refers to conventional bifocals; that is, one segment in the lower half of the lens.

Advantages of bifocals

- Clear vision over both distance and segment portions (Contrast this with Progressive Addition Lenses).
- Wider reading area than PALs.
- More convenient than separate distance and near single vision lens spectacles.

Disadvantages of bifocals

- Visible junction of distance portion and segment. Indicates patient's age, and reflection from the junction can be irritating, especially to first time wearers.
- Reading portion only in lower half of lens which is not convenient when needing near vision in upwards gaze or primary position gaze.
- Smaller segment diameters have limited width of field of view compared with single vision readers.
- In patients over 55 years of age, lack of an intermediate portion can be annoying, as when looking in shop windows, for example.

From the cosmetic point of view, round segments are less visible than D-shaped segments, curved top (C-shaped) segments, or the most visible E-type segment. This latter type of bifocal, first marketed by and still available from the American Optical Company under their trade name Executive, whilst having the most visible segment top does have other superior qualities such as a full width reading field of view and no image jump at the segment top. A large proportion of patients are not bothered by reflections from the segment top or by its visibility, so the advantages of the E-type bifocal must be uppermost in the dispenser's mind when considering bifocals and when advising patients of their relative merits.

On the question of round segments, they are sometimes described as i*nvisible bifocals* when, in their most common form, the junction of the segment with the distance portion is simple an *edge*. An edge is defined in mathematics as the intersection of two surfaces and, as such, is therefore a line. Little light is reflected from this edge and this is the reason for the use of the exaggerated soubriquet *invisible* bifocal. Compare this with the E-type or D-type where the segment top is a narrow flat surface. It is from this surface that light is reflected and renders the segment more visible than a round type. Occasionally, a patient may be wearing a small round segment, say R25, indicating a 25 mm diameter round segment, and be persuaded to change to a D-segment, with its wider field of view. Beware: it is not unknown for such patients to reject the D-segment bifocal on the grounds that reflected light from the segment top is noticeable.

Bifocals must satisfy a number of mechanical, cosmetic and optical requirements:--

- Ideally, the lenses should be no heavier than single vision lenses and should have a barely visible dividing line between the distance and near portions.
- The near portion should be permanently fixed to the main lens.
- There should be no sudden change in the prismatic effect at the uppermost point on the dividing line.
- The differential prismatic effect at the near visual points should be kept within acceptable limits.
- The near portion (the segment) should be sufficiently wide for the patient's particular needs.

Needless to say, not all of these conditions can be met simultaneously and each design is a compromise.

Important optical principles of bifocals

Calculations of Adds, depression curves in fused bifocals, transverse chromatic aberration, and the precise details of the segment surfaces are commonly taught in lecture programmes on bifocals. The intention here though is to concentrate on those optical principles which influence dispensing and, ultimately, mean the difference between good, bad, and indifferent dispensing of bifocals. The following list indicates the topics we shall discuss under this heading of *optical principles of bifocals*.

❑ Segment diameter and field of view.

❑ Lateral and vertical placement of the segment in the spectacle frame.

❑ Near Vision Effectivity Error and the prescribed Add.

❑ Position of the distance optical centre in bifocals.

❑ Vision in the segment top zone.

Dispensing Bifocal Lenses

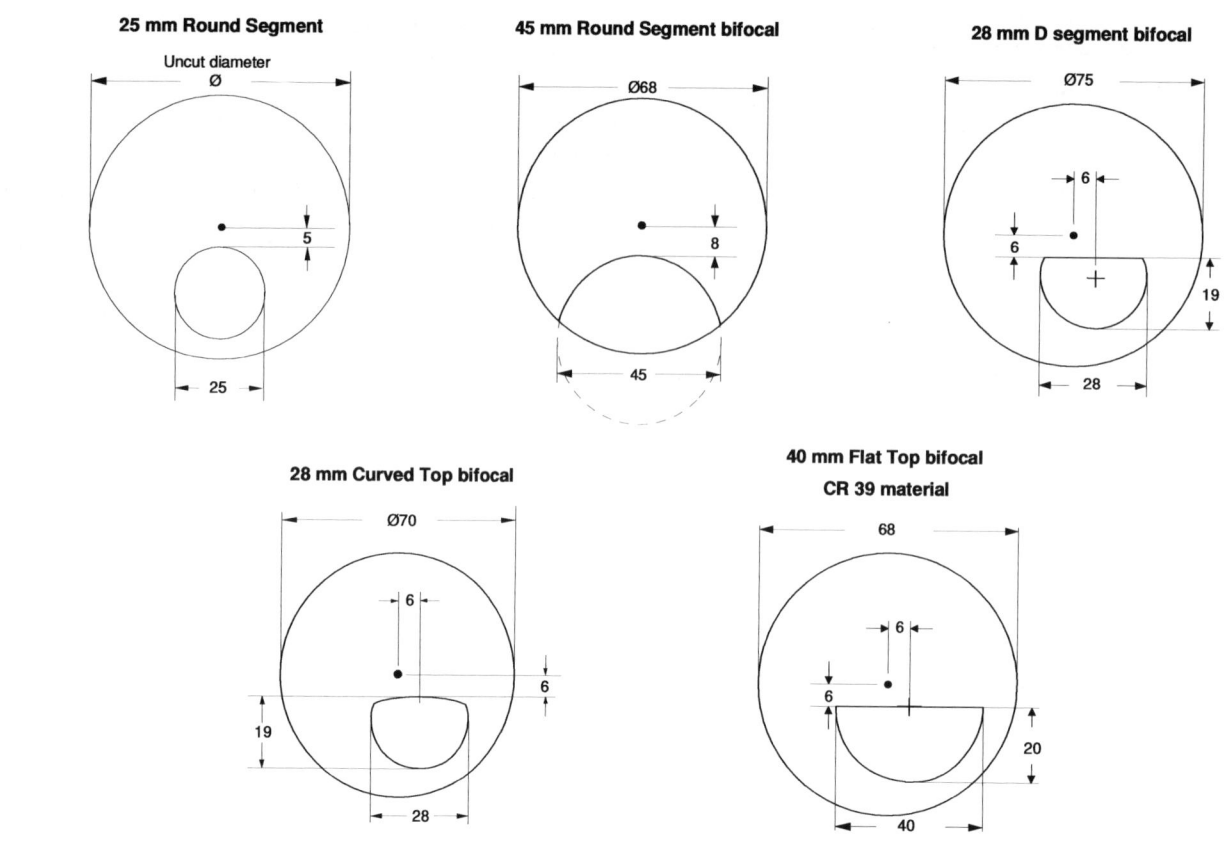

Fig. 3 These diagrams illustrate how the diameters of various segments are defined. Each diameter is indicated in millimetres as the horizontal dimension of the segment, which is indicated by the value shown at the bottom of each diagram. Note the 40 mm flat top segment bifocal, which has not been mentioned before.

Notice the decentred segments in the case of the D, C, and flat top bifocals. This enables smaller Near Centration Distances to be obtained from the uncut than would otherwise be possible if the segment were not decentred.

❑ Segment diameter

As already stated, the Executive bifocal, and its imitators the E-type bifocals as they are generically known now, has the widest lateral field of view in near vision because the segment occupies the full width of the lens aperture in the lower part of the spectacle frame. With other bifocals the lateral field of view is proportional to the segment diameter. In this latter context, it is worth noting how the segment diameter is defined for the various segments. Figure 3 illustrates the definitions for R25, R45, D28, C28 segments, and a previously unmentioned 40 mm flat top segment.

Flat top segments are generally best as far as width of field of view is concerned. This is because immediately the visual axis crosses into the segment, on looking downwards, very nearly the full width is available for clear vision. Compare this with a round segment, as illustrated in figure 4. In this figure the depth of the shaded area is 10 mm, a useful depth giving at 40 cm reading distance about 13 cm vertical linear field of view in the author's case. It at first seems surprising how some patients can adapt to R25 segments when we consider the extra infraduction required compared with flat top bifocals, but this amount of infraduction is about the same as that required in PALs. The author's horizontal field of view with a D25 is about 30 cm, about 1½ times the width of an A4 page. This should be contrasted with

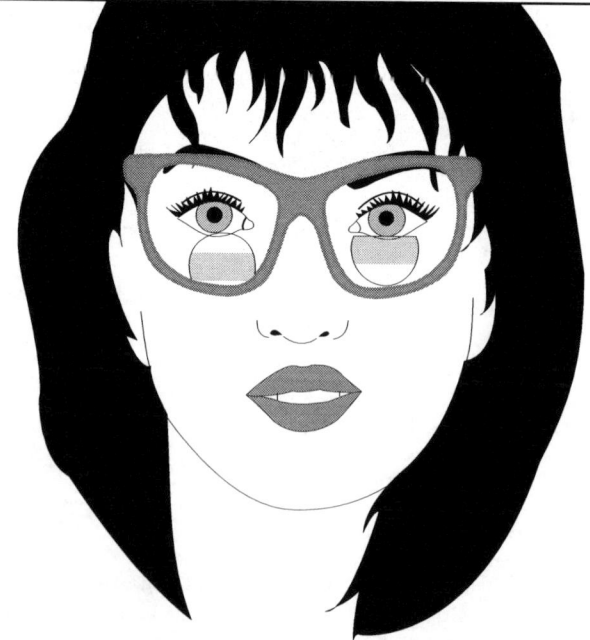

Fig. 4 R25 and D25 segments compared for width of segment and lateral field of view. Compared with a D-segment, in the round segment it is necessary to move the visual axis further into the segment to obtain a useful horizontal field of view. For example, the grey shaded area is 10 mm deep, but notice how in the R25 the same area is some 6 to 7 mm further into the segment, thus causing the patient to use a lower part of the segment. This involves greater infraduction of the eyes and the need to raise the head position somewhat awkwardly.

the corresponding field of view with modern PALs, which is about two-thirds of this amount! A linear field of view of 30 cm at a working distance of 40 cm is more than adequate when one considers that it involves about 20° ocular rotation either side of the forward gaze position. More than this is uncomfortable for the extraocular muscles if undertaken for any length of time. So, the purpose of larger diameter D-segments is really to put the edges of the segments out of the full field of view, rather than to extend the fixation field of view. From the author's personal wearing experience, even a 30 mm segment was not wide enough to avoid the temple edges of the segment being annoyingly noticeable. However, I have worn E-type bifocals without being appreciably troubled by the segment top.

☐ Lateral and vertical placement of the segment

Segment inset for coincident fields of view

Because the eyes converge to fixate an object point at the reading distance, each bifocal segment has to be inset from its respective distance centration point; see figure 5. The problem with bifocal segment inset involves making the eyes look through the centres of the segments when fixating a point on the median line* at the requisite working distance. Figure 5 indicates how this inset is calculated and Table 1 lists the results using paraxial theory to calculate the insets. The inset of the bifocal here, making the right and left fields of view coincide through the bifocal segments, is the horizontal displacement OQ of the segment centre from a vertical line through the distance optical centre of the lens. From figure 5, it is apparent that $\tan \theta$ is given by OQ/s, but OQ is the bifocal inset, so we can write:

$$\text{bifocal inset} = s \tan \theta.$$

Using paraxial optics for refraction at the lens, the image point is taken to be a distance h' from the optical axis of the lens, and the object point a distance $h \ (= -p)$ from the axis. Then, from the magnification expression,

$$h' = h\frac{L}{L'} = -p\frac{L}{L'} \quad \text{since} \quad h = -p$$

and $\quad \tan \theta = -\dfrac{h'}{l'-s} = -\dfrac{(-p(L/L'))}{l'-s} = \dfrac{p(L/L')}{l'-s}$

We can now substitute for $\tan \theta$ into the expression for the bifocal inset and obtain:

$$\text{bifocal inset} = \frac{spL}{1-sL'}.$$

Writing $s = 1/S$ and $L' = L+F$, and substituting for s and L' in the last expression, we have

$$\text{bifocal inset} = p\left(\frac{L}{L+F-S}\right)$$

which gives the inset in terms of the mono-PD (p), the object vergence (L), the distance correction (F), and the dioptric value (S) of the fitting distance†. Table 1 was obtained from this equation.

Table 1 Inset necessary to make the right and left visual fields coincide through the segments, as a function of object distance, mono-PD, and the distance Rx. 35 cm object distance. Values rounded to nearest 0.5 mm.

Dist. Rx	Mono-PD								
	28	29	30	31	32	33	34	35	36
−20.00	1.5	1.5	1.5	1.5	1.5	1.5	1.5	1.5	2.0
−16.00	1.5	1.5	1.5	1.5	1.5	2.0	2.0	2.0	2.0
−14.00	1.5	1.5	1.5	1.5	1.5	2.0	2.0	2.0	2.0
−12.00	1.5	1.5	1.5	2.0	2.0	2.0	2.0	2.0	2.0
−10.00	1.5	1.5	2.0	2.0	2.0	2.0	2.0	2.0	2.0
−8.00	1.5	1.5	2.0	2.0	2.0	2.0	2.0	2.0	2.0
−6.00	1.5	2.0	2.0	2.0	2.0	2.0	2.0	2.0	2.0
−4.00	2.0	2.0	2.0	2.0	2.0	2.0	2.0	2.5	2.5
−2.00	2.0	2.0	2.0	2.0	2.0	2.5	2.5	2.5	2.5
0.00	2.0	2.0	2.0	2.0	2.5	2.5	2.5	2.5	2.5
+2.00	2.0	2.0	2.5	2.5	2.5	2.5	2.5	2.5	2.5
+4.00	2.0	2.5	2.5	2.5	2.5	2.5	2.5	3.0	3.0
+6.00	2.5	2.5	2.5	2.5	2.5	3.0	3.0	3.0	3.0
+8.00	2.5	2.5	2.5	3.0	3.0	3.0	3.0	3.0	3.0
+10.00	2.5	3.0	3.0	3.0	3.0	3.0	3.0	3.5	3.5

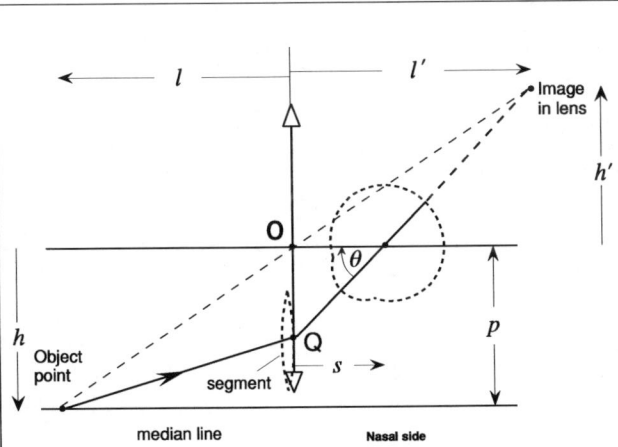

Fig. 5 The inset OQ of a bifocal segment, shown schematically. This inset ensures that the centre of the segment is correctly positioned to view a chosen object point on the median line. p is the mono-PD, the distance of the centre of the pupil from the median line in distance gaze. θ is the rotation of the eye, and s is the fitting distance. F is the power of the distance correcting lens.
Note that θ is negative, making the inset OQ come out negative in this diagram. A positive value is obtained by multiplying by -1.

For other working distances the inset values differ, of course, greater inset being expected for shorter working distances, and vice versa. At the time of writing, the author computed the values for 30 and 40 cm working distances, but did not feel that much would be gained by putting them in print. The main reasons for not printing them are that in practice the above table is generally ignored and for other working distances the geometrical inset is usually sufficient. Geometrical inset considers the placement of the geometrical centre of the segment only in relation to the mono-PD and the near centration distance, as indicated in the next section.

---

* *Median line* — the horizontal line which bisects the line joining the centre of rotation of right and left eyes.

† The right hand side of this equation has been multiplied by -1 to make the inset come out positive.

Geometrical inset of the bifocal segment

The segment insets in Table 1 were to make the fields of view coincide through the segments. However, it is common practice to use the geometrical inset, as calculated from the PD and the *near centration distance*. The *near centration distance* (NCD), the distance between the near centration points, is less than the PD since the eyes converge for near. Its relationship to the PD is shown in figure 6. This relationship is unaffected by different mono-PDs. If the segment centre is set on the vertical line through the Near Centration Point, then the inset involved is called the *geometrical inset*. Geometrical inset is calculated simply from the relationship

$$\text{geometrical inset} = \tfrac{1}{2}(PD - NCD).$$

Table 2 gives the NCD for different working distances.

Table 2 Near Centration Distance (NCD) as a function of interpupillary distance (PD) and working distance. Results to the nearest millimetre.

| | \multicolumn{7}{c}{Working distance (cm)} |
PD	20	25	30	35	40	45	50
54	48	49	50	50	51	51	51
56	49	51	51	52	52	53	53
58	51	52	53	54	54	55	55
60	53	54	55	56	56	57	57
62	55	56	57	58	58	58	59
64	56	58	59	59	60	60	61
66	58	60	61	61	62	62	63
68	60	61	62	63	64	64	65
70	62	63	64	65	66	66	66
72	63	65	66	67	67	68	68
74	65	67	68	69	69	70	70
76	67	69	70	71	71	72	72

Although Table 2 can be used in dispensing, many practitioners simply measure the NCD. Nonetheless, the values given do show what to expect: because the NCD is smaller with shorter working distances, the inset will be greater. For a given working distance, the inset will be greater with larger PDs, again because the eyes have to converge more.

If we use the 35 cm working distance from Table 2, and calculate the geometrical insets for the PDs which match those in Table 1, then the results compare as follows:

PD	56	58	60	62	64	66	68	70	72
				Insets					
Table 2	2.0	2.0	2.0	2.0	2.5	2.5	2.5	2.5	2.5
Table 1 Rx									
-20.00	1.5	1.5	1.5	1.5	1.5	1.5	1.5	1.5	2.0
-12.00	1.5	1.5	1.5	2.0	2.0	2.0	2.0	2.0	2.0
-6.00	1.5	2.0	2.0	2.0	2.0	2.0	2.0	2.0	2.0
0.00	2.0	2.0	2.0	2.0	2.5	2.5	2.5	2.5	2.5
+4.00	2.0	2.5	2.5	2.5	2.5	2.5	2.5	3.0	3.0
+8.00	2.5	2.5	2.5	3.0	3.0	3.0	3.0	3.0	3.0
+10.00	2.5	3.0	3.0	3.0	3.0	3.0	3.0	3.5	3.5

In the range from minus lenses to medium plus powers, the convention of making the separation the geometrical centres of the segments equal to the NCD is sufficiently accurate, as we can see from the above table. It is only in the higher plus powers that Table 2 becomes inaccurate. If a similar comparison is done for other working distances, this observation is generally true. That is, except for distance Rx powers of about +8.00 D and over, it is sufficiently accurate to use the geometrical inset when dispensing bifocals.

Calculated from the values in Table 2, Table 3 gives the geometrical insets which can be used in practice for prescriptions in the minus range and below +8.00 D in the plus range.

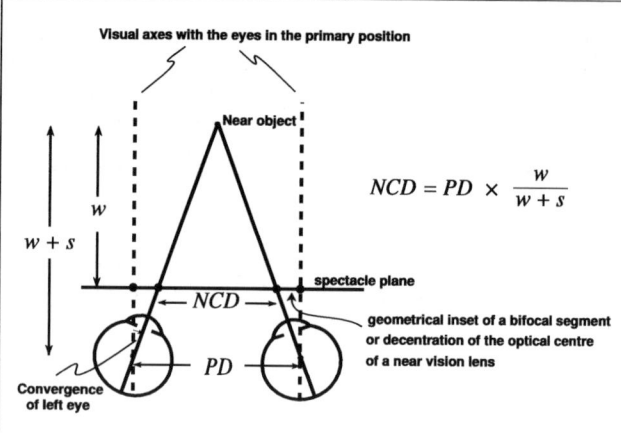

Fig. 6 The eyes are shown converging on a near object point. The Near Centration Distance (*NCD*) is seen to be a function of the working distance (*w*), the fitting distance (*s*), and the interpupillary distance (*PD*). The outer bold points in the spectacle plane are the distance centration points, and their separation is equal to the *PD*. The inner points are the near centration points, their separation being the *NCD*.

$$NCD = PD \times \frac{w}{w+s}$$

Table 3 Geometrical inset for bifocal segments. Results to the nearest millimetre.

| | \multicolumn{7}{c}{Working distance (cm)} |
PD	20	25	30	35	40	45	50
54	3.0	2.5	2.0	2.0	1.5	1.5	1.5
56	3.5	2.5	2.5	2.0	2.0	1.5	1.5
58	3.5	3.0	2.5	2.0	2.0	1.5	1.5
60	3.5	3.0	2.5	2.0	2.0	1.5	1.5
62	3.5	3.0	2.5	2.0	2.0	2.0	1.5
64	4.0	3.0	2.5	2.5	2.0	2.0	1.5
66	4.0	3.0	2.5	2.5	2.0	2.0	1.5
68	4.0	3.5	3.0	2.5	2.0	2.0	1.5
70	4.0	3.5	3.0	2.5	2.0	2.0	2.0
72	4.5	3.5	3.0	2.5	2.5	2.5	2.0
74	4.5	3.5	3.0	2.5	2.5	2.0	2.0
76	4.5	3.5	3.0	2.5	2.5	2.0	2.0

Vertical placement of the bifocal segment

The segments must be located at a position below the pupils such that the eyes can easily view reading and close work material with a comfortable eye/head postural relationship. There is some confusion amongst practitioners as to the method of positioning the segment top position relative to the eye. The author comes across a relatively large proportion of students in practice who position the top of

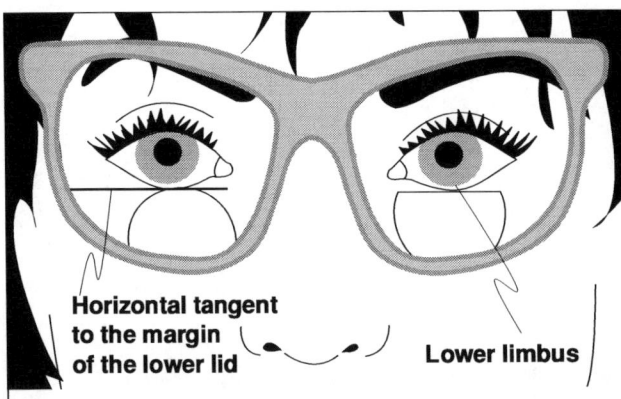

Fig. 7 A not uncommon, although incorrect method sometimes used in practice where the segment top is placed level with the horizontal tangent to the margin of the lower lid. Adapted from figure 1, different segment shapes are retained simply for illustration purposes.

the segment level with the margin of lower lid, as shown in figure 7. This method of segment top placement fails to recognise the wide variation in lower lid position relative to the pupil centre.

A method for determining the segment top position must take into account the compromise between distance field of view above the segment and the near vision field of view through the segment. When walking, for example, the patient must be able to see pavement edges or stairs

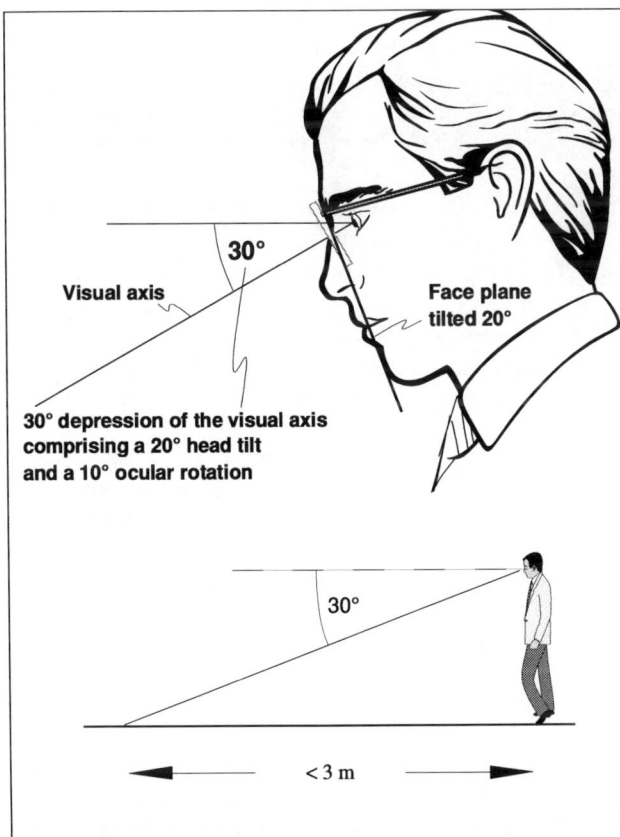

Fig. 8 Bifocal wearers approaching steps will tend to tilt the head forwards when they need to view the steps with the distance portions of their lenses. A 30° depression of the visual axis will allow them to fixate the ground at less than 3 metres distance, quite adequate for making a position judgement prior to reaching the steps.

through the distance portion of the lens. Figure 8 illustrates the geometry required to obtain an average figure for the segment top placement. Based on practical experience, the figure assumes that a 30° depression of the visual axes, comprising a 20° forward head tilt and a 10° downwards ocular rotation, is comfortable and sufficient for making distance judgements as when approaching an obstacle on foot. Simple triangulation shows that for a range of eye to ground heights the subject can fixate the ground at less than 3 metres distance, which is just about right for judging one's step at a pavement edge or a flight of stairs.

The 10° ocular rotation causes the visual axis to intersect the lens about 5 mm below the pupil centre. Since the lower limbus, figure 7, is about 5½ mm below the pupil centre, placing the segment top no higher than this allows the above head and eye position to occur without the segment intruding into the direction of gaze. Now, when the lower lid margin is at the level of the lower limbus with the eyes in the primary position, then using either the lower lid or the limbus will obviously result in the same segment height measurement, but lower lid margin positions vary from about 3 mm below the lower limbus to about 2 mm above, a range of 5 mm. Since we measure in ½ mm steps when determining the segment top position, this intersubject variation amounts to a range of 10 possible fitting positions. On the other hand, the lower limbus only varies over a range of about ½ mm distance from the pupil centre and therefore constitutes a better basis for determining the segment top position. One further point, for those students using the lower lid criterion, inspection of a number of fellow students' lower lid positions will show that about one-third of them have an asymmetry in the lid margin positions, thus making the lower lid an even worse choice for a basis of segment top positioning.

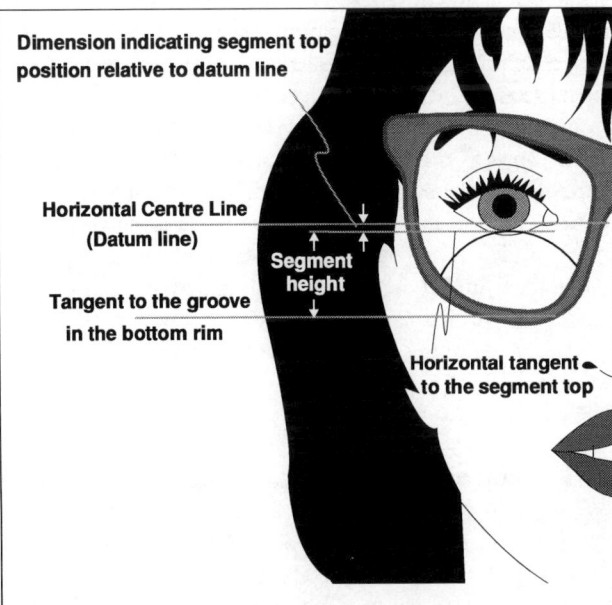

Fig. 9 The definition of segment height and the segment top position in the spectacle frame. It is the segment top position which the practitioner should write on the prescription laboratory order.

Because flat top segments give a useful width immediately the visual axis enters the segment, it is possible to place the segment top 1 to 2 mm lower than the lower limbus with D and E-type segments. This offers a deeper field of view in the distance portion without compromising the head/eye posture for reading — it is still considerably better than with a small round segment. Curved Top (C) and Round (R) segments should have their segment top placed at the level of the lower limbus.

Definition of segment height

There is some confusion amongst practitioners concerning the segment height measurement. This probably arises from a failure to consult British Standards on the definition of segment height. Figure 9 shows the height and the more important segment top position. It is the segment top position which should be included in an order to the prescription laboratory.

The segment height is defined as the distance between the tangents to the top of the segment and to the lowest point on the lens.

☐ **Near Vision Effectivity Error (NVEE)**

On pages 25 and 26, in the single vision section, we have already dealt with this effectivity problem which arises from the fact that the form of the spectacle lens differs from that of the trial lens. There we concluded that with near vision lenses of +8.00 D or more, it is necessary to adjust the ordered power to account for an effectivity power weakness experienced by the patient. The table on page 26 gives the required adjustments. Of course, with bifocals this adjustment is to the Add only.

The lens manufacturer Zeiss is unusual in this respect in that this company adjusts the supplied lens Add to account for NVEE. Quoting Zeiss' booklet *Spectacle Lens Information* (July 1993), "The near portion power . . . is computed for the beam path the spectacle wearer actually has. The addition corresponds to the value prescribed." That is, the Add is computed for the same effectivity at the vertex sphere as the patient experienced with the trial lenses. This means that the range of clear vision through the segment will correspond to that measured at the eye examination, which is obviously desirable. We shall deal with this topic in more detail under 'Measurement of the Addition in Bifocals' later.

☐ **Position of the distance optical centre in bifocals**

O_D is the symbol for the optical centre of the distance portion of a bifocal. Measured by dotting the position of O_D on the focimeter, the *drop* is the distance between O_D and the (horizontal) tangent to the segment top; see figure 10. The drop can be varied during the surfacing of the non-segment side of the lens, and can therefore be specified by the dispenser.

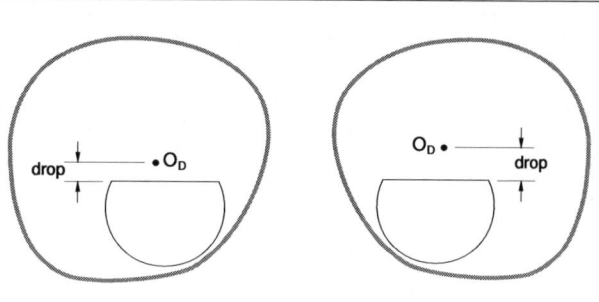

Fig. 10 Illustration of the meaning of the term *drop*. It is the distance from the optical centre O_D of the distance vision portion to the level of the segment top. In this case, the right and left drops are shown unequal, which means there will be a differential prismatic effect in the lens, assuming there is power in the distance Rx. This prismatic effect is experienced over the segment area as well.

In single vision lens theory, we have noted that the vertical placement of the optical centre depends on the pantoscopic tilt of the frame in most cases; see page 9. Thus, for best distance vision performance with bifocals, and with a 10° pantoscopic tilt, say, the distance portion optical centre O_D ought to be ordered with about a 2 mm drop. In practice, one tends to leave this to the prescription laboratory who will often work about a 2 mm drop as standard. However, it should be noted that this is uncertain and it may be prudent for the dispenser to quote the drop required with high powered bifocals. Thus, the distance optical centre will be located vertically by the *drop* and horizontally by the mono-PD for each lens. A drop of 2 mm places O_D close to the lower limbus and we would therefore expect the spectacles to need a 10° pantoscopic tilt, or thereabouts.

One particular case where the dispenser must quote the drop is when ordering a replacement or a new bifocal lens in a frame where the other lens is not to be changed. If the drop in the new lens is not the same as in the retained lens, then differential prism will be introduced. Where this involves ½$^\Delta$ of vertical differential prism or more, then the spectacles may give rise to asthenopic symptoms.

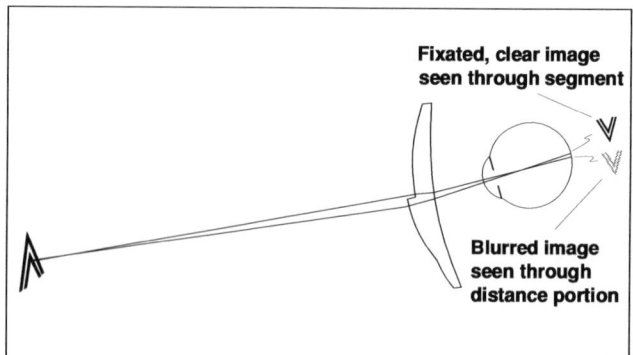

Fig. 11 Vision at the top of the segment is prone to 'confusion'. There is some overlap of the pencils of rays which can enter the eye through the distance and segment portions. With most bifocals there is also a possible image jump caused by the sudden introduction of a prismatic effect at the top of the segment.

☐ Vision around the segment top zone

Immediately above and below the segment top there is some overlapping of the fields of view through and above the segment, in general. Figure 11 illustrates the principle.

There are four problems associated with the top of the segment. These are:

1. Overlapping images formed by narrow pencils of rays through the distance and segment portions adjacent to the top of the segment, caused by the different prismatic effects in this zone. When alternately fixating just above and just below the segment top, the differential prism gives rise to image jump in cases where the segment optical centre O_s is not at the segment top.
2. These images have a different focus, one through the distance and one through the reading power.
3. They are slightly different in size, because of the difference between the two powers.
4. Light reflected from the segment top further degrades the retinal image.

Whilst these effects may disturb some patients, and be the reason for the occasional patient discontinuing with bifocals, it is surprising how few patients complain of these effects. Perhaps the only times the author has heard complaints about the segment top are in those few cases where a round 25 mm diameter segment has been replaced with a D-segment at a subsequent dispensing. Then it is the reflection from the segment top which is complained about. With solid bifocals, anti-reflection coating will solve the reflection problem.

It is well known that *image jump* is eliminated by using a bifocal in which the segment's optical centre is placed at the segment top, thus removing the sudden introduction of a prismatic effect in addition to that already there due to the distance power. The most common form of *no-jump bifocal* is the Executive bifocal from American Optical. Not quite all E-type bifocals are no-jump, so be warned.

Bifocals in Anisometropia

Although the majority of anisometropic subjects exhibit some aniseikonia with spectacles, and little or none with contact lenses†, when it comes to dispensing bifocals they are already used to wearing single vision spectacle lenses, so there is no additional problem from the point of view of aniseikonia. However they will be compelled to use a region well below the distance optical centres which may not be their usual practice with single vision lenses. Hence, we must investigate the potential problem of vertical differential prism in the reading portion of bifocals.

Vertical differential prismatic effect in spectacles, when the visual axes intersect the lenses away from the optical centres, causes the eyes to execute different degrees of infra- or supraduction. Vertical disjunctive movements are limited, the vertical fusional reserves or amplitudes being usually in the range 2^Δ to 4^Δ only. Although some patients can adapt to as much as 3 dioptres of vertical anisometropia, meaning they have comfortable binocular vision with spectacles, where symptoms do arise, the degree of ocular discomfort seems to bear little relationship to the amount of vertical imbalance (Rubin, 1950). Since the eyes have a limited vertical vergence amplitude, vertical differential prism may give rise to symptoms or, in some cases, prevent binocular vision. There is considerable intersubject variation in the tolerance for induced vertical differential prism but, as a general rule, Duke-Elder (1970) suggested that vertical differential prism of less than 1^Δ at the near visual points (NVPs) is unlikely to give rise to symptoms of asthenopia.

Prism adaptation

At first, one might expect, for example, that 2^Δ base up differential prism before the RE would induce the need for 2^Δ base down compensation prism in the spectacles. That is, one might expect there would be an induced right hyperphoria. However, several studies have found some anisometropic subjects with as much as 5^Δ of vertical differential prism at the NVPs who experience no symptoms and who have little or no measurable hyperphoria. This phenomenon is called *prism adaptation* and refers to the response of the oculomotor system to the presence of differential prism. For example, suppose an orthophoric subject suddenly has 1^Δ base up placed before the right eye. Immediate measurement of his vertical phoria will show 1^Δ of apparent right hyperphoria. That is, 1^Δ base down is required in front of the right eye to neutralise the 1^Δ base up and shift the image onto the centre of the macula. However, after a short period of binocular vision with the prism, most subjects show orthophoria when measured with the 1^Δ base up RE in situ. That is, the right eye remains infraducted when the eyes are dissociated for the phoria measurement. If the 1^Δ base up RE is removed, immediate measurement of the phoria shows 1^Δ of right hypophoria, indicating a hypertonic condition of the right depressor/left elevator muscles. The adaptation or hypertonicity takes about 10 minutes to decay and vertical orthophoria returns.

Such motor adaptation to differential prism is fairly rapid. Henson and North (1980) found an average of 1.5^Δ adaptation to 2^Δ base up in front of the RE occurred in a little more than 3 minutes. That is, on average, they recorded only about 0.5^Δ of right hyperphoria with the prism after 3 minutes wear. In a further experiment, Henson and Dharamshi (1982) induced anisometropia using a -1.50, a -3.00 and a -4.50 dioptre soft contact lens on one eye. The subject then wore a spectacle correction. They found that adaptation to the vertical phoria induced by looking above or below the optical centres increased gradually over 2 to 3 hours. The rate of adaptation was smaller as the anisometropia increased. For the 1.5 D anisometropia, the adaptation was almost complete, but adaptation was less as the anisometropia increased. They concluded that this oculomotor adaptation was identical to that required of naturally occurring anisometropes wearing spectacles and that, within a little time, their vertical phorias would not vary when looking up and down through different parts of their spectacle lenses.

† See *Introduction to Visual Optics*, 1994 edition, page 510.

Bifocal spectacle correction

Where the anisometropic patient is compelled to look through NVPs which introduce vertical differential prism, as with bifocals or Progressive Addition Lenses, the question of prism adaptation is raised. What amount of vertical differential prism can be tolerated? An answer to this question was sought as long ago as the nineteen-forties. Ellerbrock and Fry (1948) fitted 47 anisometropic subjects with two pairs of spectacles, one pair without and the other pair with prism compensation (slab-off or bi-centric lenses). 18 subjects reported no difficulty with their uncompensated lenses but, despite prism adaptation, 29 subjects reported that they were more comfortable with the prism compensated spectacles. Another study on 50 patients, by Ellerbrock and Fry, was reported by Elvin (1954) and again about 60% of the subjects preferred the slab-off prism compensated lenses.

What then are the practical points regarding anisometropic spectacle wearers, as far as vertical differential prism is concerned? Patients using single vision lenses can, if they have symptoms, adjust the head and/or any reading material in order to look more nearly through the optical centres and reduce the differential prismatic effect. Positioning the optical centres about 5 mm below the pupil centres in single vision lenses, a standard practice anyhow, allows the patient to read with the visual axes not too far from the optical centres. Bifocal and PAL users are compelled to use the reading portion of their lenses and the question of prism-compensation must first be raised by the prescriber. The fact that Ellerbrock and Fry found 60% of subjects preferred prism compensated spectacles suggests that 60% of anisometropic bifocal wearers should have some form of prism compensation. Unfortunately, it is not possible to decide absolutely who can or cannot tolerate vertical differential prism. Allen (1974) reported one of the two presbyopes in his group of 20 anisometropic subjects needed slab-off lenses to relieve asthenopia, despite the fact that he exhibited complete prism adaptation. With prism compensation this patient also reported "the print appeared sharper", presumably because the binocular acuity was better with perfectly in-register retinal images (Tunnacliffe and Williams, 1985). *Prism adaptation does not therefore mean that a patient is necessarily comfortable with uncompensated differential prism.*

Finding the patient who needs prism compensation

What can we do to try and find the 60% of those patients who would benefit from prism compensated lenses? For an anisometropic patient who is about to have his first bifocals dispensed, if a vertical fixation disparity is present when viewing the test target through the NVPs of his single vision lenses, but not when viewing the target through the optical centres, then one should further consider the effect of prism compensation. The same test can be applied with the anisometrope already wearing uncompensated bifocal lenses, where they observe the near fixation disparity test through the segments of their present bifocals. If there is no vertical fixation disparity when viewing through the segments, and the patient has no symptoms which can be ascribed to vertical differential prism, then prism compensation is unlikely to be required. However, the final arbiter is the actual effect of prism compensation. This test is available to the dispenser, even in the absence of fixation disparity information. Remembering that the patient must be observing print at the resolution limit, if adding the compensating prism elicits a response of "better", meaning that the acuity is better, then this suggests the retinal images are maintained in better register and prism compensation will be beneficial. If in doubt, through lack of information, it is better to prism compensate the bifocals, when 1^Δ or more of vertical differential prism exists at the NVPs, at least in the case of first-time bifocal wearers.

Prism compensated lenses and other approaches

The methods of eliminating the differential prism at the NVPs in bifocals, multifocals and PALs are dealt with in text-books on ophthalmic lenses. Alternatively, it may be better not to use bifocals in some circumstances. The various approaches for tackling the problem are listed below:

1   **Single vision lenses** for relatively lengthy periods of close-work, supplemented by bifocals for general use. The single vision lenses can be decentred downwards to allow the patient to use areas of each lens closer to the optical centre. For each millimetre decentration downwards, the pantoscopic tilt will need to be increased 2°.

2   **Unequal bifocal round segments** (there is generally insufficient difference in the vertical differential positioning of the segment centres of D-segments to use this type, although Sola Optical now has a 40 mm Flat Top which can be combined with their D35 to produce $½^\Delta$ compensation per dioptre of Add). The larger round segment has its optical centre lower down and therefore introduces more base down prism than does the smaller segment. The larger segment is used to neutralise the vertical differential prism by adding prism to one lens. In the case of myopic anisometropia, the lesser myopic eye will need the larger segment. In hypermetropic anisometropia, the higher powered lens introduces more base up prismatic effect at the NVP, so this lens will need the larger base down effect of the larger segment.

3   **Prism segment bifocals or slab-off (bi-prism).**
    In prism segment bifocals, the vertical differential prism is neutralised by incorporating the neutralising prism in the segment. In slab-off lenses, prism is effectively removed over the lower portion of the lens, resulting in a horizontal visible edge across the front surface. With full-aperture straight-top bifocals this is cosmetically unnoticeable, being coincident with the top of the segment.

4   *Bonded prism segments.* These are CR 39 lenses where the compensating prism is incorporated in the segment and bonded to a single vision main lens.

5   *Franklin split bifocals.* This is a lens, made in upper distance and lower near vision portions which are usually bonded together. Franklin bifocals are essentially distance and near single vision lenses which are cut in two and bonded together along the straight edge. Different centrations of the two parts is easily achieved, so any vertical differential prism at the NVPs is eliminated. When neatly executed, Franklin split bifocals look very similar to E-type bifocals.

6   Fresnel prism segments (see below and in Chapter 10 of *Introduction to Visual Optics*).

7   Contact lenses!

Where prism-compensated lenses are to be dispensed, there are several choices, besides unequal round segments. Table 4 lists various makers and suppliers in the UK market. Note that one could also supply slab-off and Franklin split forms to neutralise the vertical differential prism in single vision form.

Table 4 Lenses available for vertical differential prism compensation

Supplier	Lens Type
	Single Vision
Norville	Glass and CR 39 slab-off
	Fused Bifocals
Norville	D-segment slab-off
Zeiss	Duopal C28, C25 (1.6), C30 (1.6) slab-off
	Glass Solid Bifocals
Lentoid	30 mm Round prism segment
Norville	Franklin Split
Rodenstock	Ardis 25 mm Curved Top prism segment and slab-off
Rodenstock	Excellent full-width straight-top, prism segment or slab-off
	Plastic Bifocals
Norville	D, E and Round segment slab-off, and Franklin Split
	Glass Trifocals
Norville	Slab-off on any type
	Progressive Addition Lenses
Norville	Slab-off on all CR 39 lenses
Zeiss	Slab-off on Lantal Gradal HS and Top, Gradal Top, Gradal 3 and Gradal RD

Trial prism compensation with Fresnel prisms

Fresnel prisms are thin polyvinyl chloride sheets, about 1 mm thick, which can be cut to fit over the reading area. Since they reduce visual acuity by about 1 to 2 rows of letters on the Snellen chart, they should be used only for temporary experimentation, using one in front of each eye. This removes the patient's objection to reduced acuity in one eye alone which would be more objectionable if prism were used in front of one eye only. The effect of prism compensation on the comfort of binocular vision when reading can be judged by the patient before permanent lenses are dispensed. One advantage of this type of prism compensation is that a blind experiment can be run in which the patient does not know when prism compensation is occurring. This is done by having both Fresnel prism bases up or down for a period, then one up and one down for a similar time. In the latter case the vertical differential prism is neutralised. The patient then reports the effect on symptoms during the two periods. If the patient is symptom-free in the prism compensated period, but not during the uncompensated trial, then one can confidently dispense prism compensated lenses.

Prism compensation with unequal segments

Methods of calculating the prismatic effect at the NVP are considered in ophthalmic lenses text-books. In practice one tends to use a table for this purpose. The prismatic effects in the table have been calculated by one of the standard methods, of course. Below is a table which assumes that the visual axes are to intersect the lenses at point 10 mm below and 2 mm in from the optical centres. The prismatic effects obtained are described in the table heading.

Table 5   Vertical prismatic effect at the NVP, 10 mm down and 2 mm in from the distance optical centre due to a +1.00 D cylinder. All base directions are UP. Reverse the base direction for minus cylinders. Values for other cylinder powers can be obtained by multiplying by that cylinder power.

Axis	RE	LE	Axis	RE	LE
5	1.00	0.97	95	0.00	0.02
10	1.00	0.93	100	0.00	0.06
15	0.98	0.88	105	0.01	0.11
20	0.94	0.81	110	0.05	0.18
25	0.89	0.74	115	0.10	0.25
30	0.83	0.66	120	0.16	0.33
35	0.76	0.57	125	0.23	0.42
40	0.68	0.48	130	0.31	0.51
45	0.60	0.40	135	0.39	0.60
50	0.51	0.31	140	0.48	0.68
55	0.42	0.23	145	0.57	0.76
60	0.33	0.16	150	0.66	0.83
65	0.25	0.10	155	0.74	0.89
70	0.18	0.05	160	0.81	0.94
75	0.11	0.01	165	0.88	0.98
80	0.06	0.00	170	0.93	1.00
85	0.02	0.00	175	0.97	1.00
90	0.00	0.00	180	1.00	1.00

The vertical prismatic effect at the NVP of a lens can be obtained by considering the spherical component and the cylindrical component separately. The cylinder's contribution will be found from the table, but the spherical components can be found from the well-known Prentice's Rule which gives the prismatic effect as $P = c |F|$, where c is the distance from the optical centre to the NVP in cm, and F is the lens power, here the power of the sphere. Because the distance $c = 1.0$ cm here, the spherical component's contribution to the prismatic effect at the NVP is numerically equal to the sphere power. The base direction will be *up* for a plus sphere and *down* for a minus sphere; see figure 12.

As *an example* of its use, consider the anisometropic prescription

R. $-1.00 / -2.25 \times 35$ L. $-3.00 / -3.75 \times 120$.

Due to the spheres, the prismatic effects at the NVPs, 10 mm below the optical centres, are:

R. 1^{Δ} base down   L. 3^{Δ} base down.

The prismatic effects due to the cylinders, obtained from Table 5, are:

R. $2.25 \times 0.76 \Rightarrow 1.71^{\Delta}$ base down
L. $3.75 \times 0.33 \Rightarrow 1.24^{\Delta}$ base down.

Adding the respective spherical and cylindrical contributions, the resultant vertical prismatic effects are:

R. 1^{Δ} base down + 1.71^{Δ} base down = 2.71^{Δ} base down and
L. 3^{Δ} base down + 1.24^{Δ} base down = 4.24^{Δ} base down.

The vertical differential prismatic effect between the two NVPs is therefore $4.24^{\Delta} - 2.71^{\Delta} = 1.53^{\Delta}$ base down left lens.

With round segment solid bifocals, it now remains to decide on the segment diameters to neutralise this vertical differential prism. A simple formula will be found in *Worked Problems in Ophthalmic Lenses*, for those who wish to check the derivation. The difference (Δd) in segment diameters is given by where ΔP is the vertical differential prismatic effect.

In the current example, suppose the patient is to have prism compensated bifocals and the *Add* = +2.50, then the difference between round segment diameters must be

$$\Delta d = 20 \frac{\Delta P}{Add} = 20 \times \frac{1.53}{2.50} = 12.24 \text{ mm}.$$

Round segment diameters are available in solid bifocals in the sizes 25, 30, 38 and 45 mm. Any two with a difference most nearly equal to 12.24 mm will suffice to neutralise the vertical differential prism. 25 and 38 come nearest, although 30 and 45 are very nearly as good. In the present example, we need to add extra base down to the lens providing the smaller base down effect, so the larger segment will be placed in the right lens.

Note that using Sola's 40 and 35 mm D-segments, producing $\frac{1}{2}^{\Delta}$ base down more in the larger segment would provide *Add* $\times \frac{1}{2}^{\Delta} = 2.50 \times \frac{1}{2} = 1.25^{\Delta}$ base down right neutralising prism, which would be alright, being only about $\frac{1}{4}^{\Delta}$ short. The difference in segment diameters would be barely noticeable and therefore cosmetically acceptable.

Dispensing Bifocal Lenses

Choice of Patient for First-time Bifocals

As with any complex spectacle lens, there is no absolutely certain way in which the practitioner can be sure that a patient is suitable for bifocals. Given this situation, a patient considering bifocals for the first time is always taking some gamble on his/her ability to adapt to them. Following advice from the practitioner, it is the patient who must decide whether or not to try bifocals and, consequently, it is the patient's responsibility if there is a failure to adapt. This, of course, assumes that the bifocals have been correctly dispensed.

Nonetheless, the practitioner should try and ensure that the prospective bifocal patient's gamble is not too great, and this is done by assessing the patient's suitability for bifocals. There are certain guidelines which can be followed.

❶ The patient's visual needs should include the requirement for clear distance and near vision.

❷ For conventional single segment bifocals, the patient's near vision tasks must involve only infraduction of the eyes. Patient's with near visual tasks above the normal reading level will need to consider separate single vision pairs, occupational bifocals (double D-segments, say), or nowadays the newer occupational progressive lenses (near/intermediate vision progressives).

❸ Bifocals must be available in the patient's prescription, and this can be determined from the *Ophthalmic Lens Availability* manual, or manufacturers' data.

❹ The patient must be prepared to spend an unspecified time adapting to bifocals. They will need to adapt to the visibility of the segment top and to the blur encountered on looking down at the floor, especially on descending stairs. Most patients report feeling reasonably at ease with bifocals in about 2 to 4 weeks, although some report taking longer.

Many patients have been warned at previous examinations that they will soon have to face the decision about correction

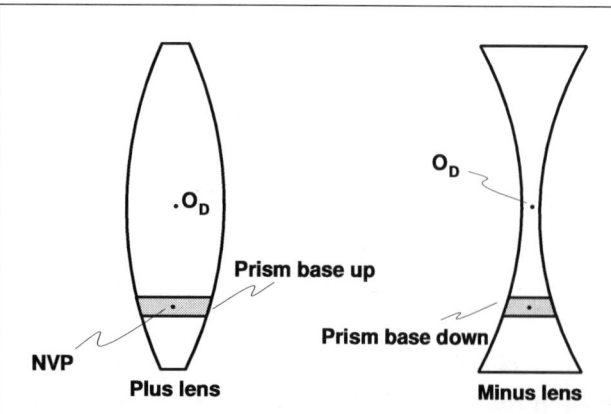

Fig. 12 Vertical prismatic effect due to the spherical component of a prescription lens. The distance from the optical centre (OC) to the near visual point (NVP) is 1.0 cm. The prismatic effect is base up with plus spheres, by inspection of the diagram, and base down with minus spheres.

for presbyopia. Such patients often state that they have come for bifocals. However, the practitioner should inform the patient of the alternative choices: distance and near single vision lenses, PALs, or OPALs. The practitioner should never get into the situation where he/she makes the choice for the patient, because if the patient fails to adapt to bifocals then blame can be directed at the practitioner, in which case the patient will expect any extra financial outlay to fall to the practitioner. *Trying bifocals is the patient's risk, not the practitioner's.*

Some patients should be advised against bifocals. These include:

❑ Previously failed wearers of bifocals, unless one can be sure the bifocals were incorrectly fitted, say.

❑ Patients who express doubts about them or who recount and believe stories of other people's difficulties with bifocals. Some of these may well be suitable provided they realise that tales about difficulties with bifocals are much exaggerated since all the successful bifocal wearers rarely talk about them. Only unsuccessful wearers complain and tell their stories, so these are the only bifocal stories abroad.

❑ Patients who suffer from depression (check the medication entry on the Rx card to see if they are being treated with anti-depressants). Such patients are unlikely to be able to cope with the initial adaptational problems of two foci within the one lens aperture.

❑ Patients whose job is unsuitable for bifocals, either because of the blur when looking at the floor, or the position of a near vision task is too high. Specialist bifocals may be suitable, but the gamble with adaptation is greater than with conventional bifocals.

The practitioner must spend considerable time explaining the properties of bifocals, especially the head/eye positioning for close work, the fact that the floor will be slightly blurred even with a low first-time Add, and the effects of 'confused' vision at the top of the segment. It should also be explained that near vision with the eyes in an elevated position will not be possible, so all those DIY jobs above eye-level will be out of the question with bifocals. If some close work tasks cannot be undertaken through the segment, this indicates that a supplementary single vision close-work pair of spectacles might be necessary. One thing must be clear to the practitioner: when considering the presbyopic patient, there is no single type of lens suitable for all visual tasks, and patients who regularly do any near vision task requiring fixation above the segment level will need some other form of supplementary correction. For the odd, occasional, momentary above-eye-level requirement, lifting the spectacle frame off the nose is not an unusual thing to see bifocal wearers doing, but this is only feasible for a few seconds. Some cases with elevated near vision tasks might benefit from double-D bifocals, bifocal with a further reading segment at the top; see figure 1 on page 62 at the beginning of this section on dispensing bifocals.

It all sounds terribly depressing, but we must not forget that millions of people successfully wear bifocals and the success rate with them is over 90% of those who try them!

Established wearers of bifocals

If a patient already wears bifocals, then maintaining the same type of bifocal with the same segment top position is unlikely to cause any wearing problems. This assumes there has not been a large change in refractive error, such as caused by index myopia in one eye compared with the other, thus introducing anisometropia. It is generally true to say that if the segment type in the current spectacles has been perfectly satisfactory, and there is no complaint about the segment top position, one can confidently order the same again.

With medium to high powered lenses it is always important to maintain good lens form (best form). Certainly, one must not supply a form which will degrade the quality of vision in oblique gaze, compared with the current spectacles. That seemingly simple little device, the optician's lens measure, is a vital piece of equipment in this respect, and this applies just as importantly to medium and high powered lenses of other types.

Choice of Conventional Bifocal

The choice depends on the patient's visual needs and the price he/she can afford to pay. Sometimes the best optical solution is more than the patient can afford, and in that case the patient must be advised that he/she is not getting the best. With the first-time bifocal wearer, the whole range of bifocals available should be discussed. On the other hand, with an experienced bifocal wearer it may be that he/she is already wearing a good design — one with a flat top or curved top. We have already mention that small round segment bifocals require more infraduction for the same width of field of view as a D-segment of similar diameter. Also, if someone is upgrading from an R25 to a D-segment, do not forget to warn them about the increased reflection from the segment top. Like almost all choices in spectacle lens dispensing, changing a lens type for an improvement of one characteristic often involves deterioration of another, and compromises and judgements have to be made. Unfortunately, there is no substitute for experience, and the practitioner learns most of the pitfalls by expensive mistakes. Hopefully, they are not made repeatedly.

The factors which are to be considered in choice of a conventional bifocal type are:

1   Segment diameter.
2   Segment top shape (C, D, E, and R-type).
3   Jump or no-jump.

The larger the diameter, the wider the field of view through the segment. Table 6 lists the types of bifocals available, both white and photochromic, and in glass and plastics.

Dispensing Bifocal Lenses

Table 6 Segment types and diameters available

Glass lenses

 Fused bifocals
  White R 25, 26, 28, 32
       C 25, 28, 30, 32
       D 25, 26, 28, 35

  Photochromic C 25, 26, 28
         D 25, 28, 35

 Solid bifocals
  White R 22, 30, 38, 40, 45
       E-type
       Upcurve

  Photochromic R 30, 38
         E-type

Plastic lenses

  White R 24, 25, 28, 38, 40, 45
       C 25, 26, 28, 40
       D 25, 28, 35, 40, 45
       E-type
       Seamless R28

  Photochromic D 28, 35

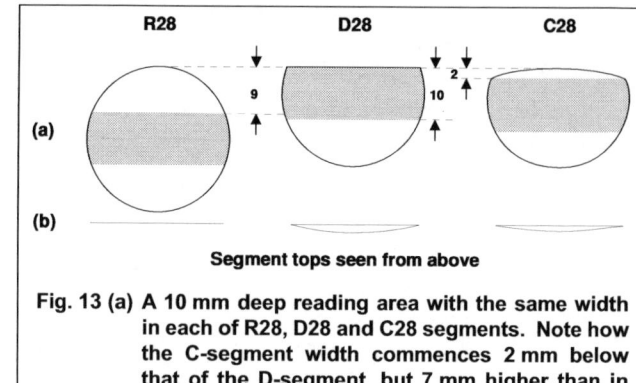

Fig. 13 (a) A 10 mm deep reading area with the same width in each of R28, D28 and C28 segments. Note how the C-segment width commences 2 mm below that of the D-segment, but 7 mm higher than in the R28 segment. The C-segment, with a less noticeable segment top than a D-segment, is a good compromise.
(b) Being less wide than the D-segment's, the top edge of the C-segment is less noticeable.

Segment top shape influences two things: the immediate width of segment available, and the confusion zone at the segment top. Clearly, a flat top is desirable for a good usable width of segment, the E-type obviously being best in this respect since the whole width of the lens is available for close-work. Flat top segments, however, have wider edges at the distance portion/segment junction which reflect more light than other segment shapes. Glazed *demonstration lenses* are essential when explaining this cosmetic feature of bifocal lenses; a picture tells a thousand words!

Comparing 28 mm R, D and C segments, figure 13 illustrates the fields of view positions for a 10 mm depth at the widest portion of each segment. Although a round segment reflects the least light from the segment top because it has a *knife edge*, as we have seen from figure 4, page 54, the width of the uppermost portion of the segment is not as great as in a D-segment of the same diameter. A curved-top (C) segment is a good compromise between round (R) and D-segments, in these two respects. We have already mentioned that a D-segment can be fitted 1 to 2 mm lower than round small round segments, simply because the segment top shape confers an immediately useful portion of segment at the top.

Jump and no-jump at the segment top

To avoid the introduction of a sudden change in prismatic effect as the visual axis crosses into the segment at the top, the optical centre of the segment needs to be at the segment top. This necessarily produces an edge rather than the line junction seen in round segments. Hence, no-jump bifocals have a visible segment at the upper margin. Once again, this illustrates the fact that the dispenser, and therefore the patient, is faced with a set of compromises when deciding upon spectacle lenses.

Aspheric Bifocals in the low to medium power range

These are relatively recent introductions to the ophthalmic lens product range, at least in the 'normal' power range. They have a front aspherical surface only in the distance portion, conveying the same optical advantages as for single vision lenses. Thus far, only a few manufacturers make them, as can be seen from Table 7 below.

Table 7 Available aspheric bifocals in the low to medium power range

Cosmolux C28 in 1.6 index glass	Rodenstock
Cosmolit C28 in CR 39	Rodenstock
Spectralite C28 and D28	Sola
Kodak C28 and D28 1.56 index plastic	Signet Armorlite

In the first four cases, the vertex A_0 of the aspherical surface is 3 mm above the segment top, see figure 14, whilst in the Kodak lenses it is 4 mm. For the lens to perform to its design criteria, the optical axis of the aspherical surface must pass through the eye's centre of rotation. In the first four lenses, placing the segment top at the lower limbus level will position A_0 about 2½ mm below the pupil centre, so the frame will need fitting with a 5° pantoscopic tilt when aspheric bifocals are dispensed. With the Kodak lenses the pantoscopic tilt will need to be about 3°.

Lenticular and high powered aspheric bifocals

Occasionally, one needs high powered lenticular bifocals, of which a few are available, although the minus range is very limited. However, one can always bond a segment to a main single vision lens. Norville Optical Company have this

Dispensing Bifocal Lenses

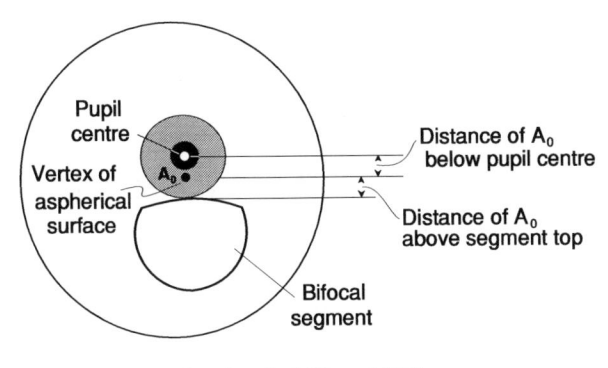

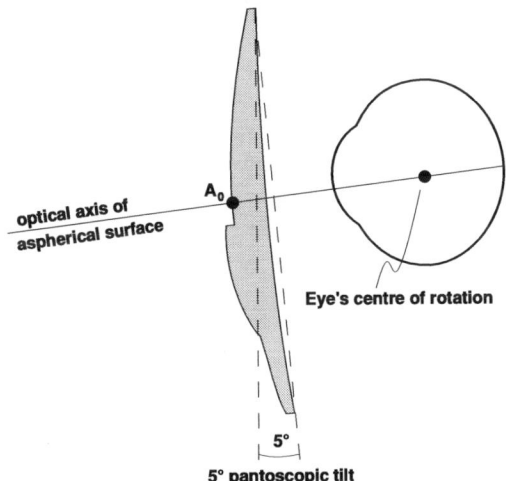

Fig. 14 Determining the pantoscopic tilt for aspheric bifocals. A_0 is the vertex of the aspherical front surface of the distance portion. The distance of A_0 above the segment top is obtained from the manufacturer's data, and in the four of the six lenses currently available it is 3 mm. This places A_0 about 2½ mm below the pupil centre. The pantoscopic tilt is 1° for each 0.5 mm that A_0 is below the pupil centre with the eyes in the primary position of gaze, resulting in a required pantoscopic tilt of 5° with these lenses. For those lenses where A_0 is 4 mm above the segment top, it will be about 1½ mm below the pupil centre and thus determine a 3° pantoscopic tilt.

facility and it is worth consulting them. Figure 15 illustrates types of lenticular bifocals available.

Occupational and Special Bifocals

There are several types of bifocals, some with two segments, which are designed to be used only in special circumstances. Since these circumstances are usually dictated by the visual requirements of a job, such bifocals attract the soubriquet *occupational bifocals*. Generally, these bifocals are only suitable for the job in question, and this means that the patient will need other spectacles for ordinary use. Figure 16 illustrates the range of occupational bifocals currently available.

Bonding segments to a single vision main lens, mentioned above in connection with minus lenticular bifocals, also applies to unusual items like having a high powered segment bonded in the upper temple quadrant of the frame lens shape, for someone who wishes to inspect some very small detail from time to time.

Bifocals with high Adds

Most manufacturers offer their bifocals with Adds from 1.00 to 3.50. A few do 0.50 and 0.75 Adds, and a few go as far as 4.00. Over 4.00 dioptres the range is very limited. Zeiss have one C25 lens in glass with Adds to 6.00. The Adds are 0.75 to 4.00 in the normal stock range, but Adds of 4.50, 5.00, 5.50, and 6.00 are available to special order. Called Duopal C25, it is a fused bifocal in 1.6 index glass.

Sola make a CR 39 lens called the LVA (low vision aid) Bifocal with Adds 4.00, 5.00, 6.00, 8.00, 10.00, 12.00, and 16.00. The segment is an R25.

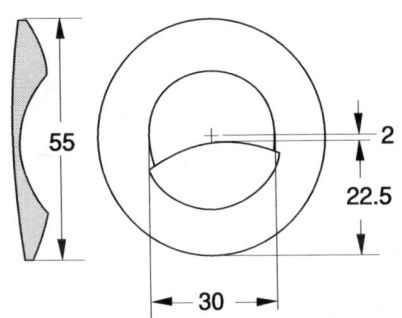

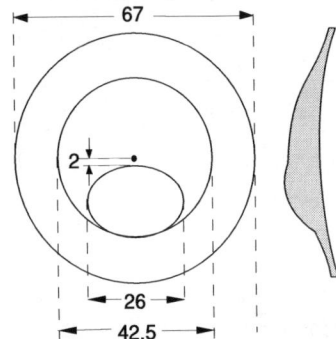

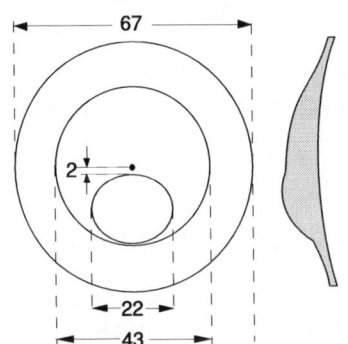

Fig. 15 Types of lenticular bifocal. Others are available — consult the *Ophthalmic Lens Availability* file.

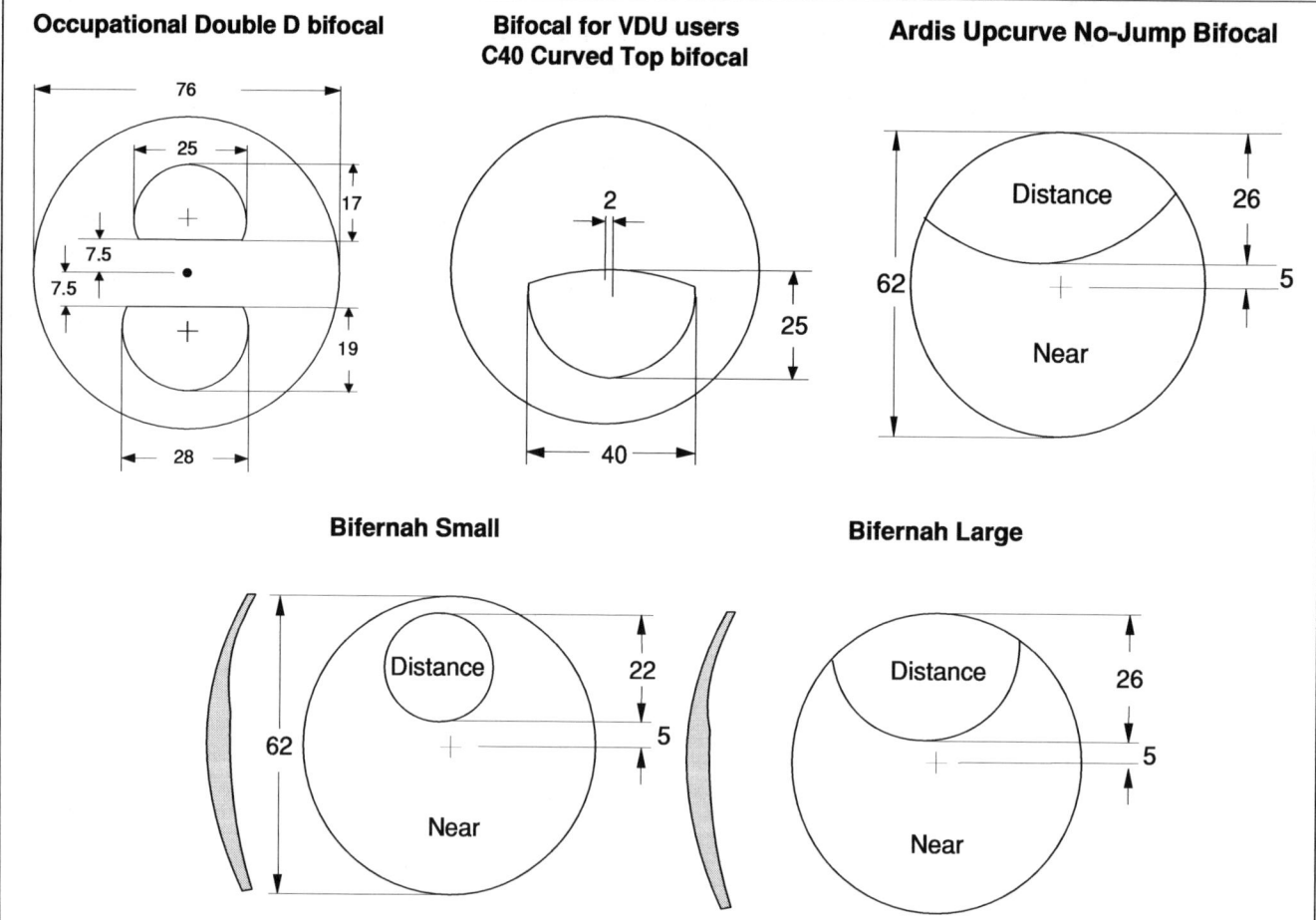

Fig. 16 Occupational bifocals. Details of the power ranges of these lenses can be found in the *Ophthalmic Lens Availability* file. The Double D lens is available with both segments having the reading power, when it is known as a 'bifocal'. It is also available with the upper segment having 60% of the near Add, when it is called a 'trifocal'. The C40 VDU user's lens will be ordered with the intermediate Rx at the top for focus on the monitor screen. This can be done with any conventional bifocal, too.

Front and Back Surface Segments

Generally speaking, glass fused bifocal lenses have the segment in the front surface and glass solid bifocals have round segments on the back surface and E-type (Executive) on the front surface. Plastic lenses all have front surface segments. Zeiss did, until recently, have several fused bifocals with back surface segments. However, only Rodenstock has any back surface segments in glass lenses remaining from old designs, namely *Ardis* Solid R40 and *Excellent* E-type.

Jalie has shown, by computer ray traces, that plus lenses have a better optical performance with front surface segments, the opposite being true of minus lenses.

The Smart Seg Progressive Bifocal

We mentioned this unique lens on page 62 and also in figure 2 on page 63. The author has worn this lens and it has the unique property of providing a progression with absolutely no noticeable surface aberrational astigmatism. The distance portion presents clear vision over the whole width and the reading area is much wider than with a conventional PAL. Sola recommend that the segment top should be fitted 3 mm below the pupil centre. This means that the segment top is some 2½ mm higher than the lower limbus, and patients must be warned of this fact. The author's only problem with this lens was that the 30 mm diameter segment was narrow compared to the Executive bifocals being worn at that time. I did not find the segment top too much of an intrusion into the distance visual field, probably because the first 12 mm below the top is the progressive zone, and the thickness of the top edge is relatively narrow, a result of the small starting addition power.

Segment Top Positioning vis-à-vis the Eye

There are a number of different bifocal fitting situations we should consider:

1. Conventional fitting
2. VDU use
3. Juvenile stress myopia and accommodation control
4. Double D segments
5. Upcurve bifocals.

The positioning of segments is largely determined from the collective experience of practitioners, or from wearer trial experiments in the case of something new like the Smart Seg. It is generally true to say that low fitting bifocals are more a cause of complaint than high fitting ones. The author has seen one asymptomatic patient with R24 segments fitted with the segment top at the pupil centre level, and no amount of persuasion could make her consider this to be wrong. She had adapted to it. On the other hand, fit the segment 1 mm below someone's previous fitting and that person will often complain of having to raise the segments when reading, or of having to hold the head in an uncomfortable backwards tilted posture. If a patient has adapted to some out-of-the-ordinary segment top position, it is often unwise to alter it, and any alteration should only be undertaken after close consultation with the patient.

1 Conventional fitting

Figure 17 shows what might be considered the consensus opinion on 'normal' fittings with round and C-segments positioned with their segment tops at the lower limbus, and flat tops about 1 to 2 mm below the lower limbus. These would be the positions in the absence of any other constraints, the most common constraint on segment top position being those cases who have adapted to some other position.

Figure 18 shows how patients fitted with a large vertex distance should have their segment tops lower than usual. Patients with a large vertex distance, say 15 or 16 mm, might have their segments fitted about 1 mm lower than the average. This approximation is calculated by allowing the same depression of the eyes for a vertex distance of 10 mm and using similar triangles, as in figure 18, with fitting distances of 25 and 30 mm.

2 VDU use

VDU users who need bifocals will require an intermediate Rx in the upper portion, often focused for a distance between 50 and 80 cm, the range of distances reported by computer users for the eye-to-screen distance*. This distance will need to be measured by the patient in the workplace. The segment top position for most users turns out to be similar to the conventional position, but it is worth asking the patient to measure the position of the bottom of the screen relative to eye-level. Then, at the dispensing a simulated screen position can be adopted and the patient or practitioner marks a dummy lens in the frame with the segment top position required. This will be the maximum height of the segment such that the screen can be seen through the upper intermediate portion above the segment.

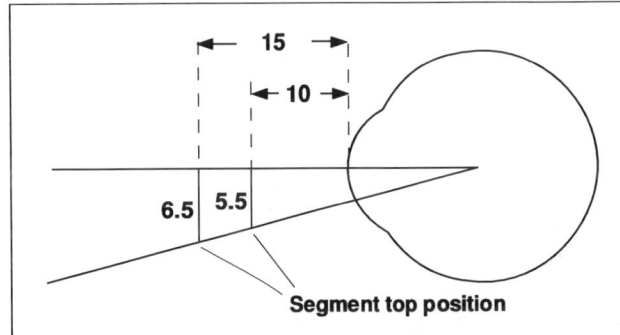

Fig. 18 Bifocals with a large vertex distance, 15 mm say, should be fitted 1 mm lower than the standard position, otherwise the segment will encroach into the distance field of view more than usual.

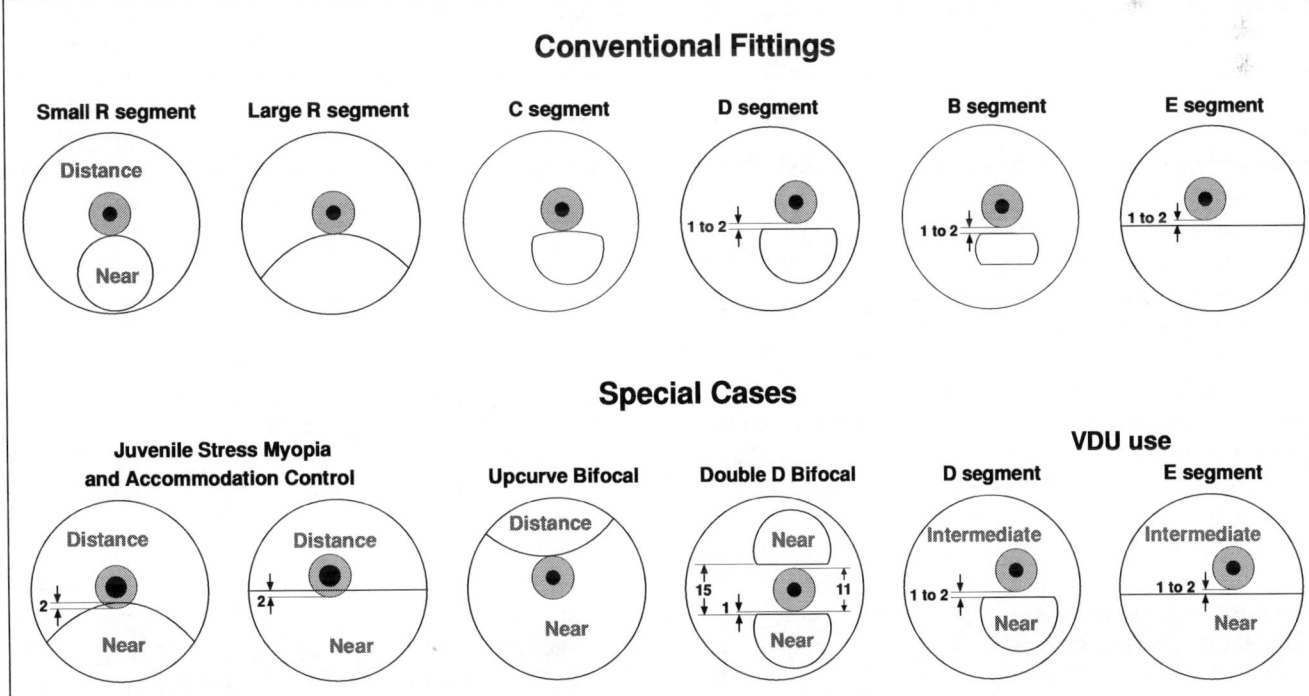

Fig. 17 Upper row: normal fitting position for the segment top. Lower row: special cases.
These fittings are guidelines for the dispenser, but there will be a fair proportion of cases where variation from the guidelines will be necessary. For example, not all VDU users have the monitor at the same height; in order to determine the segment top position with some precision, the dispenser should ask the patient to measure the distance to the monitor, and the height of the upper and lower edges of the screen relative to the patient's eye level.

* Larger screens have allowed longer eye-to-screen distances in recent years.

3 Juvenile Stress Myopia and Accommodation Control

In both these cases, the segment tops are usually set 2 mm above the lower limbus, the idea being to ensure that the child does not use the upper portion of the lens for close-work. This might happen if the spectacles work very loose over a period of time, a not unusual circumstance arising from the rough and tumble of play.

4 Double D Segments

It has to be said that these lenses are very rarely fitted. The upper segment can have the full near vision Add or 50% of this, which in the latter case makes it a trifocal! The segments are 15 mm apart so, if the lower segment is fitted 1 mm below the lower limbus, the straight edge of the upper segment will be about 3 mm above the upper limbus.

5 Upcurve bifocals

These are also infrequently used, the only suppliers at the current time being Rodenstock and Norville. Although one can think of a 'standard' position of the segment bottom, as shown in figure 17, perhaps the best approach is to mark the outline of the segment on the patient's old spectacle lens. By trial and error it is possible for the patient to decide the required position of the segment. For this purpose, a ½ mm thick ink-line is easily noticeable by the patient, despite its being very blurred. The blurred line appears quite wide and it is therefore a good idea to ask the patient to use the centre of the blurred line image when making judgements about the line position.

Head and eye position during measurements

When measuring the PD, or mono-PDs, or the segment top position, it is assumed that the patient's eye being measured is in the primary position. That is, the head is erect and the eye is fixating straight ahead. If the head should turn about a vertical axis by just 2°, then one mono-PD will be measured 1 mm larger and the other 1 mm smaller. If the head is tilted forwards or backwards by 2°, then the segment top will be located 1 mm too high or 1 mm too low, respectively. These errors are determined in the same manner as the relationship between pantoscopic tilt and vertical optical centre position. A head tilt or rotation of 2° introduces a 1 mm error in mono-PD and segment top position measurements. Hence, great care must be taken to ensure that the head is erect during these measurements.

Ordering Bifocals

With experience, ordering becomes a matter of routine, but as with all routines mistakes can be made if the routine becomes habitual. To minimise the occurrence of costly ordering errors, it is a wise precaution to have every order checked by a second person. Even then errors seem to escape detection and orders are incorrectly executed, to the detriment of the practice in terms of cost and delays.

For a laboratory to execute an order efficiently, certain data are essential. The order for bifocals should include the following:

- The *distance prescription*, including *any prescribed prism*. The distance prescription is as for single vision lenses. Where the upper portion of the lens is for intermediate use, as with VDU bifocals, then this upper portion's power will be the distance Rx plus the intermediate Add.

- The *Add* is the difference between the upper portion and lower portion powers. In a distance/near bifocal, the near vision portion through the segment will have a power equal to the distance Rx plus the near vision Add.

- *Bifocal type, segment diameter, segment top position* and *inset*. The bifocal type includes fused or solid when the lens is in glass, but it is not necessary to specify this for plastic bifocal lenses since they are all solid except in the rare case where a bonded or cemented segment is used. The type of segment needs to be specified: B, C, D, E, R, Upcurve, etc.

  Some practitioners specify the segment height, but because of the occasional misunderstanding about the definition of this parameter it is better to order the segment top position relative to datum line (HCL). This latter measurement is the one required by the laboratory when setting the uncut for machining.

  We have said that geometrical inset will suffice except for high plus powers (see pages 65 and 66).

- The *PD* or *mono-PDs*, where the latter are different. With high power lenses it is important to specify the mono-PDs in order to ensure the lens performs to its best form design criterion of having the optical axis in the distance portion pass through the eye's centre of rotation.

- *Lens material*, including *tint, anti-reflection coating* and *other processes*. Anti-reflection coatings differ. One manufacturer's coating may have a better transmittance than another's. These can be compared in one of the tables on page 3 of the *Ophthalmic Lens Availability* file. This table lists AR coating and hard coat combinations. Mid-index plastics are softer than CR 39 and many come with a multiAR coat/hard coat combination as standard.

- *Frame style, colour, measurements* and *the manufacturer's name.*

- To match an existing lens, the *drop* and the *form* of the lens should be quoted when ordering only one bifocal lens.

- The *drop to match the pantoscopic tilt*. This is necessary on high powered lenses, at least, in order to correspond with the pantoscopic tilt. For flat-topped segments fitted 1 to 2 mm below the lower limbus, a *standard* drop of 2 mm would place the optical centre of the distance portion about 5 mm below the pupil centre and would correspond to a 10° pantoscopic tilt.

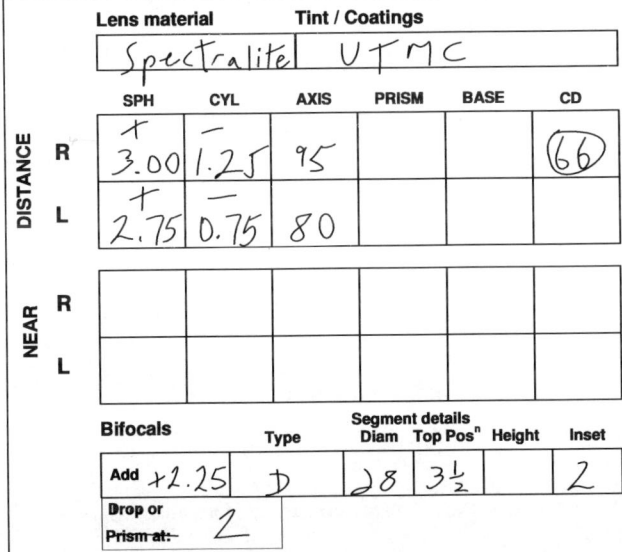

Fig. 19 Example of a routine bifocal order. In Spectralite material this lens is an aspheric and this fact could be mentioned on the order.
Note the placement of the plus or minus signs: this is permissible when there is a shortage of space in the boxes, which is not unusual.

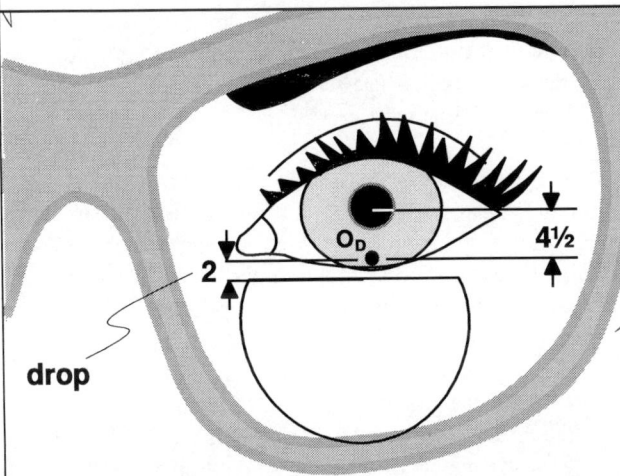

Fig. 20 Assuming the segment top position is 1 mm below the lower limbus and the Visible Vertical Iris Diameter (VVID) is 11 mm, with a 2 mm drop the optical centre (O_D) of the distance portion is 4½ mm below the pupil centre. The pantoscopic tilt will need to be adjusted to close to the usual 10°.

Figures 19 and 20 illustrate some of the data from *a fairly routine bifocal order*. Note the drop is ordered as 2 mm, but this is the standard position for the optical centre or for prescribed prism. If you use a single Rx laboratory, check with them to see if they require this information. If they always use this drop or prism reference point then there will be no need to mention it on orders for a pair of bifocal lenses. However, on an order for one bifocal lens, either to replace a scratched or broken lens, or because there is a prescription change in one lens only, then it is essential to state the required drop or prism reference point to match the retained lens. To match the ordered drop, the pantoscopic tilt is adjusted at the collection when the effect on vision can be checked for subjective response. That is, the patient is asked to comment on the effect of slight adjustments to the pantoscopic tilt whilst viewing a Snellen chart and reading material, and the tilt is adjusted to that value affording the best vision.

Ordering prescribed prism, where it is the same in the distance and near portions, simply requires one entry in the prism box for each lens on the order form. There will normally be one entry for each lens since the prism is usually split equally between the lenses, as shown in the figure 21. In this example, suppose the segment tops have been fitted 1 mm below the lower limbus, as in figure 20, except that the point marked O_D is now the prism reference point. The prism has been ordered at 2 mm above the segment top and note that the optical axis/centre of rotation condition cannot be satisfied — the optical centres will have been moved by the prisms! Just as in any other case where the optical centres are at the centration points, pantoscopic tilt is adjusted in practice at the collection.

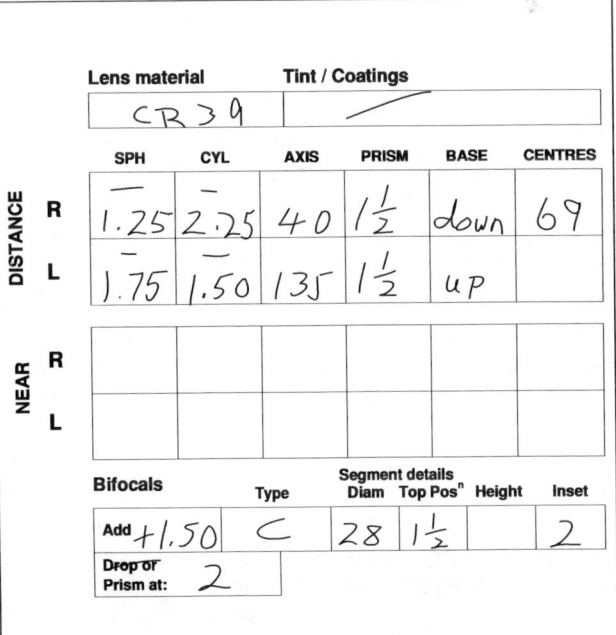

Fig. 21 An order for bifocals which includes prisms. Note that the prism will be effective over the whole lens, including the near vision portion.

Dispensing Bifocal Lenses

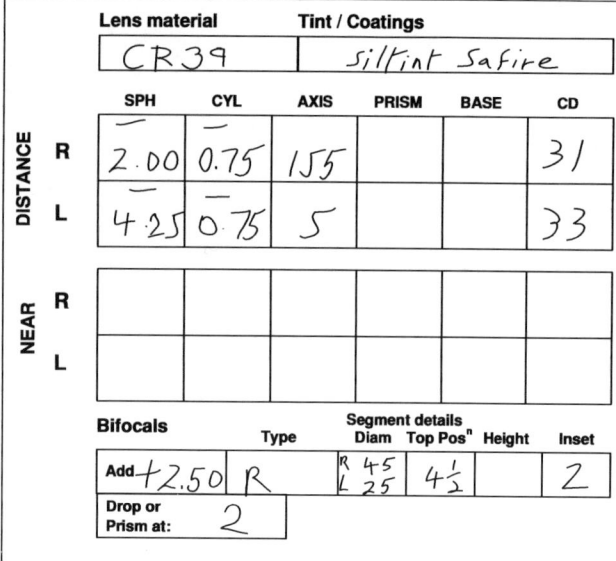

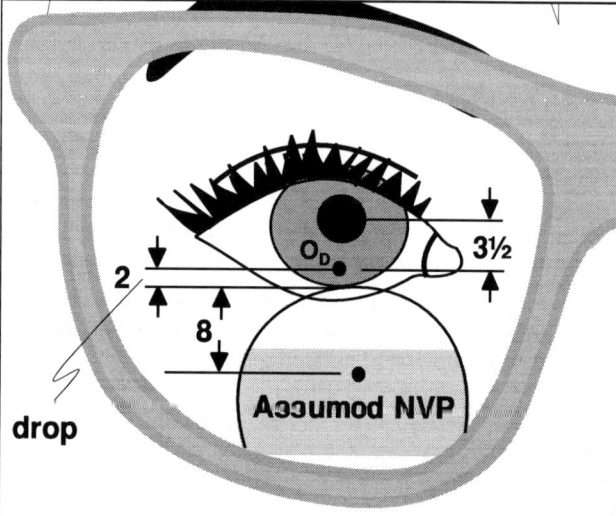

Fig. 22 A bifocal order for unequal diameter round segments to compensate for the vertical differential prism at the NVPs in this anisometropic case.

Fig. 23 Assuming the NVP is 10 mm below the distance optical centre O_D, ordering a standard 2 mm drop places O_D 3½ mm below the pupil centre, so the pantoscopic tilt will need to be 7°. This is determined by adjustment for the best distance vision at the time of the collection.

Figures 22 and 23 relate to an example of prism compensation in anisometropia using unequal diameter round segments. Calculation of the segment diameters is from the method using Table 5 and the description on pages 71 and 72. Here, as shown in figure 23 with a 2 mm standard drop, the round segment top is fitted at the lower limbus and the Near Visual Points (NVPs), assumed 10 mm below and 2 mm in from O_D in the calculation of the unequal segment diameters, will be about 13½ mm below the pupil centre. The average distance of the NVP below pupil centre is 11 mm, but 13½ mm is about right for a reasonable width of reading area in the R25 segment (see figure 4 on page 64). This distance to the NVP from pupil centre is close to values assumed in PAL design, so it is not unusually large.

Notice how the standard 2 mm drop produces a pantoscopic tilt close to the conventional 10°. Any slight adjustment to

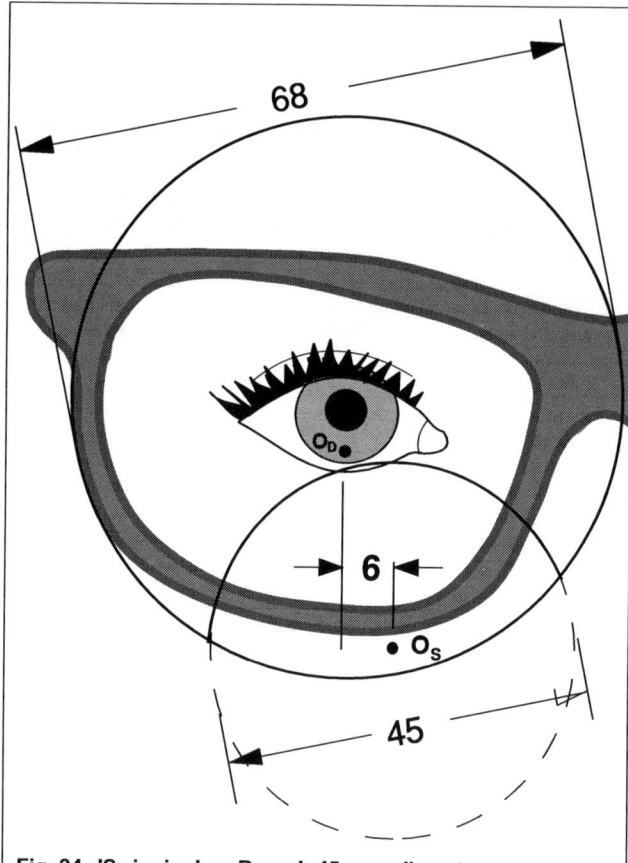

Fig. 24 'Swinging' a Round 45 mm diameter segment to give a 6 mm inset. The extra 4 mm produces *base in prism* which is calculated using Prentice's Rule in the form *prismatic effect* = $0.4 \times Add$.

give the best visual acuity can be made when the spectacles are collected.

Another non-standard order is the use of **R45 segments to obtain a small amount of base in prism for near** only; see figure 24. If the Add is sufficiently high, say 2.50, 4 mm extra inset will produce 1^Δ base in prism in the near portion. This is only possible on a large round segment because the extra inset can be obtained by 'swinging the segment' inwards before surfacing the non-segment surface, and at the same time retaining a reasonable amount of segment to look through. It is a useful ruse for obtaining 1^Δ base in R & L in the segment.

Split Bifocals consist of upper and lower portions made of single vision lenses cut and bonded along a horizontal edge. At first glance they resemble E-type bifocals. Closer scrutiny reveals their optical difference lies in the fact that the prismatic effects in distance and near portions are different. In fact, this is the reason for using split bifocals nowadays. For example, suppose the distance portion of each lens required 1^Δ base in, but the reading portion of each lens required 3^Δ base in. One would normally glaze split bifocals with these prismatic effects at the junction so that at this level there is no vertical prismatic effect. Since there is no vertical prismatic effect in either portion at the junction, there is no sudden vertical change in prismatic effect as the visual axis crosses from one portion to the other. Alternatively, the dispenser could specify the levels at which the prisms are to be effective in each portion of the lens.

Verification of Bifocals

This refers to the checking procedures to determine the accuracy of the finished spectacles after they have been received from the Rx laboratory. Every aspect of the order must be checked. That is, the frame and lens details must be checked against the Rx card details. Before the order was sent to the laboratory it is wise to have double checked all the details, and as a precaution it is better to verify the spectacles against the Rx card details rather than the order form since this method presents a further opportunity to spot any error which might have been incurred in writing the order form. This procedure assumes that the Rx card details are correct in the first place, and only at the collection will errors in segment height measurements, centration, and so on be discovered if the data on the Rx card is wrong. Recall from page 31, at the initial consultation the dispensing optician must check the validity of the data on the Rx card, thus hopefully spotting any errors there before they get to the order.

Measurement of the Addition in Bifocals

Power measurements on bifocal lenses refer to vertex power measurements made on the focimeter. For the majority of manufacturers, the measurement of the Add depends on whether the segment in on the front or back surface of the lens.

> For *front surface segments* the manufacturer defines the Add as the difference between the front vertex powers measured over the segment and the distance portions.

> For *back surface segments* the Add is the difference between the back vertex powers measured over the segment and the distance portions.

Whilst these Add measurements are precise, they take no account of the fact that the Add required is really the difference between the vergences measured at the vertex sphere. The focimeter reads vertex power which involves parallel rays leaving the spectacle lens when set to read the vertex power. But in near vision there are no parallel rays at the reading lens when in use and what the eye experiences in terms of vergence change is not quite what the focimeter indicates. If the vertex distance is kept at the same value when determining the distance and near prescriptions during the test procedures, then to match the power performance of the trial lenses we really need the Vertex Sphere Addition. The German company Zeiss call this the Practical Addition and actually do compute it with their bifocal lenses and progressive lenses, but this means that the Add measured on the focimeter does not then correspond with the Vertex Sphere Add which has been supplied. Zeiss then measure the Add, using back vertex measurements, and issue the dispenser with a correction value to determine the Vertex Sphere (Practical) Add, the one the dispenser really needs because this is the prescription Add. Each bifocal type and each Add value will produce slightly different effectivities at the vertex sphere which can be determined by a computer

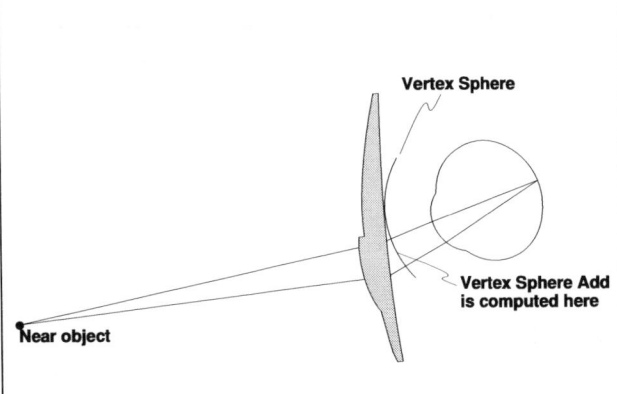

Fig. 25 The Vertex Sphere Add, or the Practical Add as it is called by Zeiss, is the value required to match the power performance of the trial lenses used in the eye examination. Zeiss use lenses with this computed Add value to match the prescription Add. They issue the dispenser with the uncut lens packets which indicate the measured Add. If this measured Add is then precise, the bifocal lens will perform to specification when used in conjunction with the eye.

ray trace through the segment from a near object, see figure 25. From this type of analysis, Zeiss determine *the correction value (K)* to be applied to the measured Add. These correction values turn out to be about −0.25 D for medium to high powered minus lenses, 0.00 D for lenses of low plus or minus power, and up to +0.75 for high plus powers. If you order Zeiss bifocals it means you should not apply a Near Vision Effectivity Error adjustment since this will be done by Zeiss. The relationship between the measured Add, the correction value, and the Vertex Sphere Add (Rx Add) is:

measured Add = Rx Add + correction value.

For example, using values in Zeiss' tables, if the Rx Add is 2.00, and for a +7.00 distance Rx in a CR 39 C25 bifocal, the measured Add should be

$$\begin{aligned}measured\ Add &= Rx\ Add + correction\ value \\ &= 2.00 + 0.50 \\ &= 2.50\ .\end{aligned}$$

If the measured Add does not read 2.50, and the error is outside tolerances, then the power is incorrect. Zeiss actually make it easier than the above example suggests; they send the uncut lens packets which simply state the Rx Add and the measured Add so that it is not necessary to state the correction factor. The measurements are made with the back surface of the lens on the focimeter lens rest.

Power, axis, centration, and prism tolerances

Manufacturers operate a set of engineering tolerances which allow them to deviate slightly from the ordered data, but these tolerances are agreed as being below the thresholds of noticeable image degradation by the patient. Making

Dispensing Bifocal Lenses

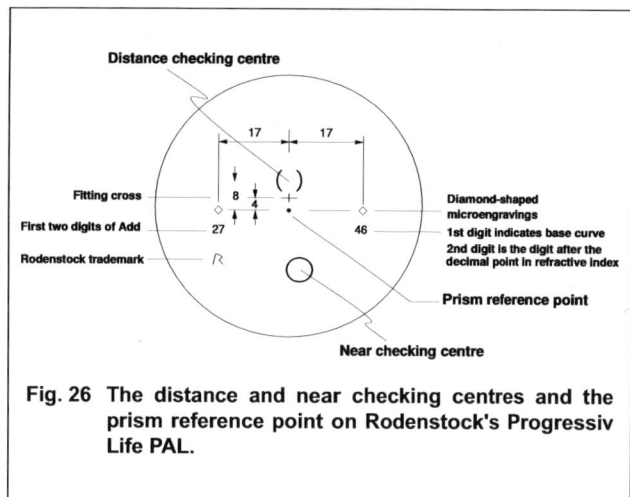

Fig. 26 The distance and near checking centres and the prism reference point on Rodenstock's Progressiv Life PAL.

A reference point on a lens is defined as a point at which the prescription requirements are to apply. In the case of single vision lenses, with the exception of pre-decentred uncuts, there will be only one reference point for the back vertex power and any prismatic effect and this is usually at the centre of the uncut. This will coincide with the centration point specified in the order when the lens has been glazed into the frame. With progressive addition lenses there are three reference points: the distance and near checking centres, and the prism reference point, see figure 26. We are probably most familiar with these since when progressive lenses are returned from the laboratory they have these regions painted on them.

In bifocals, the reference point is that specified by the manufacturer. British Standards is not forthcoming with a definition in this respect, stating that unless otherwise stated by the manufacturer, the two locations on the surface of measurement shall be on a straight line drawn through the reference point and equidistant from that point, with one being within the segment area and the other within the major area.

For completeness, a summary of the **power tolerances on glazed spectacle lenses** is given in Tables 7(a) and (b) for single vision, bifocals, trifocals, and progressives. Note that there is a tolerance on each meridional power, and a tolerance on the cylinder power.

spectacles is like any other engineering job, we must specify tolerances on the accuracy and precision of the work. A tolerance is defined as follows:

Definition of a tolerance — the difference between a measured value and the corresponding value stated in the prescription order.

Because of the effects of form and thickness of lenses on vergence and prism measurements, manufacturers refer to points on the lens where measurements should be taken.

Table 7(a)	Power tolerances for single vision, bifocal, and trifocal lenses				
Higher absolute power	**Tolerance on each meridian**	**Tolerance on cylinder power**			
		Up to 0.75	1.00 to 4.00	4.25 to 6.00	Over 6.00
0.00 to 3.00	± 0.09	± 0.09	± 0.12	± 0.18	—
3.25 to 6.00	± 0.12	± 0.12	± 0.12	± 0.18	± 0.25
6.25 to 9.00	± 0.12	± 0.12	± 0.18	± 0.18	± 0.25
9.25 to 12.00	± 0.18	± 0.12	± 0.18	± 0.25	± 0.25
12.25 to 20.00	± 0.18	± 0.18	± 0.25	± 0.25	± 0.25
Over 20.00	± 0.25	± 0.25	± 0.25	± 0.25	± 0.25

Table 7(b)	Power tolerances for progressive addition lenses[†]				
Higher absolute power	**Tolerance on each meridian**	**Tolerance on cylinder power**			
		Up to 0.75	1.00 to 4.00	4.25 to 6.00	Over 6.00
0.00 to 3.00	± 0.12	± 0.12	± 0.18	± 0.18	—
3.25 to 6.00	± 0.12	± 0.12	± 0.18	± 0.18	± 0.25
6.25 to 9.00	± 0.18	± 0.18	± 0.18	± 0.18	± 0.25
9.25 to 12.00	± 0.25	± 0.18	± 0.18	± 0.25	± 0.25
12.25 to 20.00	± 0.25	± 0.18	± 0.25	± 0.25	± 0.25
Over 20.00	± 0.50	± 0.25	± 0.25	± 0.25	± 0.25

† Note that British Standards uses the name Progressive Power Lenses which could arguably mean that a minus lens increases in power over the progression zone!

Power Tolerances on the Addition

(a) ±0.12 for a lens with a meridian of higher absolute power in the distance portion up to ±9.00 D.

(b) ±0.18 for a lens with a meridian of higher absolute power in the distance portion greater than ±9.00 D.

Cylinder axis tolerances are shown in Table 8(a) for single vision, bifocal, and trifocal lenses, and in Table 8(b) for progressive addition lenses.

Table 8(a) Cylinder axis tolerances for single vision, bifocal, and trifocal lenses

Cylindrical power (D)	Tolerance (degrees)
0.25 to 0.50	± 5
0.75 to 1.50	± 2½
over 1.50	± 1½

Table 8(b) Cylinder axis tolerances for progressive addition lenses

Cylindrical power (D)	Tolerance (degrees)
0.25	± 7
0.25 to 0.75	± 5
1.00 to 1.50	± 3
over 1.50	± 2

Tolerances on lens positioning and optical centration

Single vision, bifocals, and trifocals

After neutralising any prescribed or thinning prism, the tolerances on the position of the optical centre (or, for multifocal lenses, the distance optical centre) shall be:

(a) horizontally: the sum of 0.12^Δ and 1.0 mm
and (b) vertically: the sum of 0.12^Δ and 0.5 mm.

To calculate in millimetres the equivalent of a tolerance expressed in prism dioptres (D), use the equation

$$\text{tolerance (mm)} = \frac{\text{tolerance}(^\Delta) \times 10}{\text{lens power (D)}}$$

Progressive Addition Lenses

(a) horizontally: the sum of 0.12^Δ and 1.0 mm
and (b) vertically: the sum of 0.12^Δ and 0.75 mm.

Pairing of Tolerances on all Lenses

The tolerance on the total prismatic error between the two reference points of a pair of lenses, due to individual errors each within the tolerance specified above shall be:

1.0^Δ horizontally and 0.25^Δ vertically.

Note that the above requirements do not preclude the need to satisfy the individual tolerances.

Planos and plano-cylinders

Any prism in a plano lens or in the axis meridian of a plano-cylinder shall be of prism power not greater than 0.12^Δ.

Prism Base Setting Tolerances

Table 9 gives the tolerances on base setting directions in degrees.

Table 9(a) Prism base setting tolerances for single vision, bifocal, and trifocal lenses

Power ($^\Delta$)	Tolerance (degrees)
0.25 to 3.00	± 5
3.25 to 6.00	± 2½
over 6.00	± 1½

Table 9(b) Prism base setting tolerances for progressive addition lenses

Power ($^\Delta$)	Tolerance (degrees)
0.25 to 1.50	± 8
1.75 to 3.00	± 6
3.25 to 6.00	± 5
6.25 to 9.00	± 4
over 9.00	± 3

Prism Power Tolerances

Table 10 gives the tolerances on prism powers.

Table 10(a) Prism power tolerances for single vision, bifocal, and trifocal lenses	
Power ($^\Delta$)	Tolerance ($^\Delta$)
0.25 to 2.00	± 0.12
2.25 to 10.00	± 0.25
over 10.00	± 0.50

Note the additive tolerances for differential prism applied to lens pairs still applies:

1.0^Δ horizontally and 0.25^Δ vertically.

Table 10(b) Prism power tolerances for progressive addition lenses	
Power ($^\Delta$)	Tolerance ($^\Delta$)
0.25 to 1.50	± 0.12
1.75 to 6.00	± 0.25
6.25 to 9.00	± 0.37
over 9.00	± 0.50

Segment dimension and positioning tolerances

The segment diameters, heights, and geometrical insets shall not differ by more than ±0.5 mm each from the prescription values. The previous standard also stated that the segment heights should not differ by more than 0.5 mm.

Subjective Characteristics of Spectacle Lenses

Lens Pairs

The right and left lenses of a pair should be reasonably matched for shape, size, form, and weight and, except where necessary for matching purposes, should not be substantially thicker than is required for mechanical stability.

Material and Surface Qualities

In a 30 mm diameter central zone around the reference point the lens should not exhibit any defects (such as bubbles, inclusions, scratches, pits, marks or other defects deriving from fabrication) which could impair the vision.

Outside this zone, small isolated defects are acceptable.

Inspection of the lens should be by a dark/light boundary method and by the naked eye. Room illuminance should be about 200 lux. The principle of dark ground observation will be found in chapter 16, *Optics*, by Tunnacliffe and Hirst.

Glazing

Bevelled lenses:

The bevel should be smooth, regular, free from chips and starring, and reasonably free from facets. There should be a safety chamfer at the peak and at each edge where necessary.

When mounted, the lenses should not differ significantly from the strain shown in the unglazed lens. No gaps should be visible between the edge of the lens and the rim. The halves of joints should close without undue force and without leaving a noticeable gap.

Rimless and other lenses:

Flat-edged lenses should present a smooth finish with a neat safety chamfer at each edge. Holes for rimless fittings should be drilled at the correct distance from the edge according to the type of mounting. Slots and grooves should be accurately positioned. Brow bars should be adjusted to follow the edge of the lens. The ends of screws should be neatly finished.

All lenses should show no significant strain when viewed with a strain-tester.

Setting of round lenses

Except thermally toughened glass, the setting position should be indicated by permanent marks next to the joint and on the back surface:

(a) On the right lens, a single dot.
(b) On the left lens, two dots.

Listing of British Standards Publications

The British Standards Institution publishes a number of detailed standards dealing with spectacles. The following list will allow you to consult the literature when required.

BS 679 : 1989		Filters, cover lenses and backing lenses for use during welding and similar operations.
BS 1542 : 1982		Equipment for eye, face and neck protection against non-ionising radiation arising during welding and similar operations.
BS 2092 : 1987		Eye-protectors for general use.
BS 1727 : 1987		Sun glare eye protectors for general use.
BS EN 1836: 1997		Personal eye protection Sunglasses and sunglass filters for general use.
BS 2738 :		
1989	Part 1	Spectacle lenses. Specification for tolerances on optical properties of mounted spectacle lenses.
1989	Part 2	Spectacle lenses. Specification for tolerances on optical properties of uncut finished lenses.
1991	Part 3	Spectacle lenses. Specification for the presentation of prescriptions and prescription orders for ophthalmic lenses.
BS 3172 : 1987		Screw threads for spectacle frames.
BS 3199 : 1992		Measuring system for spectacle frames.
BS 3521 :		
1991	Part 1	Terms relating to ophthalmic optics and spectacle frames. Glossary of terms relating to ophthalmic lenses.
1991	Part 2	Terms relating to ophthalmic optics and spectacle frames. Glossary of terms relating to spectacle frames.
BS 5043 : 1973		Book holders, magnifiers and prismatic spectacles for use as reading aids in hospitals and the home.
BS 6625 :		
1985	Part 1	Spectacle frames (amended 1991 & 1992). Specification for general requirements.
1992	Part 2	Spectacle frames. Specification for marking.
BS 7017 : 1988		Reference wavelengths for optics and optical instruments.
BS 7028 : 1988		Selection, use and maintenance of eye-protection for industrial and other uses.
BS 7394 :		
1991	Part 1	Complete spectacles. Specification for ready-to-wear near-vision spectacles.
1994	Part 2	Complete spectacles. Specification for prescription spectacles.
BS 7522 :		
1992	Part 1	Low vision aids. Specification for hand and stand magnifiers, including magnifiers with an integral source of illumination.
1993	Part 2	Low vision aids. Specification for spectacle magnifiers and similar devices.

These standards are available from:
> The British Standards Institution
> 2 Park Street
> London W1A 2BS

They are also available in college and university libraries.

Dispensing Trifocal Lenses

Introduction

Trifocal lenses, or trifocals, derive their name from the fact that there are three distinct power zones within the lens aperture. Examples of trifocals can be seen in figure 1 below, where there are distance, intermediate and near power regions within the lens. Figure 2 shows a Double D segment where the segment powers are either both for near vision or the lower one for reading and the upper one for intermediate use. With the exception of a concentric round segment, with an 8 mm deep intermediate portion, a D835 trifocal in a mid-index plastic by Signet Armorlite, and Norville's Flat Top S1435, the selection shown in these figures is all that is available in the UK.

In the UK, it is the experience of practitioners that few trifocals are worn. Perhaps one reason for this was due to almost 40 years of National Health Service dispensing, from 1948 to 1986, where trifocals were not among the Health Service lenses available. Further, trifocal lenses are expensive and there was, in the past, undoubted reticence on the part of practitioners to consider these lenses. Now that modern design progressive addition lenses (PALs) are more easily accepted by patients, perhaps trifocals will for ever remain the little known entity they have always been. Nonetheless, a few people do wear trifocals and a practitioner will need to dispense them occasionally. It may seem surprising, but patients who wear trifocals do come back and request them again, so there must be some advantage over bifocals or PALs.

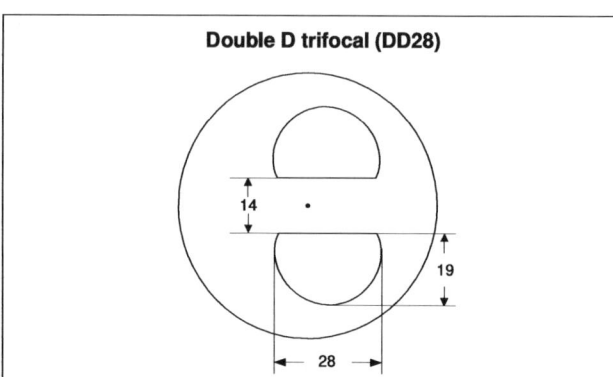

Fig. 2 Two D segments each with a near vision power or the upper one may have an intermediate Add.

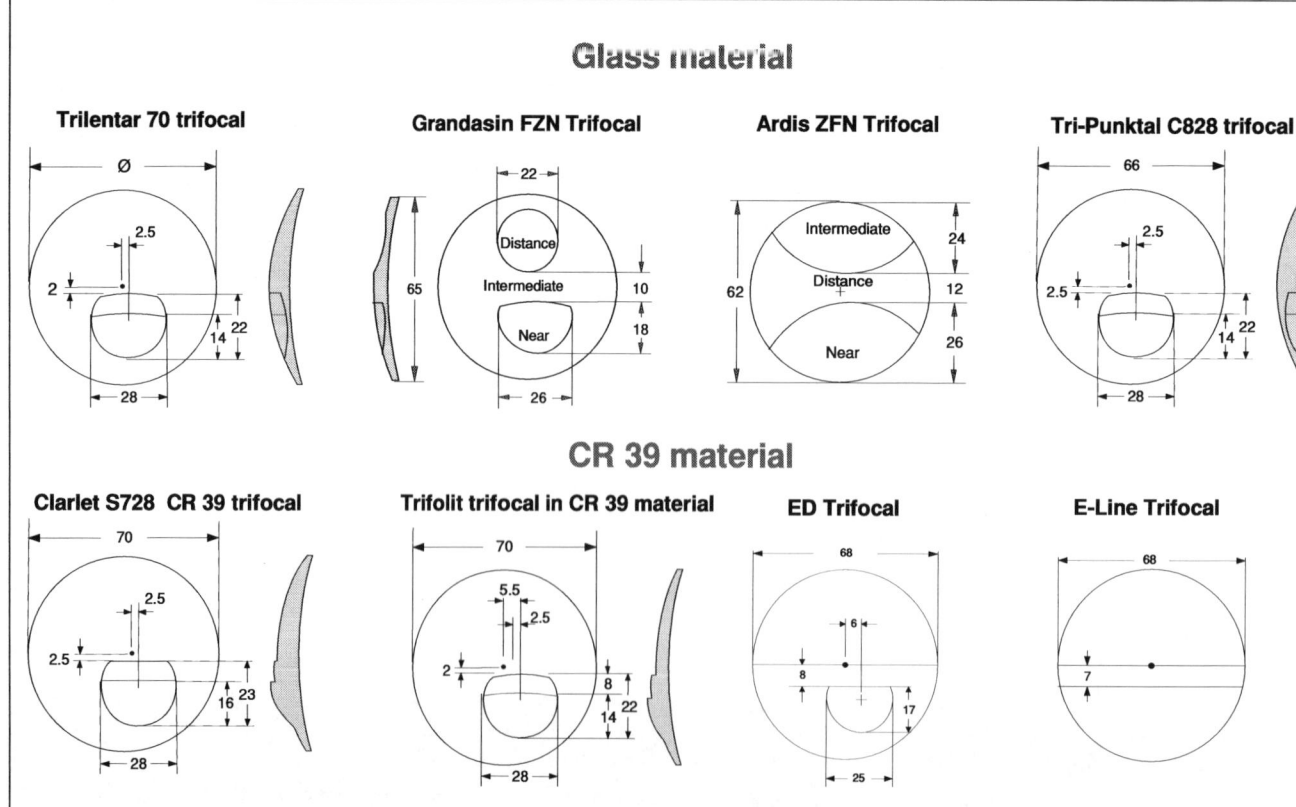

Fig. 1   Examples of trifocal lenses. Except for a round concentric segment trifocal and Signet Armorlite's D8×35 trifocal, Norville's Double D and Flat Top S1435, the above set of lenses covers the trifocals currently available in the UK. As from 2003, E style trifocals are no longer made but there may be stocks of blanks still available.

Ranges of clear vision through bifocals at ages 45 and 55 years

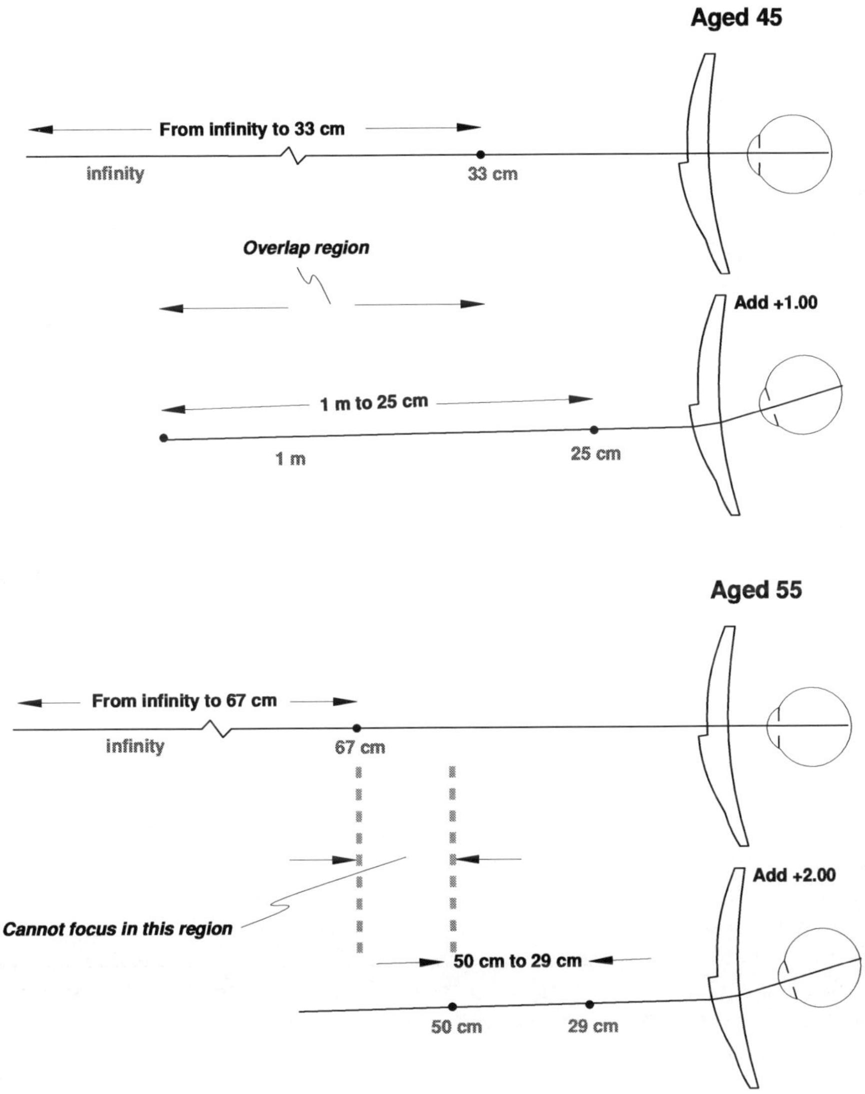

Aged 45

From infinity to 33 cm
infinity — 33 cm

Overlap region

1 m to 25 cm
1 m — 25 cm

Add +1.00

Aged 55

From infinity to 67 cm
infinity — 67 cm

Cannot focus in this region

50 cm to 29 cm
50 cm — 29 cm

Add +2.00

Fig. 3

In early presbyopia, 'aged 45' in the diagram, the ability to focus 3 dioptres through the top of a bifocal lens produces an artificial near point at 33 cm from the lens. The range of clear vision through the segment is from 1 m to 25 cm. There is therefore a region from 1 m to 33 cm where the patient can focus through either region and it is easily imagined that the patient can comfortably manage intermediate range visual tasks, even allowing for the fact that for the artificial near point calculations we are assuming full accommodation. If the patient were doing an intermediate distance task for lengthy periods, then bifocals may not be suitable, but only on the grounds that the segment might be too low.

In the lower part of the diagram, the patient is assumed to be 55 years of age and to possess only 1.5 dioptres of accommodation, measured by the push-up-to-blur method. We see that the patient cannot focus the range from 67 cm to 50 cm, even with full accommodation in the distance portion of a bifocal, and this is when an intermediate correction might be found necessary. In fact, this will occur before 55 years of age since the patient will not be able to comfortably apply full accommodation for more than a very short while. Hence, we find that an intermediate correction may become necessary at about 50 years of age.

Advantages of trifocals

❏ They present an intermediate focus for patients over 50 years of age who would otherwise have an intermediate range which could not be focused through bifocals.

❏ The intermediate zone is very much wider than that in PALs.

❏ They have a full width distance portion compared with PALs.

❏ They have a wide reading zone compared with PALs.

Disadvantages of trifocals

❏ The segment top is fitted about 3 to 4 mm above the lower limbus and this interferes with the distance field of view.

❏ The reading portion is about 2 mm lower than in a flat-top bifocal, thus making the patient depress the eyes further than in a bifocal when reading.

❏ Intermediate and reading zones have visible demarcations.

The need for an intermediate correction

In early presbyopia the patient has sufficient accommodation in reserve to be able to focus intermediate distances through the upper, distance portion of bifocals. However, over 50 years of age, and certainly by the age of 55, this is not possible, and the patient either tolerates the intermediate blur problem or seeks a solution. A typical complaint by the bifocal wearer in mid to late presbyopia is that looking in a shop window is difficult. These patients complain that they cannot get near enough to see though the segment and the vision between 50 cm and 100 cm is not clear through the distance portion. Figure 3 illustrates the problem experienced in the middle fifties[†]. The legend with this diagram also explains the problem in more detail.

[†] The range of clear vision through the distance and near portions of the bifocal, that is, between the artificial far and near points, is calculated by a standard method in visual optics.

General Purpose and Occupational Trifocals

Trifocals for general use have an intermediate portion with a 7 or 8 mm depth. The field of view depends on the power and diameter of the lens, the diameter here being considered is the depth of the intermediate portion on the lens. That is, we are considering the vertical linear extent of the patient's field of view through the intermediate portion of the lens. The field of view will also be greater when the lens is fitted closer to the eye. In any event, it is not possible to quote a single linear vertical extent of clear vision for the intermediate portion as a general case, but as a rough guide one would expect a 10-15 cm vertical extent of the field at about two-thirds of a metre distance[‡].

Occupational trifocals have a deeper intermediate portion. In figure 1, Rodenstock's *Grandasin* and *Ardis* trifocals have 10 and 12 mm deep intermediate portions, respectively. In occupational trifocals, this extra depth of intermediate portion severely restricts the usefulness of the distance portion to little more than occasional use in which the head must be tilted forwards to look straight ahead.

The Intermediate Add on Trifocals

Unless otherwise stated, the intermediate Add will be 50% of the near vision Add. This is certainly true of all the general purpose trifocals currently available in the UK, although Rodenstock's *Ardis ZFN* occupational trifocal comes with intermediate Adds in any power. Until recently, the US manufacturer Buckbee-Mears had an outlet in the UK for their trifocals with Adds 40%, 50%, 60%, and 70% of the near vision Add. In the USA there is a much larger trifocal lens wearing population, in that case probably reflecting the absence of a restricting health service on the range of lenses.

Fitting trifocals

General purpose trifocals are fitted with the centre of the intermediate portion at the level of the lower limbus, as shown in figure 4 for the right eye. These lenses have 7 or 8 mm deep intermediate zones so the lower margin of this zone will be 3½ or 4 mm respectively below the lower limbus. This placement of the intermediate segment is a consensus opinion based on experience. With what few trifocals the author has had occasion to dispense, this method has *always* proved satisfactory, so the consensus appears to be justified, at least in my experience.

In fitting the trifocal in this manner the reading portion will be up to 3½ or 4 mm lower than in a bifocal, assuming the bifocal segment top was placed at the lower limbus level. Of course, if previous bifocal lenses had been worn lower than this then the difference between the reading zone levels in bifocals and trifocals would be less noticeable. For example, if the patient had previously worn D28 bifocals fitted 2 mm below the lower limbus, then the top of the trifocal reading area would be only 1½ mm lower still. The patient should be warned of this slightly lower reading

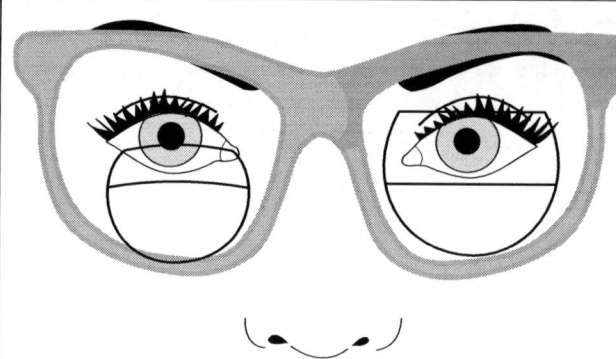

Fig. 4 In front of the right eye, the segment position with general purpose trifocals. The centre of the intermediate portion is placed at the level of the lower limbus, with the eye in the primary position of gaze as usual.

In front of the left eye is Norville's 35 mm diameter Dsegment occupational trifocal with a 14 mm deep intermediate portion. Note that lower margin of the intermediate zone has been placed at the same level as in the general purpose trifocal. This would be open to discussion with the patient, and probably subject to simulation by marking intermediate segments on the patient's existing glasses, certainly in a first-time wearer of this lens.

portion but, perhaps more importantly the patient must be advised that the intermediate portion encroaches well into what would have been a distance portion in bifocals. With a 7 mm deep intermediate portion, for example, some 3½ mm above the lower limbus is going to be occupied by the intermediate segment. As mentioned earlier, though, established trifocal wearers do not seem to be perturbed by this, obviously considering the intermediate focus gain worth the distance zone loss.

Occupational trifocals have a deeper intermediate zone, usually 10 to 14 mm, and can only be worn for specific visual needs. The exact positioning of the intermediate zone vis-à-vis the lower limbus is probably best achieved by having the patient present the practitioner with all the measurements of the distances to intermediate and reading targets which occur in their occupation, and the depths and widths of these fields. If in doubt, one might place the lower margin of the intermediate area about 4 mm below the lower limbus, as shown in figure 4 for the left eye. Although it will not be exact, the patient can obtain a good indication of the field of view by drawing segments on the patient's existing spectacles with a water-based felt-tip pen and asking the patient to look at some simulated work station object, such as a desk mirror, magazine, or card of the correct size and in the correct position.

The Smart Seg alternative

For general purposes, one should not forget Sola's Smart Seg which we have described as a progressive segment bifocal. In this case, the segment top is fitted 3 mm below the pupil centre, so the segment top is not quite as high as in general purpose trifocals. It could be fitted higher if the spectacles

[‡] Source: *Clinical Optics*, by Fannin, T.E. and Grosvenor, T. (1987), page 274.

were for purely occupational use. As already mentioned, the author found this lens optically very successful but abandoned it in favour of PALs only because the temple side of the 30 mm segment was noticeable.

Split trifocals for different prismatic effects

Franklin Split Trifocals can be a very versatile alternative to the single piece lenses discussed so far. They can be made using a bifocal lens combined with a single vision lens. Even three single vision lenses have been used; see figure 5. The distance, intermediate and near vision portions can have a fair degree of freedom in the design of their depths so that such trifocals are very much individually tailored to suit the patient's needs.

Different amounts of prism can be incorporated in the two component parts of the trifocal in figure 5(a) or in the three component parts of figure 5(b).

Occupational Progressive Addition Lens alternatives

For occupational trifocals one should always consider the newer occupational progressives. The *AO Technica* has a limited distance portion, and others such as the Gradal RD from Zeiss, Rodenstock's *Office* and Essilor's *Interview* have intermediate and reading zones as wide as in 28 mm segment trifocals. The Gradal RD is suitable for walking about indoors since the far point through the upper part of the lens is at 2 metres. Indeed, these lenses may well be the death knell of occupational trifocals, with the possible exception of those where an upper half lens segment is required.

In 2003, there were eight OPAL lenses available:

Technica	American Optical
Interview	Essilor
Continuum	Norville
Office Perfalit 1.5	Rodenstock
Access	Sola
Office	Taylor
Clarlet Business	Zeiss
Gradal RD	Zeiss

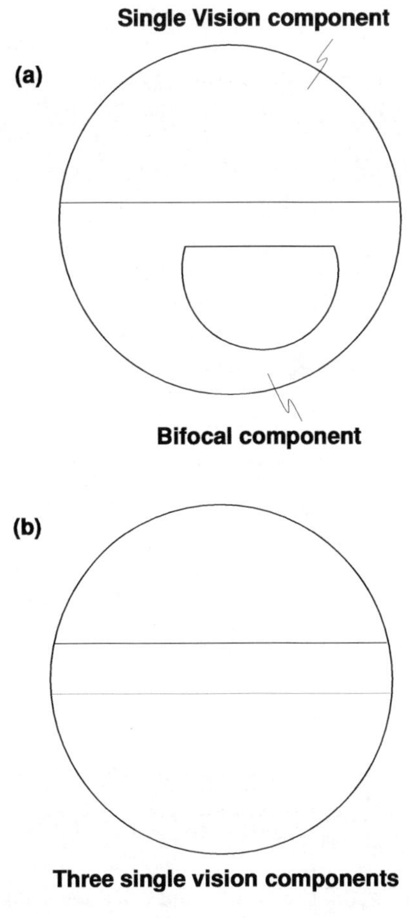

Fig. 5 Franklin split trifocals can be devised from either (a) single vision and bifocal lens components or (b) three single vision components.

The Principles of Spectacle Frame Fitting

Introduction

Fitting spectacle frames might seem to be an easy procedure which requires little or no training. After all, you just prop them on the face! This is, perhaps, the implicit analysis of those people who think little or no training is required to supply spectacles. The following brief analysis should convince the reader otherwise. Besides understanding the effects of correctly positioning spectacle lenses for the optimum performance, the dispenser should develop a skill at identifying the variations in those facial and head features which influence not only the fitting of a spectacle frame, but the very choice of frame in the first instance. Contrary to one's implicit assumption that right and left bodily features are symmetrical, a relatively large proportion of the population has one or more facial and/or head asymmetries. For a glazed spectacle frame to fit comfortably and remain in place, frame and facial features must match to a large degree. The analysis below is concerned with this aspect of frame choice and fitting.

We shall consider the following:
1 Forces retaining the frame in place on the head.
2 Matching the frame to the head.
3 Head and facial asymmetries.

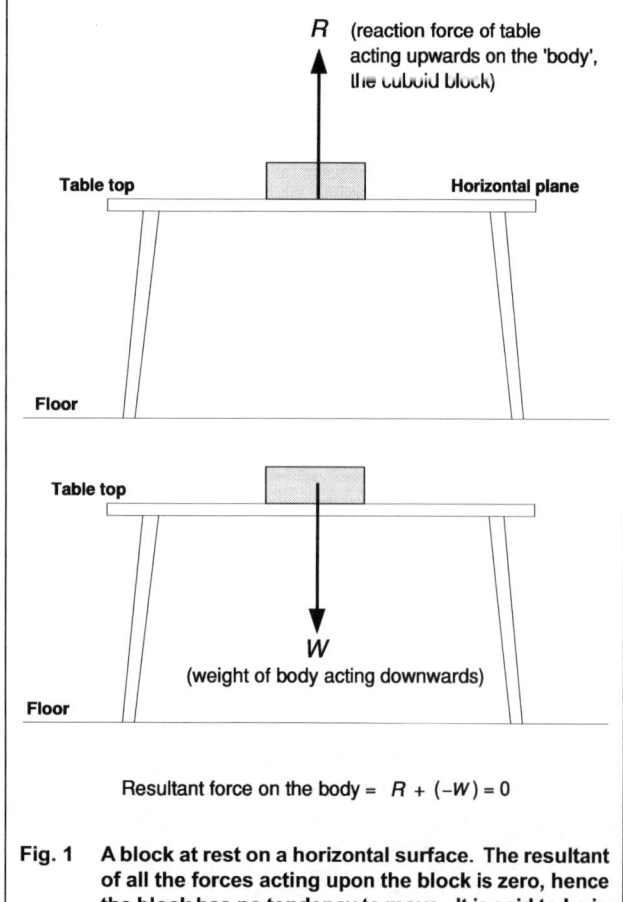

Resultant force on the body = $R + (-W) = 0$

Fig. 1 A block at rest on a horizontal surface. The resultant of all the forces acting upon the block is zero, hence the block has no tendency to move. It is said to be in static equilibrium.

1 The forces retaining the frame in place

We need to consider some elementary facts from the subject *statics*, a branch of a wider subject called *mechanics*. We need to look at the effect of the forces weight, friction, and reaction acting on the spectacle frame when it is being worn. To introduce the topic, we shall initially look at a simple system.

A body[†] in static equilibrium is acted upon by a number of forces which sum to zero. That is, for a body to be in static equilibrium, it must have a zero resultant force acting upon it. Consider a very simple case initially, a uniformly dense cuboid block at rest on the horizontal surface in figure 1. Why does it remain at rest? For a uniformly dense cuboid body, the weight (W) can be considered to act at its centre. This force (W) acting downwards on the body must be equal and opposite to the reaction force (R) of the table top pushing upwards on the body. In the equation in figure 1, the minus sign on W indicates its action is in the opposite direction to R. Hence, the resultant force is zero and the body is static.

Because forces have both magnitude and direction, they can be modelled by vectors, just like we model the addition of prisms to find the resultant prism. Hence, we can add them vectorially and when the resultant is zero the body on which these forces act will be in static equilibrium.

Consider figure 2 in which a cuboid body is in static equilibrium on a sloping surface. If the plane is imagined to be initially horizontal, the table top in figure 1 say, and then it is slowly tilted, a position will be reached where the

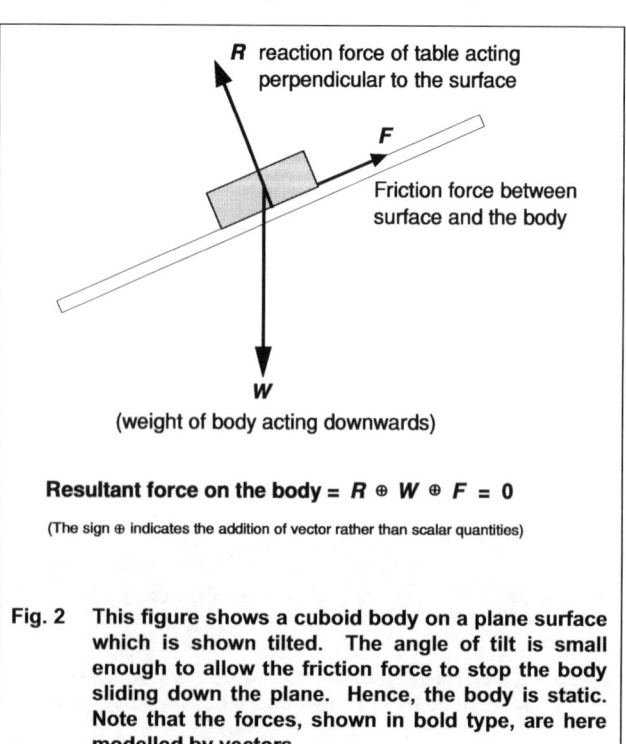

Resultant force on the body = $R \oplus W \oplus F = 0$

(The sign $\oplus$ indicates the addition of vector rather than scalar quantities)

Fig. 2 This figure shows a cuboid body on a plane surface which is shown tilted. The angle of tilt is small enough to allow the friction force to stop the body sliding down the plane. Hence, the body is static. Note that the forces, shown in bold type, are here modelled by vectors.

[†] The term body is used in mechanics to represent an object of a given mass. The weight of the body can be considered to act through a single point, its centre of gravity, which is at its geometrical centre for a body such as a cuboid with uniform density.

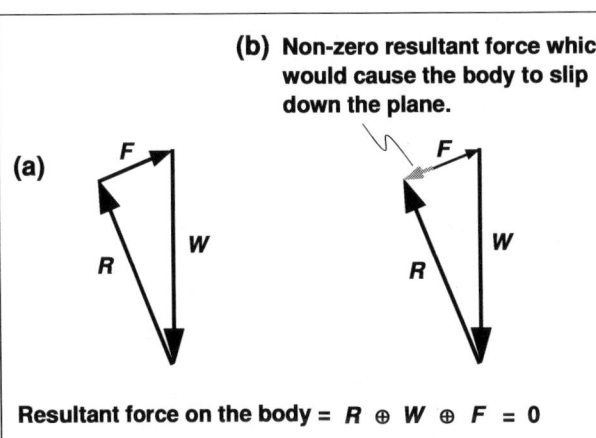

Fig. 3 (a) Vector addition of the three forces, R, W, and F acting on the body in figure 2. If the addition results in zero, then this is the same as if no external force were acting and the body remains static. That is, it does not slip down the slope.

(b) For comparison, if the friction force is too small in this example, then the component of W down the plane will be larger than F and there will be a non-zero resultant force acting down the plane. This non-zero resultant force will cause the body to slip.

body will begin to slide down the slope. However, before that situation is reached the body will remain static on the tilted plane. Under these circumstances, the three forces acting on the body add vectorially to zero, as illustrated in figure 3(a).

Using this information, we can qualitatively describe how a spectacle frame (and lenses) holds up on the head. A glazed spectacle frame is hardly a uniformly dense cuboid body, of course, but the aforementioned principles still apply. Because a pair of spectacles is not a regular solid, as a cuboid, and because its density is not uniform, most of the weight acts at the bridge, and therefore on the patient's nose. You can appreciate this latter fact from the simple experience below.

An Experience

Most of the weight of a pair of spectacles can be considered to act at the bearing surfaces of the bridge. To experience this, hold a glazed pair of spectacles as shown in figure 4 below. You should be able to feel a significantly greater part of the weight of the spectacles acting on your finger at the bridge.

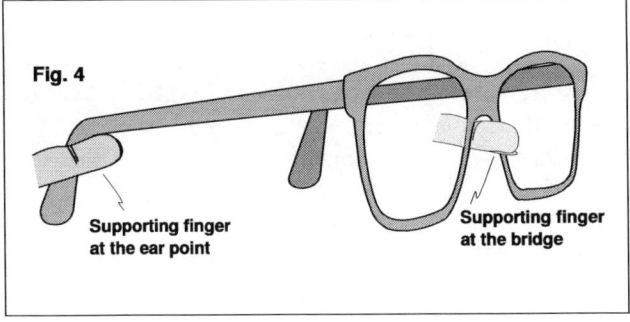

Because the majority of the weight acts upon the nose, there will be a relatively large reaction force from the nose pushing back on the bearing surfaces of the frame bridge. These bearing surfaces may be fixed or adjustable pads, or they may be the rim of the frame in the case of a saddle or regular bridge, or they may be the bearing surfaces of an insert bridge. In the case of a pad bridge there will a reaction force on each pad, and in the case of a regular bridge the resultant reaction force will be the sum of an indefinitely large number of normal (perpendicular) reaction forces acting all the way around the bearing surface of the bridge.

1.1 Pad bridges and the reaction forces

The forces considered in figure 2 were coplanar. In the case of the forces acting on a pad of a spectacle frame seated on the nose, because the nose has a splay angle it produces reaction and friction forces which cannot both be coplanar with that part of the weight acting through the pad. The reaction force R is perpendicular to the nose and can be resolved into three orthogonal components R_L, R_F, and R_U. The lateral and forwards components, see figure 5, are horizontal, and the upwards component is vertical. Only this latter one is involved in counter-balancing that part of the weight of the frame acting through the pad. (This will be a little under half the weight of the frame). There are similar components on the other pad at the other side of the nose. The two forward components (R_F), one from each pad, will tend to push the frame forwards and must be countered by backwards components established by the frame sides pressing against the head behind the ears. For simplicity, we can largely ignore the weight acting at the ear points of the sides, so the two upwards components (R_U), one on each pad, will be the main source of countering the force due to the weight of the frame.

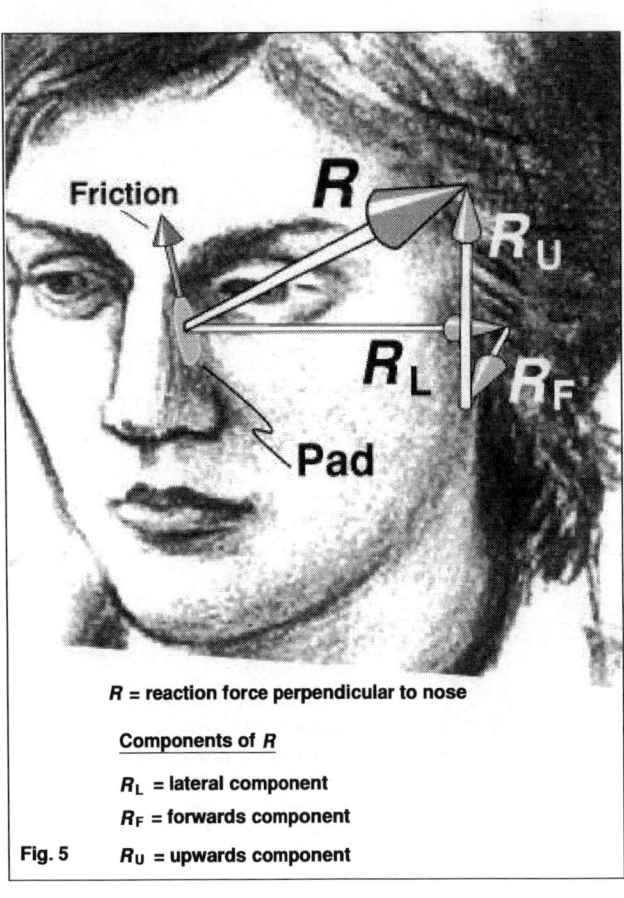

R = reaction force perpendicular to nose

Components of R

R_L = lateral component
R_F = forwards component
Fig. 5 R_U = upwards component

Principles of Spectacle Frame Fitting

There will be some friction force acting upwards on the two pads along the plane of the bearing surfaces of the nose. It is the skin which effectively pulls on the pads, and conversely, the pads pull on the skin. In those elderly patients whose skin is flaccid in this region, the friction force can pull on the skin to such an extent as to cause discomfort. This often unbearable discomfort can be avoided by fitting a regular bridge, figure 6, where the major upwards reaction is across the top of the bridge of the nose (the crest), a region of the nose where the skin is rarely flaccid.

1.2 The reaction forces behind the ears

The forward components of the reactions on the frame at each side of bridge would, in the absence of any counterbalancing force, cause the frame to slip forwards and drop down the nose. However, the frame should be fitted with a sufficiently small head width, about 10 mm narrower than the patient's head width, in order to introduce a reaction force behind each ear. In effect, the frame presses on the head and the head presses back equally, but in the opposite sense, on the frame. As shown in figure 7, it is this reaction force behind each ear which has a backwards component, and this counters the forwards component at each side of the nose. Only sufficient grip to establish this force should be applied to the frame. Any more grip and the pressure will cause pressure sores to develop behind the ears. This last point is very important: *apply only sufficient grip by the frame sides to prevent slipping.* If more than sufficient grip is applied to the sides, then the reaction forces behind the ears will have greater than necessary downwards and

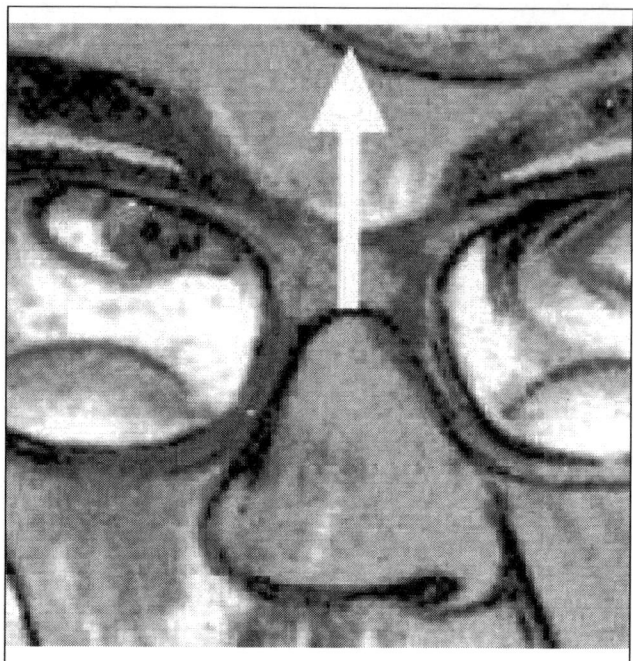

Fig. 6 In those elderly patients with flaccid skin at the sides of the nose, to avoid uncomfortable friction forces in this region it is advisable to fit a regular bridge. With a regular bridge there is a large upwards vertical component reaction which counters most of the weight of the frame. The crest of the nose does not tend to develop flaccid skin with age, and therefore this type of patient is more comfortable with a regular bridge compared with a pad bridge design.

backwards components which will cause increased upwards and forwards components at the bridge of the nose. That is, *overtight sides will also cause increased pressure at the nose.* Hence, when a patient complains of a sore nose caused by a newly fitted pair of spectacles, besides checking the bridge fitting for pad and/or rim alignment, one should also check the fitting of the sides.

1.3 Minimising pressure

Pressure is defined as force per unit area. That is,

$$pressure = \frac{force}{area}.$$

From this we can see that increasing the area of application for a given force will reduce the pressure. Therefore, in fitting spectacles we should attempt to *fit the bridge over as large a bearing surface on the nose as is practicable.* For this reason, a regular bridge, with its relatively large bearing surface, is generally more comfortable than a pad bridge.

Also, we see from the above expression, minimising the forces involved will reduce pressures on the nose and behind the ears. Thus, we prefer to keep the weight of the spectacles to a minimum and, as already mentioned, we must only apply the minimum necessary grip of the sides on the head. The effect of excessive pressure is to produce sore areas where the frame contacts the skin. One should especially *avoid pressure on the external ear* which does not possess cushioning adipose tissue beneath the skin.

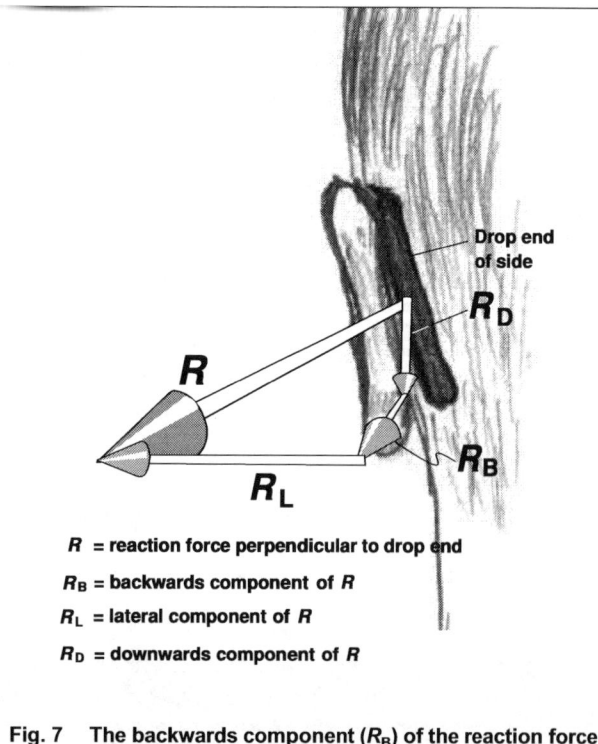

R = reaction force perpendicular to drop end
R_B = backwards component of R
R_L = lateral component of R
R_D = downwards component of R

Fig. 7 The backwards component (R_B) of the reaction force (R) is responsible for counterbalancing the forwards component at the nose, and thus preventing the frame slipping forwards. Just sufficient grip of the frame on the head should be applied to establish this force. R_D is usually relatively small.

Painful experience soon shows how a drop end pressing on the back of the outer ear will break through the skin with just a few hours wear of over-tight spectacle frame sides. Therefore, *the drop end must not contact the external ear at the back*. Rather, *it must follow the head shape down behind the ear, missing the outer ear by a millimetre or two, and gripping laterally on the head*. To maximise the contact area, the drop end should follow any bumps and hollows over the contact area. Such a fitting has been referred to as a *skull fitting*.

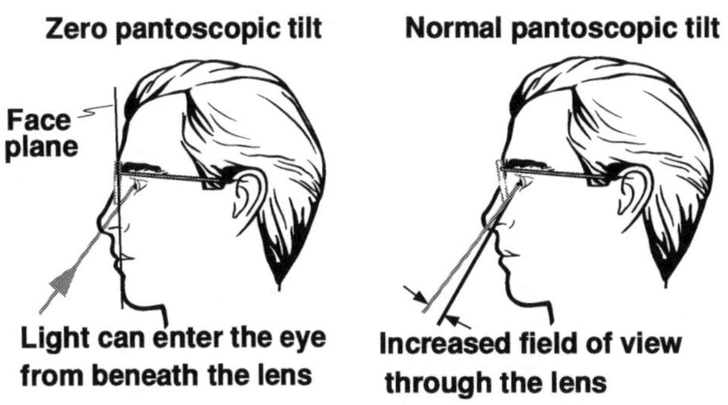

2 Matching the frame to the head

Choosing the fitting depends on several factors. Where lenses are very low powered (< 2.00 D), so that there are virtually no optical problems, then the patient is at liberty to choose the lens size from a purely cosmetic point of view. However, as the lens power increases, factors such as optical performance involving centration, pantoscopic tilt and vertex distance, all become increasingly important. Cumulative small errors can add to produce patient intolerance of new spectacles, so it behoves the dispenser to pay attention to each and every small detail. Hence, matching the frame to the head involves not only consideration of the face/head measurements, but also any over-riding prescription characteristics of the lenses. *The dispenser is there to advise the patient about frame choice and should veto choices which will not provide satisfactory fittings.* The following points should be considered at the very outset of frame choice:

(i) Interpupillary distance (PD). In the case of a patient with a small PD, large frames should be avoided to prevent excessive decentration and lens thickness; see figure 8 below. Over-large lens sizes also lead to larger frame frontal widths which make it difficult to adjust the frame to establish the necessary grip against the sides of the head behind the ears.

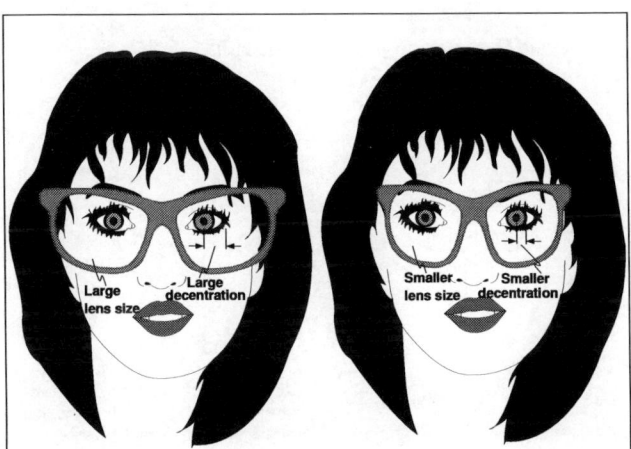

Fig. 8 Schematic illustration of how a large lens size produces the need for large decentration, which in turn produces thicker and heavier lenses.

Fig. 9 With zero pantoscopic tilt, one can see beneath the lens. With about 10° pantoscopic tilt the field of view through the lens is increased. Thus, steps are more easily seen through the lens when descending stairs, say.

(ii) Pantoscopic tilt and frontal angle: except in those cases where the pantoscopic tilt is wholly or partially determined by the lens type and fitting (lenticulars, high minus lenses, and aspheric bifocals), the frame is fitted with about a 10° pantoscopic tilt to provide the optimum field of view through the lens when looking downwards[‡]; see figure 9. You should note that the frontal angle of the nose is larger when measured in a plane where the face measuring rule is tilted 10° inwards towards the face at the bottom edge. Hence, when fitting a fixed pad or regular bridge frame, and matching the frame and face frontal angles, the frame front should be in the correct plane; that is, it should be seated on the nose with the correct pantoscopic tilt. Recall that the reason for matching face and frame frontal angles with fixed pad or regular bridge frames is to maximise the bearing surface area and therefore minimise the pressure on the nose. Of course, with adjustable pads the frontal and splay angles can be adjusted independently of the pantoscopic tilt.

(iii) Once the pantoscopic tilt is determined, then the frontal angle of the frame can be inspected with the frame in situ on the head. The intention is to match the frame frontal angle with the nose frontal angle in order to obtain the maximum possible bearing surface area. With fixed pad or regular bridges, too small a frontal angle will result in the lower rims resting on the lower part of the bridge of the nose, often where the nose consists mainly of cartilage rather than bone. See figure 10. At the same time, the frame splay angles should be inspected for a match with the facial splay angles. Unequal facial splay angles are quite common and you will need to learn how to adjust pad splay angles, not only in cases of right and left asymmetry, but also where the pad splay angles simply need to be altered to align with the nose. Again, the reason for this is to maximise the bearing surface area and minimise pressure on the nose. A pad with too little or too much splay will bear on one edge, thus causing a relatively large amount of pressure since the weight is acting on a relatively small area of the pad.

‡ *pan* = all, *scope* = view.

Principles of Spectacle Frame Fitting

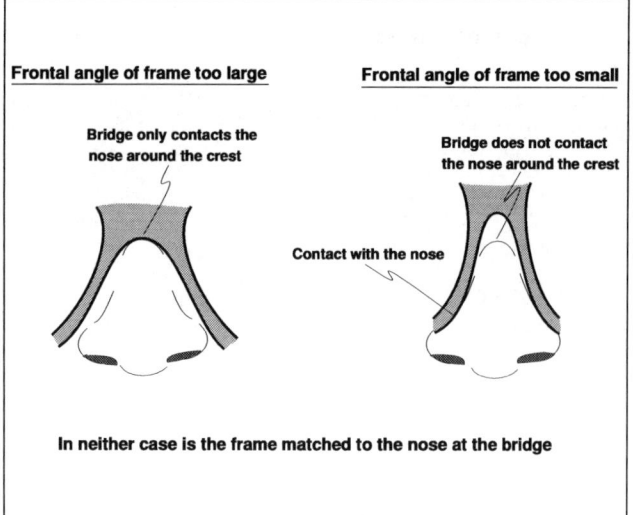

Fig. 10 Frontal angles too large and too small on fixed pad or regular bridge frames. In both cases, the bearing surface area is insufficient and pressure on the nose is therefore larger than where the frame frontal angle matches the nose frontal angle. In the case of unequal right and left facial frontal angles, adjustable pads are essential.

Remember: if during the frame selection the preceding criteria cannot be met with a frame being considered by the patient, it is the dispenser's duty to inform the patient that frame is unsuitable.

3 Head and facial asymmetries

One should always be vigilant for facial and head asymmetries between the right and left sides of the head and face. Some asymmetry is almost the rule rather than the exception. Fitting a symmetrically adjusted frame to an asymmetrical head will cause the frame front to tilt upwards at one temple if that ear is higher than the other, or project on one side if the head is wider at that side. One or both of these asymmetries may be present in any particular patient, together with frontal and splay angle asymmetries, and with eye and eyebrow height asymmetries.

3.1 Asymmetrical frontal and splay angles

We have already mentioned these, but it is worthwhile emphasising the fact that they are most easily dealt with by fitting a frame which has adjustable pads. Splay angles on fixed pad frames can be adjusted slightly, sometimes enough to solve an asymmetrical splay angle problem, but frontal angles cannot be differentially adjusted on a fixed pad frame without producing unequal lens shapes.

3.2 Head width considerations

With both symmetrical and asymmetrical heads, the sides should not touch the temples until they reach the ear points, otherwise there will be a forward acting reaction force on each side, tending to push the frame forwards; see figure 11. Hence the temple and head widths of the frame should be adjusted to provide the necessary grip but without touching the head in front of the ear points. Further description is given in the legend of figure 11.

Measured from the median plane (see *Introduction to Visual Optics*, page 311, figure 6.26), the right and left side contributions to the head width are not necessarily the same, as illustrated in figure 12 below. Fitting a frame with equal right and left side let-backs to such a head will cause the frame to fit with one lens further away from the face than the other. The remedy is to increase the let-back on the wider side of the head, possibly combined with a reduced let-back on the other side, until the front lies parallel to the face plane. In this context, you should note that if a frame with unequal let-backs is fitted to a patient with symmetrical head features, then the front will project forwards on the side needing an increased let-back. Of course, when setting up such a frame, one might increase one let-back and/or reduce the other.

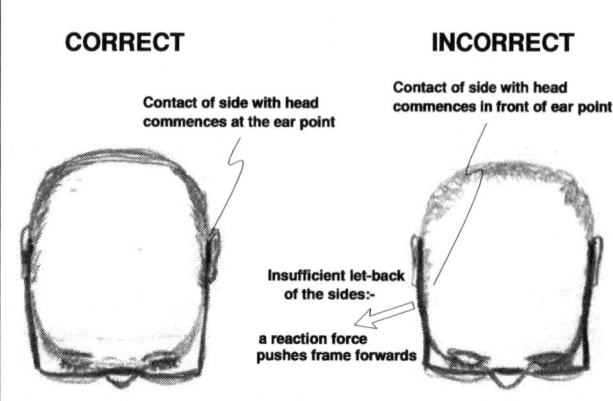

Fig. 11 The sides should not contact the head in front of the ear point. Otherwise, as shown on the right in the diagram, there will be a reaction force with a forwards component which tends to push the frame forwards. Patients complain that the 'spectacles slip down the nose', when in fact they are *pushing* forwards. The dispenser must recognise this incorrect fitting and remedy it by increasing the let-back of the sides, and shaping the sides to maintain the grip behind the ears.

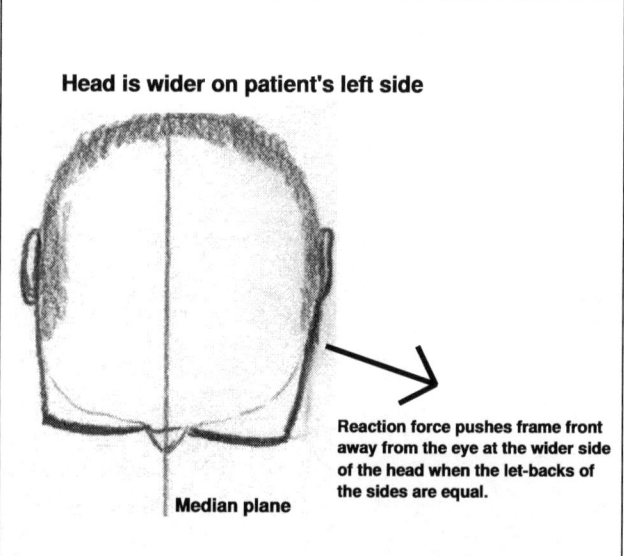

Fig. 12 The remedy in these cases of headwidth asymmetry is to increase the let-back on the wider side of the head, possibly also reducing it on the opposite side, too.

Principles of Spectacle Frame Fitting

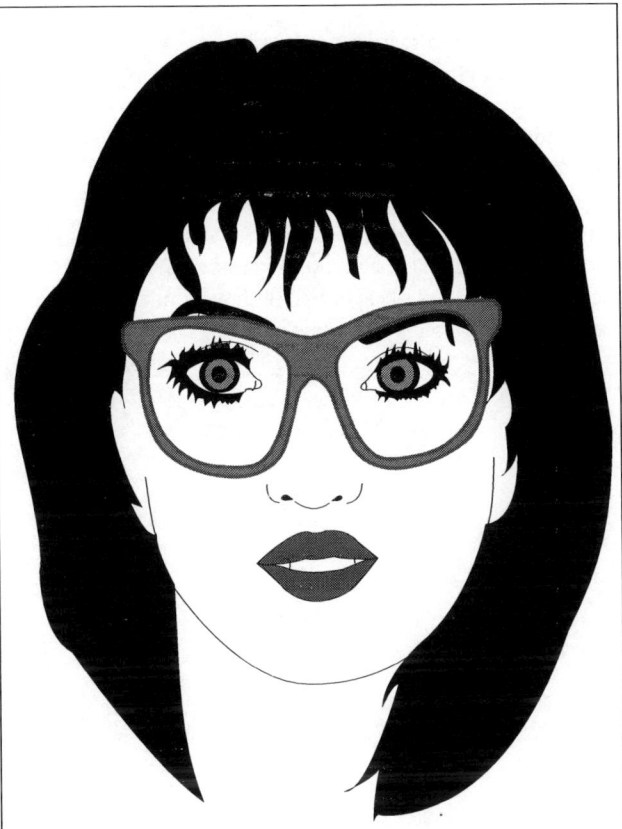

Fig. 13 Unequal ear point heights on the head will cause a frame with equal angles of side to tilt. The frame tilts upwards on the side of the head with the higher ear point. This angle of side needs reducing, or the other one needs increasing, or a little bit of both.

Conversely, a frame with unequal angles of side when placed on a subject with equal ear-point heights will also tilt, and the remedy here is to adjust the frame angles of side until they are equal and also produce the correct pantoscopic tilt.

In the case illustrated here, the frame tilts upwards on the patient's left, so the required adjustment is one of:

(i) Reduce the left angle of side to lower the left lens and raise the right lens.
(ii) Increase the right angle of side to raise the right lens and lower the left lens.
(iii) Apply some reduction to the left angle of side and some increase to the right angle of side.

In each case, the adjustment is correct when the front is 'level' and has the correct pantoscopic tilt.

3.3 Unequal ear heights

Some patients have unequal ear point heights. In such cases, a frame with equal angles of side will tilt when placed on the head; see figure 13. To level the front, the angle of side on the higher side needs reducing, or the other angle needs increasing, or a little of both, to produce a level front with the correct pantoscopic tilt.

Do not forget that the pantoscopic tilt is dependent on the angles of side, so when adjusting the latter do ensure that the pantoscopic tilt ends up correct.

3.4 Unequal lengths to bend

Another asymmetry, again not rare, occurs in patients with one ear further from the face plane than the other. Not surprisingly, this results in the need for unequal lengths to bend on the frame sides. Where the side is metal, with a plastic tip, it is often possible to lengthen or shorten one side. Where possible, shortening is achieved by removing the tip, cutting up to a maximum of 10 mm from the length of the metal side, and refitting the tip. Lengthening is achieved by drawing the tip off several millimetres and rebending the side to a longer length to bend.

Plastic sides with metal reinforcement can often be bent to a different length to bend, producing a shorter drop when the length to bend is increased and a longer drop for the converse procedure. Sometimes the longer drop can be shortened by cutting, filing, and polishing.

3.5 Hyper-brow and hyper-eye

We tend to assume implicitly that the two eyes are at the same level when the head is erect. This may not be the case, in which circumstance there is a vertical interpupillary distance (vertical PD). This should be taken into account by both the prescriber and the dispenser of spectacles, the right and left optical centres being placed at the correct positions for their respective pupil centres with the eyes in the primary position. A vertical PD is more likely to be overlooked with single vision lenses than with bifocals where, in the latter case, segment top positions should be measured separately for each eye. Different segment heights would make the dispenser look more closely for a vertical asymmetry. Similarly, with progressive addition lenses the fitting heights should be measured individually so that asymmetries are discovered when present.

Eye / eyebrow asymmetries

A further complication to the vertical setting of the optical centres of the spectacle lenses can arise when a line tangential to the eyebrows is not parallel to a line through the centres of the pupils; see figure 14. In these cases, practitioners and their patients have to decide how the spectacles are to be worn in relation to the eyes and eyebrows. If the spectacle frame is fitted so that its upper rims are equidistant from the pupil centres, and the examination was conducted with the trial frame or refractor head similarly aligned, then no special action is required from the dispenser except to confirm the position of the lenses during the examination. If, however, the frame is to be worn aligned with the eyebrows which are at different distances above the eyes, then vertical decentration will be required in one lens relative to the other. Occasionally, a patient may decide that the best cosmetic appearance is with the rim at one side between the eye and the brow when, at the other side, it lines up with the brow. Evidently, from the cosmetic point of view, each case must be dealt with according to the wishes of the patient.

Close cooperation is necessary between prescriber and dispenser, especially where a spectacle frame is to be fitted

Principles of Spectacle Frame Fitting

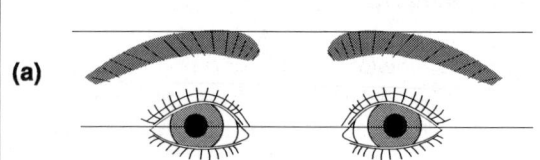
(a) The norm — eyes and brows level.

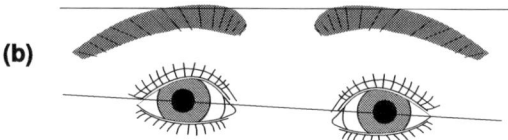
(b) Hyper eye – right eye higher than left – brows level. Make a vertical PD allowance.

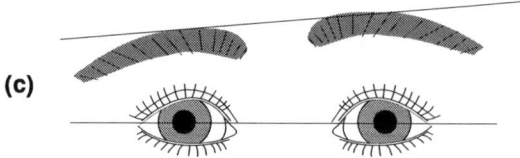
(c) Hyper brow – left brow higher than right. If frame is fitted level with eyes, no vertical centration adjustment required.

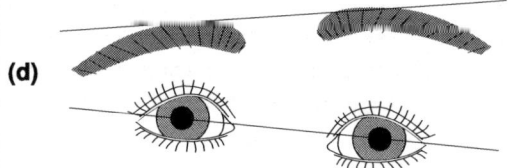
(d) Hyper RE and hyper left brow. Choose agreeable orientation of frame front, and apply vertical centration adjustment.

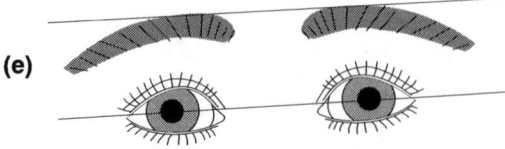
(e) Hyper LE and left brow. Frame probably fitted parallel to brows but this means it is tilted. Will need to check for possible cylinder axis adjustment.

Fig. 14 Vertical centration adjustment (positioning of the optical centres of the lenses) is necessary when the horizontal centre line in a spectacle frame is not parallel to the line through the centre of the pupils. If the frame slopes, and this differs from the trial frame orientation, an adjustment of cylinder axes will be needed.

with a tilt. If the test were not conducted with the same tilt, and the cylinder powers are significant, an adjustment to both cylinder axes will be required. The necessity for a cylinder axis adjustment can be based on cylinder axis tolerances (see page 155 in *Introduction to Visual Optics*, or page 83 of this text). Although these are engineering tolerances they may be used as a physiological tolerance. Thus, a 3° frame tilt with 0.50 D cylinders would be within the 5° tolerance, but the same tilt with a cylinder over 1.50 D would be well outside tolerance.

Dispensing Tints

Introduction

Tints are dealt with mathematically in textbooks on optics and ophthalmic lenses. Here the intention is to avoid mathematical explanations but, nonetheless, to define terms where necessary. Tints are prescribed for cosmetic purposes, for removing unwanted radiation and to modify the incident radiation at the eye. The prescribing of tints is not entirely divorced from the dispensing of tints. Except where an optometrist or and ophthalmologist prescribes a particular tint, say for dyslexia or a medical condition, the optician will often have to advise the patient on tint suitability.

1 Terminology

Tints and filters

It is necessary for the dispenser to be familiar with a range of terms used to describe the properties of tints. First of all, what is a tinted lens? The term **tint** in a general dictionary means a shade of a colour, usually a pale shade of a colour. From the point of view of spectacle lenses a *tint means a lens which appears coloured in transmitted light*. Generally this means that the lens should be viewed in white light and for observation of transmitted light a white surface should be viewed through the lens. If the lens is untinted the surface will appear white when viewed through the lens and this leads to an untinted lens being referred to as *white*, a term which is commonly used in the industry to describe untinted glass or plastics.

Tinted lenses appear coloured when they largely absorb a particular band of wavelengths in the visible spectrum which extends from about 390 nm to 760 nm[†]; see figure 1 below. *Filter*, a term which will be met from time to time in manufacturers' literature, is a device that changes the intensity and possibly the relative intensities of radiation in different parts of the spectrum before it reaches the eye. A tint is always a filter, though the reverse is not necessarily true.[‡] *Attenuation*, meaning weakening, is the term given to the reduction of light intensity caused by absorption of some of the light by the filter; see figure 2. This attenuation

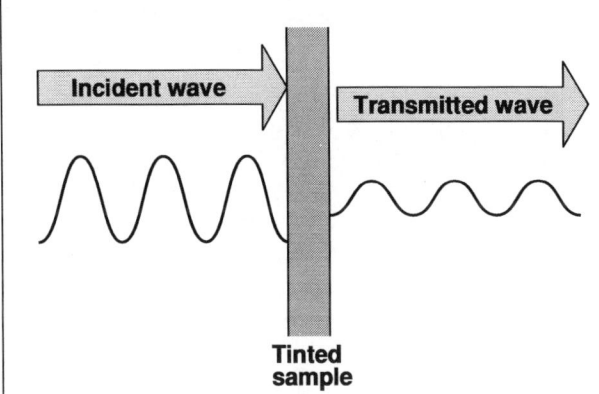

Fig. 2 The tint reduces the amplitude, and therefore the intensity of the wave which emerges from the lens. Some light (energy) is said to be absorbed and the emergent (transmitted) wave is attenuated (weakened) compared with the incident wave.

tends to apply to all wavelengths, usually to varying degrees although some filters have a band of wavelengths where much or sometimes all of the energy is absorbed.

Reflectance, transmittance and absorptance

The energy associated with the incident light at a tinted lens undergoes losses due to reflection at the surfaces and absorption within the tinted material. The tinted material may be throughout the mass of the lens, when it is referred to as a *solid tint* or infrequently as a *mass tint*, or it may be in a layer deposited on or diffused into the lens material near the surface when, not unreasonably, it is referred to as a *surface tint*. The fraction of the incident light intensity which is reflected is called the *reflectance*, that fraction which is absorbed is called the *absorptance*, and the remaining fraction which is transmitted through the lens to emerge from the second surface is called the *transmittance*. If the transmittance refers to a single wavelength, then it is called the *spectral transmittance*, whereas if it refers to the whole of the spectrum being considered it is called the *total*

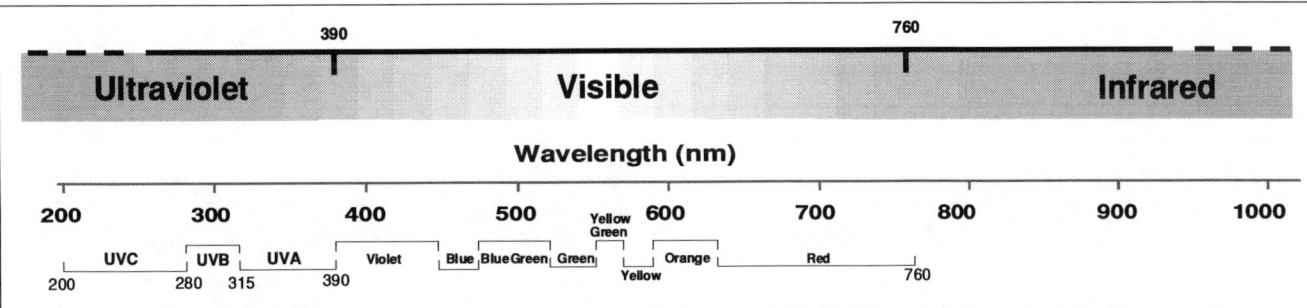

Fig. 1 The electromagnetic spectrum of concern to opticians. This is the range of wavelengths usually shown by manufacturers of tinted ophthalmic lenses. Ultraviolet radiation has shorter wavelengths than visible light and has been implicated in the formation of age related cataract, over a very long period, and in large exposures will cause inflammation of the conjunctiva and corneal damage. Infrared radiation, with wavelengths longer than those of visible light, produces a sensation of heat and can in very high exposures cause burns of the retina. *Note particularly the UVA and UVB ranges*[*].

[†] The limits of the visible spectrum are variously quoted as 380 to 400 nm at the short wavelength end and 740 to 780 nm at the long wavelength end.
[‡] If a lens absorbs only in the ultraviolet region it will not appear coloured and therefore is not a tint. However, most filters affect the visible region and produce a tint.

[*] UV and IR are abbreviations for ultraviolet and infrared (radiation).

Dispensing Tints

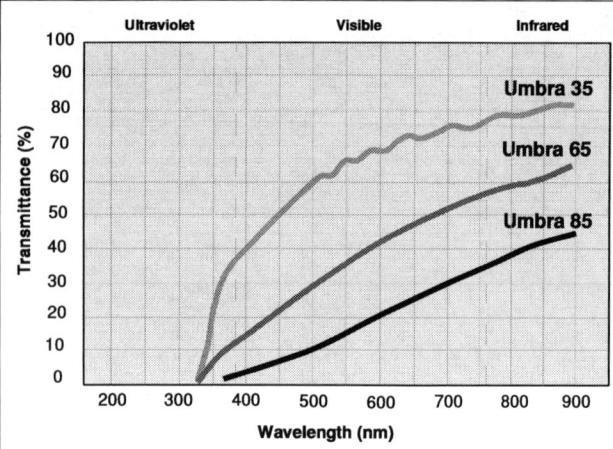

Fig. 3 Transmittance curves for three shades of Zeiss' Umbra tint. The fraction of the incident energy which is transmitted, after accounting for reflectance and absorptance, for all the wavelengths being considered is called the total transmittance and in these tints would be 65, 35 and 15% from the top curve downwards. Unless otherwise stated, *total transmittance* applies to the visible spectrum although the term can be applied to the ultraviolet and infrared regions individually. In the visible spectrum the fraction of the total incident energy which is absorbed is called the *total absorptance*. For the three tints here these would be 35, 65 and 85% from the top curve downwards indicating that the numbers applied to the tint names represent absorptances. The German firms Zeiss and Rodenstock both quote absorptances rather than transmittances, which may be sensible when we consider the filtering properties of tints.

transmittance. Unless otherwise stated, when the term total transmittance is used it refers to the visible spectrum, although it can refer to the ultraviolet and infrared regions too. A plot of the spectral transmittances for a range of wavelengths, usually although not always from about 280 nm to 800 nm, is called a *transmittance curve*, although it is often also referred to less rigorously as a transmission curve. Figure 3 shows some examples. The *total transmittance*, referring to the visible spectrum and sometimes symbolised by T_V, can be appreciated from figure 4. Suppose, for example, we represent the incident light intensity in the visible region by 100 arbitrary units, and only 25 units of this are transmitted, then the total transmittance is 25% and the total absorptance is 75%, including any losses due to reflection.

Luminous transmittance

This is often abbreviated to LT and is again a fraction but this time it involves the eye's brightness response to visible light of different wavelengths. The method of determining Luminous Transmittance will be found in ophthalmic lens text-books, but the definition is

$$LT = \frac{luminous\ flux\ transmitted\ by\ the\ lens}{luminous\ flux\ incident\ on\ the\ lens}$$

where the word luminous implies the visible spectrum is the domain for the wavelengths and the word flux means flow, referring to the rate at which light energy passes through unit area of the lens. Tints are categorised as shown in Table 1.

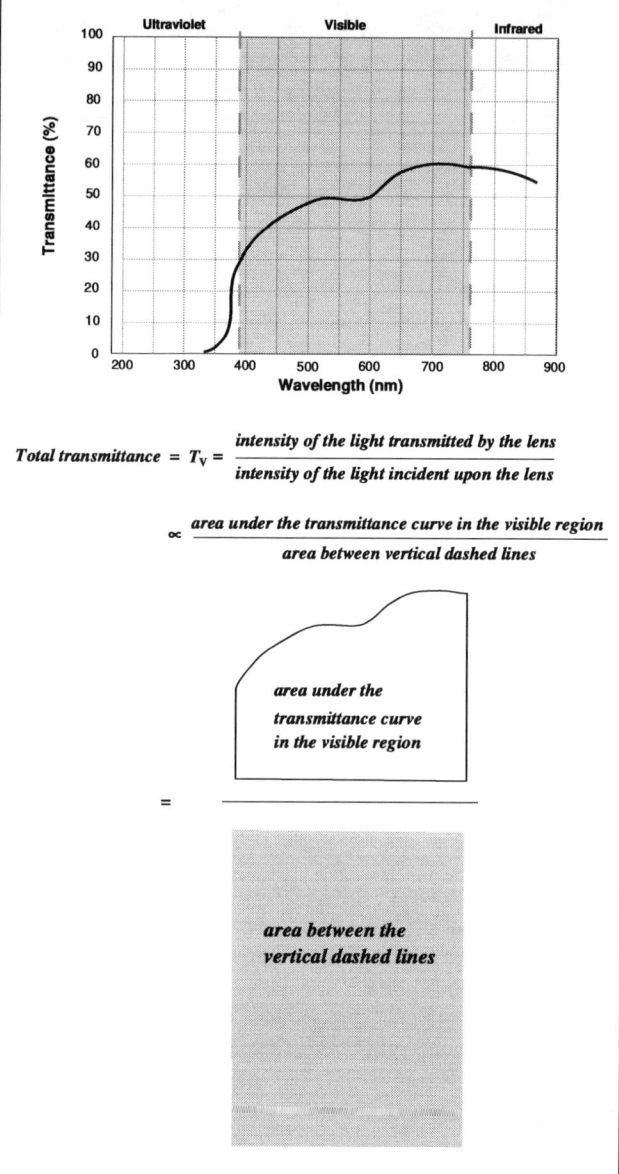

Fig. 4 A 'pictorial' representation of the meaning of total transmittance. The upper part of the figure shows a transmittance curve, the visible spectrum being between the vertical dashed lines. The intensity of the unfiltered incident visible light is proportional to the grey area whereas the intensity of the visible light transmitted through the tinted lens is proportional to the area under the curve between the limits of the visible spectrum.

Table 1 Tint categories in BS EN 1836 : 1997

Category	Luminous Transmittance (%)
0	100 to greater than 80
1	80 to greater than 43
2	43 to greater than 18
3	18 to greater than 8
4	8 to greater than 3

A high Luminous Transmittance, say 80%, indicates that a white surface will look light coloured through the tint, whilst conversely a small LT value such as 20% indicates that the surface will appear relatively dark. This darkening indication works well except for those tints which act as contrast filters[*]. So, for ordinary tints, that is non-contrast filters, if a green tint has an LT of say 40% it will generally make the environment appear as dark as say a brown tint with the same LT. Of course, a white surface would appear differently coloured through the two tints, but it would appear about as dark. This is useful when dispensing tints of different colours. As a rough guide, Table 2 indicates how the LT may be used to help select the darkness of a tint.

Table 2 Rough guide to use of Luminous Transmittance

LT	Use of tint
80% and over	Cosmetic
80% to > 43%	Comfort tints
43% to > 18%	Sunglasses for use in UK
18% to > 8%	Sunglasses for use in subtropics
8% to > 3%	Sunglasses for use on snow, sand, sea or for mountaineering

Such a guide is certainly rough, one exception immediately demonstrating this; people often wear tinted spectacle lenses as a fashion accessory – *fashion tints* – which may be any colour or combination of colours (rainbow tints, for example) and any total transmittance resulting can vary from light through to very dark lenses. Front surface highly reflecting two layer interference film[†] mirror coatings are available in silver, gold and blue colours on glass or plastics and although these are essentially sunglass tints they are sometimes worn just for fashion.

There is a case to be made for all spectacle lenses to be made ultraviolet (UV) absorbing so any tinted lens ought to satisfy this criterion, especially any lens which is to be worn as sunglasses. This is especially true for people exposed to sunlight reflected from snow.

Manufacturers vary in the way they classify their tints, quoting one of transmittance or absorptance, and possibly Luminous Transmittance. Often, the terms transmission(%) or absorption(%) will be used instead of transmittance or absorptance. For example, Essilor have used *light transmission* to indicate *total transmittance* and, in common with some other companies, a letter grading system: see Table 3. These letter gradings, together with the pictorial weather conditions, are a very attractive way of understanding the use of tints for visual comfort purposes. Some manufacturers use a number grading, different from the new standard in Table 1, but whatever the system something similar to Essilor's tabular guide applies.

[*] Contrast filters such as yellow 'night driving' tints stimulate nerve cells in the retina/brain which normally have an opponent colour response. Absorbing one of the opponent colours allows the other to drive the cell at a higher than usual firing rate and this falsely signals to the brain that the environment is bright, even though the tint is absorbing a considerable proportion of the incident light.

[†] See Optics, Tunnacliffe and Hirst, page 386.

Table 3 Essilor's guide to tints

Weather conditions	Light transmission	Code
☁	100% to 80%	A
☀☁	79% to 58%	AB
	57% to 43%	B
☀	42% to 29%	
	28% to 17%	C
☀	16% to 9%	CD
☀ 〰 ⛰ 🚗	8% to 3%	D

Classification of tints by material and form

Tints may be subdivided into fixed and variable types: a fixed tint does not change its absorption properties over time, with the possible exception of some unwanted fading, whereas a variable tint is designed to change from light to dark and back again according to the prevailing UV and visible light intensities. Variable tints are customarily called **photochromic** filters, from the Greek *photos* = light and *chroma* = colour, recognizing their light activated colour change. **Fixed tints** can be either within and throughout the glass or plastics material, when they are referred to as **solid tints** or occasionally mass tints, or they can be applied to the surface of glass as a coating or to the surface of plastics as a dye. In the latter case the dye material penetrates the surface as an evenly thick layer. Such **surface tints** have the advantage that they appear uniform (**equitint**) across the lens, unlike solid tints which vary in darkness with the thickness of the lens. Surface tints are by far the more common nowadays.

Photochromic glass is a solid tint and although most of the darkening occurs at and near the surface it will appear darker where the lens is thicker, but this does not seem to be a problem until the lens power exceeds about 6 dioptres. To produce an equitint in high power glass lenses some manufacturers bond a fixed or photochromic tint lamina to the white glass main lens; see figure 5. A more recent development, photochromic plastic can be either a solid tint or a surface dye. Probably the most common type is Transitions, a surface imbibed tint to a depth of about

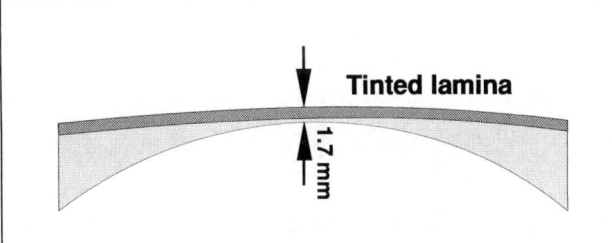

Fig. 5 A glass white lens with a tinted lamina. In the case of the Zeiss Tital Equitint lens, the lamina is 1.3 mm thick and can be a photochromic or a fixed tint.

Dispensing Tints

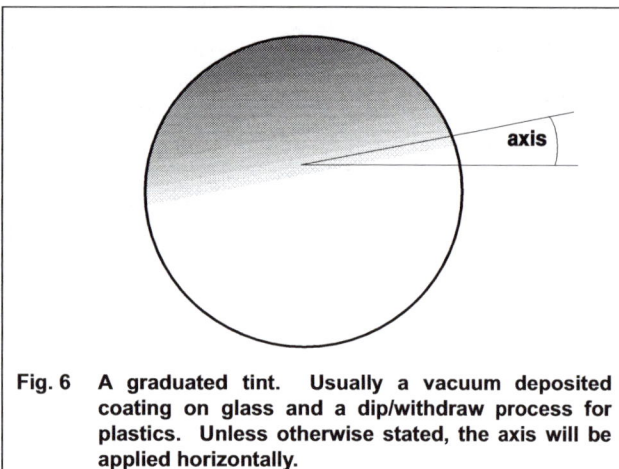

Fig. 6 A graduated tint. Usually a vacuum deposited coating on glass and a dip/withdraw process for plastics. Unless otherwise stated, the axis will be applied horizontally.

0.15 mm, although Hoya and Rodenstock both have a solid or mass photochromic plastic in their lens ranges. A further, not uncommonly used form of tint is the **graduated tint** or **gradutint**. Here the tint is applied to the lens surface in a density which gradually changes over the area of application; see figure 6 for the effect. In contradistinction to graduated tints, the more common application over the whole surface is called a **full tint**. Table 4 summarises this classification of tints.

Table 4	Summary of tint type classification
Fixed	Does not vary with exposure*
Photochromic tint	Varies with exposure
Full tint	Has uniform density over the lens
Graduated tint	Is fixed but varies over the lens

2 Properties of tinted lenses

The main physical properties of fixed, photochromic and graduated tints will be considered briefly from the dispensing point of view.

Transmittance properties

Perhaps the most important information the dispenser can have is spectral transmittance plots of all the tints he/she is likely to use. There are a number of questions one should ask oneself about a tint's transmittance curve:

- Where is the ultraviolet radiation cut-off?
- What is the total transmittance and/or Luminous Transmittance?
- What is the colour of the tint?

In addition, one would want to investigate the nature of any particular absorption characteristics in the visible spectrum and, though much less often, in the infrared region. This would be most advisable when the tints are specific such as dyslexia tints and perhaps tints for medical conditions.

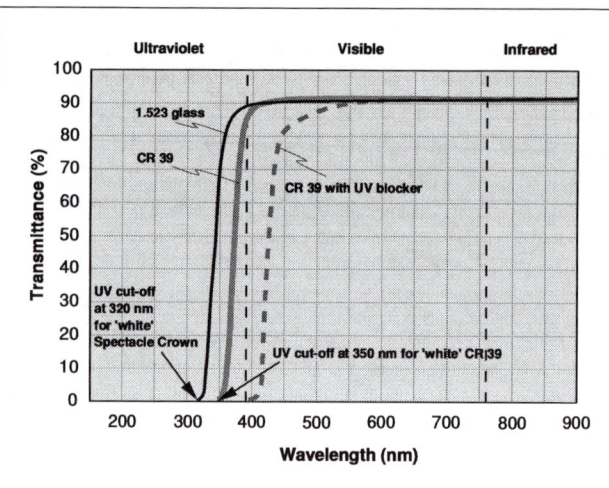

Fig. 7 UV cut-offs for white (untinted and uncoated) Spectacle Crown glass and CR 39 plastic; the reduction in transmittance in the visible region is due to some reflection at each surface. The dashed curve is a CR 39 lens treated with a UV blocker dye.

Where is the ultraviolet radiation cut-off?

The ultraviolet cut-off point is where the transmittance curve goes to zero; see figure 7. Note that white 1.523 Spectacle Crown has a UV cut-off at 320 nm and white CR 39 has its UV cut-off a little higher at about 350 nm. CR 39 can be treated with a UV filter (blocker, absorber, inhibitor) in the form of a dye so that all UV radiation is absorbed as shown by the dashed curve in figure 7. Mid- and high index plastics tend to have a UV cut-off at about 380 nm whilst white mid- and high index glasses have UV cut-offs between about 320 and 340 nm. The effect of antireflection coatings has little or no effect on the UV cut-off but does allow a little more UVA through, see figure 8, although it is not worth considering from the practical point of view.

UV cut-off and transmittance in photochromic lenses

The darkening of photochromic materials is somewhat dependent upon the ambient temperature, lenses darkening

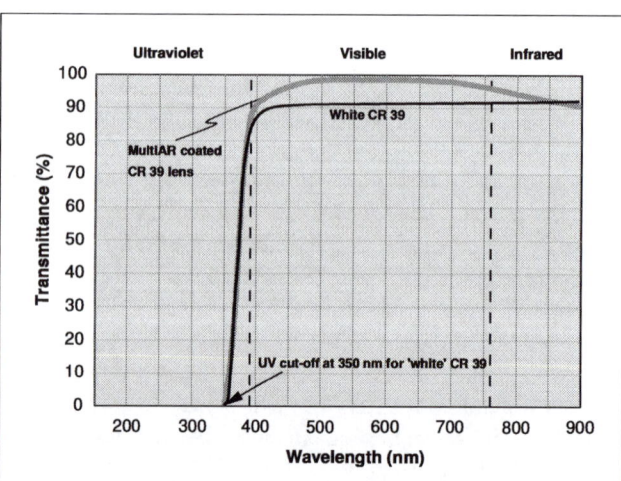

Fig. 8 Transmittance curves showing that antireflection coating makes only a little difference to the transmission in the UV region.

* Exposure (E) is defined by $E = I \Delta t$, where I is the intensity and Δt (read as delta-tee) is the exposure time: see Optics, by Tunnacliffe and Hirst, page 215.

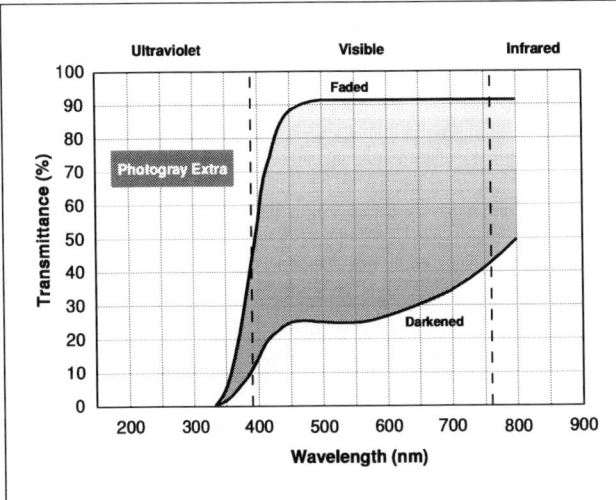

Fig. 9 Faded and darkened transmittance curves of Corning's *Photogray Extra* photochromic glass: solar simulator data with a 2 mm thick sample at 25°C.

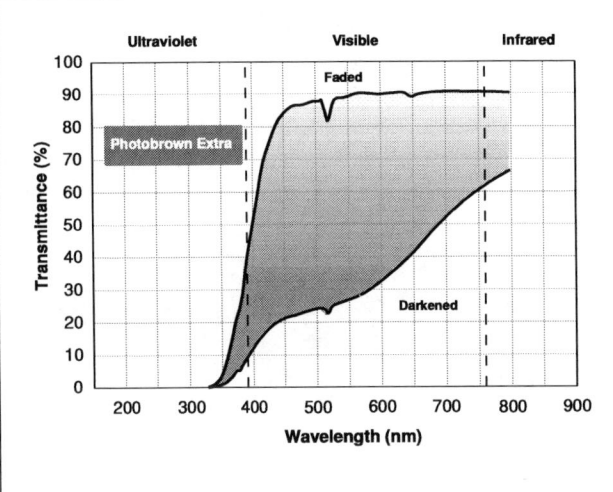

Fig. 10 Faded and darkened transmittance curves of Corning's *Photobrown Extra* photochromic glass solar simulator data with a 2 mm thick sample at 25°C.

less as the temperature increases. Most manufacturers quote the maximum darkening effect at 22 to 25°C although there is no agreed standard for the illuminant, Corning, for example, stating "Clear sunlight conditions, 25°C, 1 hour exposure/overnight faded." Figure 9 shows the transmittance curves for Corning's glass photochromic *Photogray Extra* in the faded and darkened states. Figure 10 shows the equivalent transmittance curves for *Photobrown Extra*. The UV cut-off is marginally though unremarkably higher when the photochromic glass is darker, but the UVA transmittance falls from about 8% in the faded state to about 2% in the darkened state. This degree of UV absorptance is adequate in sunglass use for most leisure and general pursuits and since the lenses darken more in cold conditions, they are suitable for skiers and mountaineers. Photobrown and Photogray Extra allow signal recognition and are therefore suitable for road users.*

The Luminous Transmittance (LT) ranges quoted at 25°C for these two glass photochromics, and for the more recent *Photogray Dark* and *Photobrown Plus* are:

	Luminous Transmittance	
	Faded	Darkened
Photobrown Extra	86%	24%
Photogray Extra	87%	22%
Photobrown Plus	84%	19%
Photogray Dark	86%	13%

The rates of change of darkening and fading for Photobrown Extra and Photogray Extra glasses are shown in figure 11 where the temperatures stated are intended to simulate outdoors (25°) darkening and indoors (20°C) fading. Both glasses begin darkening immediately on exposure to sunlight and very nearly reach their full darkness within 1 minute. They return to about 60% Luminous Transmittance in about 2 minutes under indoor lighting conditions.

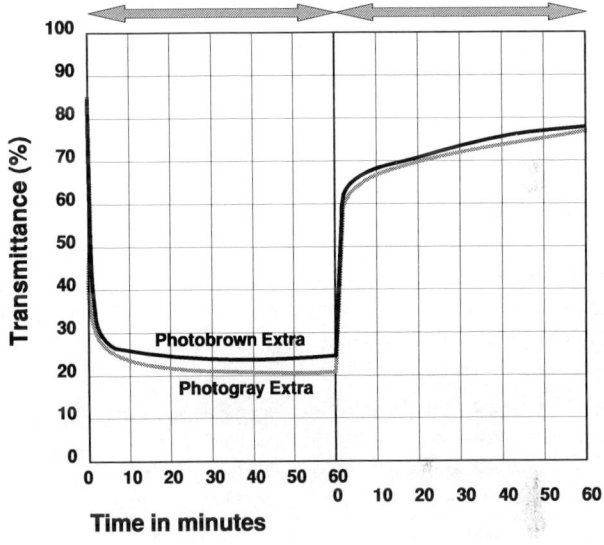

Fig. 11 Speed of the darkening and fading process for Corning's Photogray Extra and Photobrown Extra photochromic glasses.

The German firm Rodenstock has a range photochromic materials in both glass and plastic. The Luminous Transmittances (LT) quoted below are for the faded and darkened states

Photochromic glass:

    Photochromic Grey   (LT 75% to 15%).
    Photochromic Brown   (LT 70% to 15%).
    Colormatic 1.6 is brown   (LT 88% to 30%).

Photochromic plastic $n_e = 1.520$, $V_e = 51.6$, $SG = 1.22$:

    Colormatic Extra Brown   (LT 85% to 15%).
    Colormatic Extra Grey   (LT 85% to 15%).

Figure 12 shows (a) the Darkening/Fading rates (kinetics diagram), (b) the Excitation diagram showing the relative

---

* Corning produce a manual, *Optical Glasses*, which lists their white and photochromic glass properties in some considerable detail.

excitation for activating wavelengths in the UV and visible spectra and (c) the spectral transmittance curves in the fully faded and darkened states at 23°C ambient temperature for Rodenstock's photochromic plastic *Colormatic Brown* ($n_e = 1.520$, $V_e = 51.6$ and $SG = 1.22$) coated with Rodenstock's multiAR film *Solitaire*. The Excitation diagram, part (b) of Figure 12, shows that these plastic photochromics are activated mainly by ultraviolet radiation, a fact common to all glass and plastics versions.

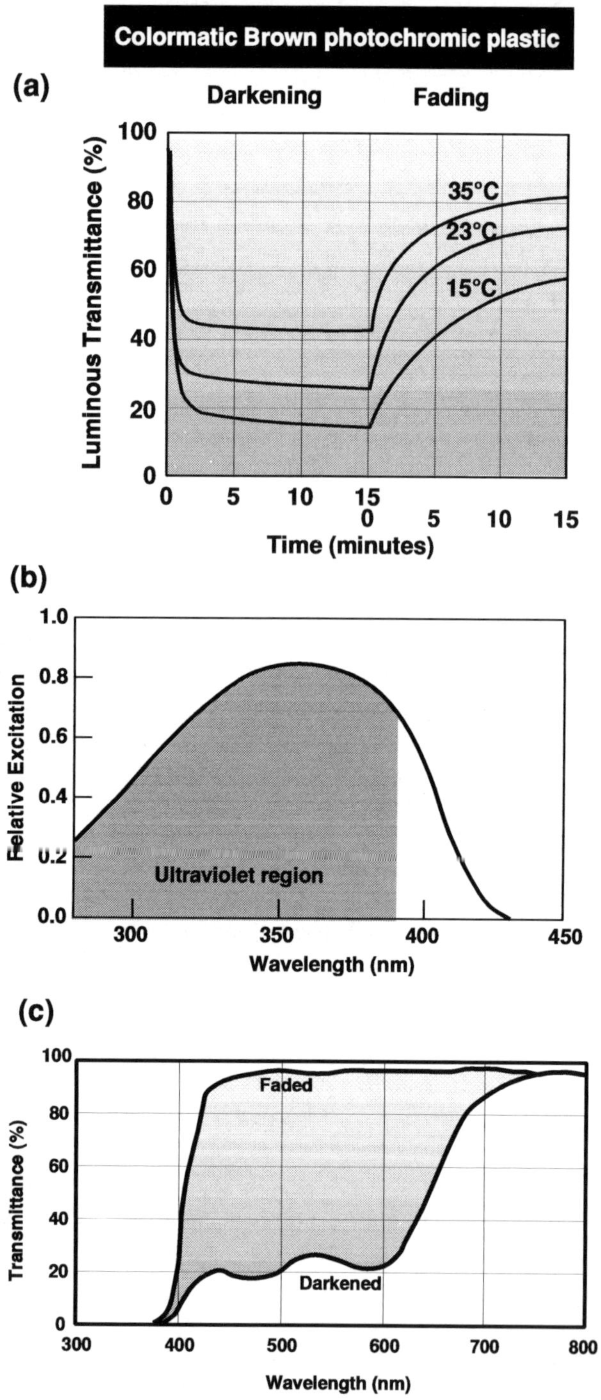

Besides 1.523 index, glass photochromic lenses come in 1.6 indices from Corning, Rodenstock and Zeiss. The absorption properties of the 1.6 index lenses are not dissimilar to their 1.523 relations. Corning's photochromic glass lenses can be ***thermally*** and ***chemically toughened***, Safety Eyewear Ltd offering chemical tempering in the UK. Norville offer their thin lens thermal tempering on Corning photochromic glasses for non-industrial use. However, one should be aware that thermally toughened photochromic glasses darken more in response to light and clear more slowly. Antireflection coating is routine but any UV absorbing coating, such as might occur with a pretinted photochromic lens, must be done on the back surface only, which would be true of vacuum coated tints on glass lenses anyhow.

Transitions, perhaps the best-known plastics photochromic material, has a Luminous Transmittance range 89% to about 16% at 23°C and is available in grey and brown tints. In both the faded and darkened states it absorbs 100% of UVA and UVB, the cut-off being at 390 nm. Because, as noted earlier, *Transitions* is a surface imbibed tint, its absorption is independent of lens thickness and it is therefore an equitint; see figure 13. A darker plastic photochromic material, *Transitions XTRActive*, has a Luminous Transmittance range of 75% when faded to 25% when darkened. Norville Optical Company have single vision, D28 and D35 bifocals, a trifocal and a progressive lens available with *Transitions XTRActive*.

Transitions[†] lenses, available in modified CR 39, Spectralite and mid-index plastics, come hardcoated and can be multi-AR coated with a hardcoat and hydrophobic coating. Some interesting practical facts about the lens are that it will not darken fully using a UV demonstration lamp and that the photochromic material 'fatigues' so that only a 3 year lifespan is guaranteed[*]. Fatiguing is caused by photo-oxidation of the photochromic molecules so that the material will not darken as much as when new. Single lens replacement may produce a tint match if the lenses are less than one year old, otherwise replace both lenses. The lenses should not be bleached or have a UV blocker applied. It is recommended that the lenses should not have additional tint applied although this is possible, brown and grey being recommended for the corresponding Transitions

Fig. 12 (a) Darkening/Fading kinetics of Rodenstock's *Colormatic Brown* photochromic plastic material.

(b) Excitation spectrum showing which wavelengths are responsible for the darkening process. The shaded area is in the ultraviolet region.

(c) Transmittance curves in the faded and darkened states at 23°C.

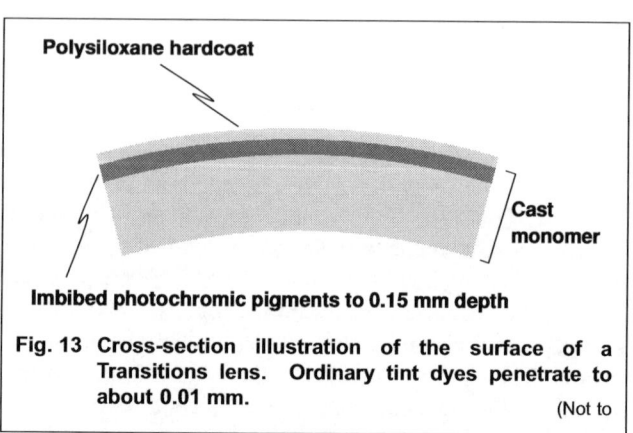

Fig. 13 Cross-section illustration of the surface of a Transitions lens. Ordinary tint dyes penetrate to about 0.01 mm.
(Not to

[†] In 2003, the latest Transitions material is referred to as Transitions Next Generation. The preceding version was Transitions III. All data here are for Next Generation.
[*] This is not a problem since people tend to change their spectacles within this time.

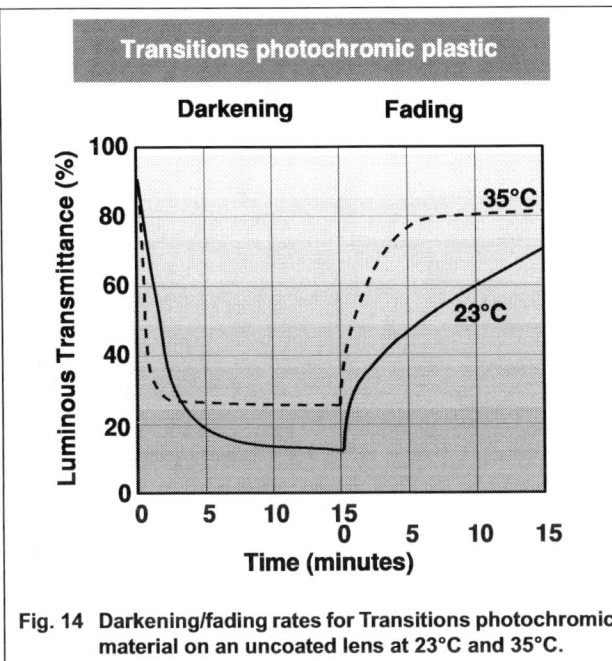

Fig. 14 Darkening/fading rates for Transitions photochromic material on an uncoated lens at 23°C and 35°C.

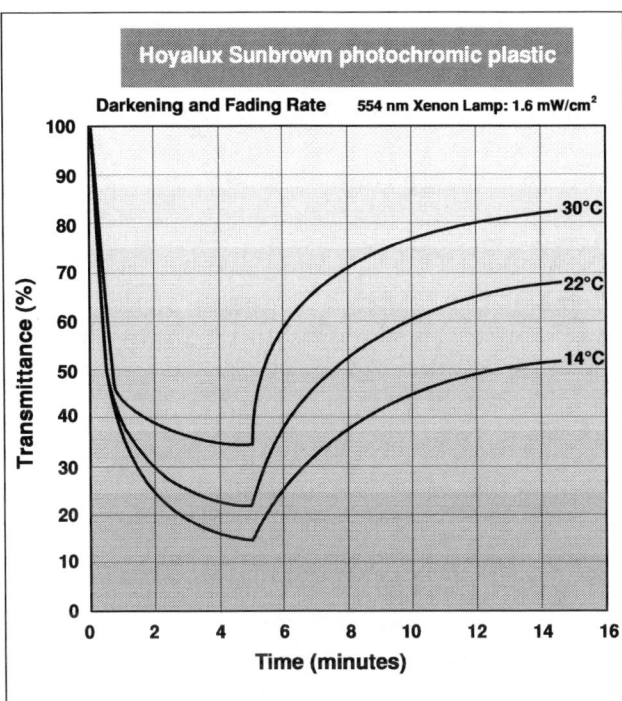

Fig. 15 The rates of darkening and fading for Hoya's Sunbrown photochromic plastic: $n_e = 1.50$, $V_e = 55$ and $SG = 1.19$. This sample was AR coated.

tint. Transitions Optical suggest some experimentation will be necessary to obtain the correct colour! It might be better to use the *XTRActive* version if a darker tint were required in the faded state, although this will not clear when fully faded having an LT of 75% then.

Antireflection (AR) coatings on Transitions lenses reduce the darkening capacity a little. At 23°C, uncoated lenses have a transmittance range 89% indoors to 16% outdoors. With multi-AR coating this may be 94%* to 20%. All photochromics are temperature sensitive and Transitions is no exception. The lenses are activated by ultraviolet radiation and so darken outdoors in sunlight but not indoors in artificial lighting. The Luminous Transmittances at two ambient temperatures are shown in the kinetics diagram of figure 14.

Hoya's photochromic plastic, **Hoyalux Sunbrown**, is a solid tint which is mainly activated at and near the surface so producing an equitint when darkened. Darkening and fading are temperature dependent and are quoted as 15% transmittance at low temperatures and 85% transmittance at high temperatures, respectively. The plotted rates are shown in Figure 15. For the plot at 22°C, *Sunbrown* appears to darken and fade at almost exactly the same rate as *Transitions* (at 23°C), although Transitions has the wider range, being slightly clearer when faded and slightly darker when fully exposed.

Photochromic lenses and driving

All photochromic lenses, whether glass or plastic, darken outdoors in sunshine to about 60% of their full darkness in approximately 1 minute. However, since photochromic lenses are activated mainly by UVA radiation *they do not darken too well inside a motor vehicle* because UV radiation is partially absorbed by the windscreen glass. This is true of both glass and plastics varieties and because patients may complain of this it is best to advise them about it. If photochromics are worn on a regular basis it may be worth considering the use of a clip-on fixed tint over the regular photochromic lenses when driving. Clip-ons may consist of either polarised (see the next paragraph) or non-polarised lenses. For driving, glass photochromics, pretinted on the back surface with a brown or grey tint of 30% absorptance may be a viable alternative, or *Transitions XTRActive*, which are darker to begin with, might be a suitable choice.

Polarising lenses

Plano sunglass and prescription polarising plastic lenses are available. These lenses have the special property that they absorb light reflected from surfaces when the 'absorption axis' is parallel to the surface. In the case of sunglasses, the absorption axis is placed horizontal so that reflections from horizontal surfaces are attenuated. For drivers on wet roads with the sun low down to the front of them, this type of filter is especially useful, as the author can testify. Norville supply single vision and bifocal polarised lenses with 15% and 40% Luminous Transmittances. A popular form of plano polarised sunlenses is the clip-on or the flip-clip, both of which clip over the patient's spectacle lenses and in some cases may be cut to shape. The flip-clip has the advantage that when going indoors, say during shopping, the tinted lenses may be flipped up so that the patient is back to untinted lenses whilst in the dimmer indoors environment. The flipped up state is somewhat idiosyncratic in appearance, but older patients tend not to care too much what others think about such an eccentric appearance. Polarised lenses for sunglasses usually have less than 5% UV transmittance with a UV cut-off at about 350 nm, somewhat similar to that for darkened glass photochromics.

Is the colour of a tinted lens significant?

Virtually any colour of tint can be manufactured. Just look at Rodenstock's tint range produced in full, along with special coatings, in Table 5. Note that Rodenstock, in common with Zeiss and Hoya, quotes absorptance as

---

* This means they appear untinted indoors after fading.

Dispensing Tints

Table 5 Rodenstock's list of tints and coatings available on their lenses.

Brown Brown vacuum tint: 15, 25, 50, 75 and 90% absorptance

Tints available on CR 39 lenses

Available with Solitaire, Solitaire Plus coating or with Duralux hardcoat.

Colour	Absorptance	Colour	Absorptance
Basic full tints (UV absorption to 350 nm)			
Rogal (light rose)	12%	Brunal (light brown)	12%
Brown	15 and 25%	Grey	15 and 20%
Green	20%	Blue	15, 25 and 35%
Amethyst	20%	Sand/Orange	15%

Standard UV full tints (UV protection up to 380 nm).
Brown UV 50, 65, 75, 85%:   Grey UV 50, 65, 75, 85%:   Grey-Green UV 75%:   Blue UV 65%

Basic graduated tints (UV absorption to 350 nm). Absorptance indicates minimum and maximum %.
Brown 10%/25%:   Grey 10%/25%:   Green 10%/25%:   Blue 10%/25%, 10%/35%
Skyline double colour graduated tint: Azure (blue/pink), Moos (green/pink), Smoke (grey/pink)
Pastella single colour graduated tint: Sand (sandy brown), Coralle (peach), River (blue-grey)

Standard UV graduated tints
Brown UV   10%/50%, 10%/65%, 10%/75%:   Grey UV   10%/50%, 10%/65%, 10%/75%:   Green UV   10%/75%

Non-standard graduated tints (UV blocker to 380 nm applied over 50% absorptance).
Not available with Solitaire or Solitaire Plus.
    Brown   70, 60, 35, 30, 20, 15, 10%   Grey   70, 60, 35, 30, 20, 15, 10%
    Green   35, 30, 20, 15, 10%   Blue   60, 50, 40, 30, 20, 15, 10%

Special Tints

Lambda 400   UV blocker; brown 12% or 75% absorptance tint.
Lambda 660   Brown 80% and 90% absorptance: for use with degenerative retinal disease. Cut-off at 660 nm.

Tints with UV protection up to 400 nm: **Nature** (Brown 75%), **City** (Grey, 75%), **Pilot** (Green, 85% absorptance)
Suncontrast (Amber 65%, Brown 75% and Green 85% absorptance)

Mirror Coatings   Gold and Blue (both including Duralux) on CR 39 with 85% absorptance

Tints for 1.6 index plastic

Brunal	Light brown 12% absorptance	**Brown**	15, 25, 50, 65 and 75% absorptance
Rogal	Light rose 12% absorptance	**Grey**	15, 20, 50 and 65% absorptance
Graduated	**Brown** 10%/25%, 10%/50%10/65%, 10%/75% absorptance	**Grey**	10%/25% absorptance
	Green 10%/50%, 10%/65%, 10%/75% absorptance		(All with UV cut-off 380 nm)

Pastella graduated (also available with Solitaire coating)   Sand (sandy brown), Coralle (peach), River (blue-green)

Tints for 1.67 index plastic

Brunal   Light brown 12% absorptance   Rogal   Light rose 12% absorptance

opposed to transmittance. Incorporating reflection with absorption, since both are energy loss mechanisms, these are related by

% transmittance = 100 − % absorptance.

For example, if absorptance is 30%, then the transmittance is 100 − 30 = 70%.

Lists like Table 5 are initially bewildering and only long use and familiarity with a manufacturer's product range will make you feel comfortable. This table is worth paying more than a cursory glance because it indicates that not all tints are necessarily available on all materials and it points to things like double colour tints, UV blockers, mirror coatings and some exotic sounding tint names, all of which the dispenser is expected to encompass along with other manufacturers' product ranges.

So, what does the colour tell you about a tint's characteristics? Well, firstly, and probably most importantly, it tells you nothing about any UV absorption by the lens. You need to look at the transmittance curve for this, or at the manufacturer's quoted figures. However, the colour of a tint does have some use. For example, if the tint appears green then it not only reflects predominantly green light but it also transmits mainly green light and through such a tint a white surface will appear green. In a green tint, blues and reds will be transmitted less and may therefore appear darker*. That is, the relative colour values will be changed. Where a tint has a roughly horizontal transmittance curve in the visible spectrum it will appear grey and grey tints are said to be *neutral filters*. That is, they do not upset colour discrimination so that judging colour matches in such jobs as textile design, colour mixing in the paint industry, and recognising colour codes in electronics are unaffected by the tint. Figure 16 illustrates hypothetical transmittance curves of a variety of coloured tints.

Hence, grey tints will preserve colour discrimination, the need for which must be elicited from the patient. For drivers it is important that traffic signal recognition is not upset; this means that sufficient green and red must be transmitted by the tint. Since police lights on cars are blue one might suggest that sufficient blue should be transmitted too, so we are back to a neutral tint preferably. Otherwise, it is a matter of personal preference what colour the patient chooses when cosmesis is the only consideration. Incidentally, all the photochromics mentioned pass the International Standards Organisation (ISO) Traffic Signal Recognition requirements.

3 Uses of tinted lenses

Tints are used to reduce the amount of visible light and ultraviolet and infrared radiation reaching the eye. Intense visible light causes visual discomfort for most people especially when there are light coloured surfaces to reflect a high proportion of the incident light. Intense visible light which creates visual discomfort is called glare. Excess visible light scatters within the eye and reduces the image contrast, especially in older eyes where water spaces develop in the eye's lens and act as scattering sources. Ultraviolet radiation, and to a lesser extent infrared radiation, is potentially hazardous to the eye. Evidently, tints reduce and/or prevent

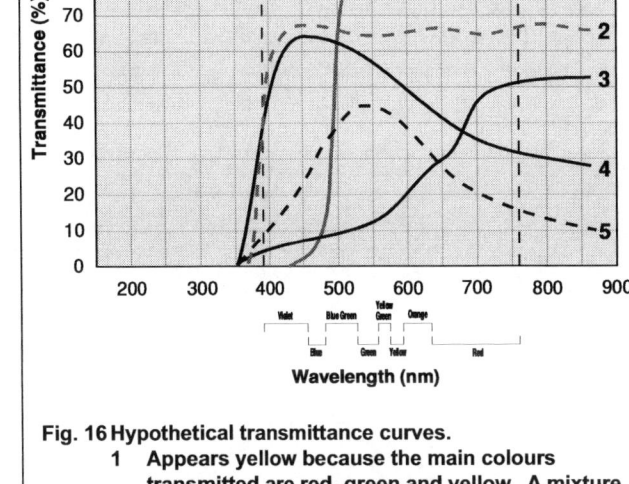

Fig. 16 Hypothetical transmittance curves.
1   Appears yellow because the main colours transmitted are red, green and yellow. A mixture of red and green lights produces subjective yellow, so the tint appears yellow.
2   Appears grey – neutral. All colours are transmitted in roughly equal amounts.
3   Appears brown due to preponderance of low intensity red, yellow and orange.
4   Appears blue due to the preponderance of blue in the transmitted light.
5   Appears dark green because of the preponderance of green in the transmitted light, but dark because this is relatively low in intensity (low transmittance).

unwanted radiation from reaching the eyes and in the process allow more comfortable and safer vision. The purposes for which tints are prescribed and dispensed, in probable order of frequency in routine optometric practice, are:

1   Cosmetic appearance (cosmesis).
2   Visual comfort – reducing the intensity of the visible part of the spectrum for general or occupational use.
3   Sunglasses† – with much attenuated visible light and for UV absorption.
4   Tints for dyslexia and migraineurs.
5   Contrast filters for sports and driving.
6   Industrial filters for UV and IR absorption, usually with a dark tint.
7   Filters for medical conditions.
8   Special occupational filters.

Cosmetic, fashion and comfort tints

Cosmetic tints are generally very light tints with Luminous Transmittances about 80 to 85% and often, though not exclusively, in 'warm' colours of pink or brown. These are the #1 grade lenses of say Essilor and Siltint. Warm colours are often considered to be cosmetically enhancing, as opposed to grey, green and blue light tints which can actually make the skin around the eyes look uncomplimentarily dark — this is especially true if the skin is already darker around the eyes. Occasionally cosmetic tints will be chosen as Gradutints, with about 50% transmittance at the darkest upper part of the lens fading to 10% transmittance, or thereabouts. Cosmetic

---

*   Even an appreciation of simple coloured light effects is a little tricky and beyond the scope of this text. See *Optics*, by Tunnacliffe and Hirst, pages 169 - 173 for an introduction.

†   Historically, lenses were all made from glass and the term sunglasses is often used today even when the lens material is plastics.

Table 6 UV absorbing tints

For general use, a tint will be regarded as UV absorbing when its transmittance does not exceed 10% at 380 nm and attenuates at shorter wavelengths. For complete UV absorption in plastic lenses use a UV blocker combined with a tint to reduce the Luminous Transmittance, or note that most 1.6 and 1.7 index plastics are intrinsically UV absorbing. Other UV absorbing lenses are:

Fixed tint	**Colour**	**Supplier**	**Comment**
UV-IR tints	Various	BPI	CR 39 (uncoated and hardcoated)
Greyray	grey	Norville	Glass material tint
B25 and B35	brown	Norville	Coating on glass or dye on CR 39
	yellow, orange, tan, red	Norville	Material tint in plastics
PLS	green	Norville	Coating on glass or dye on CR 39
F18	green	Norville	Coating on glass
F28			
Nature	brown	Rodenstock	Dye on 1.5 index plastics
City	grey	Rodenstock	Dye on 1.5 index plastics
Pilot	green	Rodenstock	Dye on 1.5 index plastics
Versil 2 and 4	green	Siltint	Coating on glass or dye on CR 39
Skylet	brown	Zeiss	Dye on CR 39 (3 tints — *fun*, *road*, and *sport*)
Umbra 85%	brown	Zeiss	Coating on glass
Umbral	brown	Zeiss	Plano sunglasses
Photochromic glass (fully exposed)			
CPF tints	brown	Corning	
Photobrown Extra	brown	Corning	
Photogray Extra	grey	Corning	
Photobrown 16	brown	Corning	
Photogray 16	grey	Corning	
HC-Photosolar	brown	DESAG	Zeiss Umbramatic 16 and Rodenstock Colormatic 1.6
Photochromic Grey	grey	Rodenstock	
Photochromic Brown	brown	Rodenstock	
Umbramatic Brown	brown	Zeiss	
Umbramatic Grey	grey	Zeiss	
Photochromic plastic (fully exposed)			
Sunsensors	brown	Corning	LT range 85% to 20%. UV cut-off at 385 nm.
Sunsensors	grey	Corning	LT range 86% to 17%. UV cut-off at 385 nm.
Sunbrown	brown	Hoya	LT range 85% to 25%. Absorbs 99% UVA and 100% UVB.
Sungrey	grey	Hoya	LT range 85% to 18%. Absorbs 99% UVA and 100% UVB.
Transitions Next Generation	brown	Transitions	LT range 89% to 17%. UV cut-off at 390 nm.
Transitions Next Generation	grey	Transitions	LT range 89% to 15%. UV cut-off at 390 nm.
Transitions XTRActive	grey	Transitions	LT range from 75% to 25%. Absorbs 99% of UV.

tints are, as the name suggests, simply for appearance and not particularly for visual comfort. As such the dispenser may allow the patient free reign in choosing the tint. Darker tints, nominally sunlenses, are sometimes worn as a fashion accessory and may be mirrored to accentuate the appearance of the lens. These lenses are usually good UV absorbers and double as sunlenses too. It is worth checking that the lenses do absorb UV because wearers of dark fashion tints will certainly expect them to absorb UV radiation.* Fashion sunglasses often spend more time pushed up onto the top of the head where UV absorption or any other optical or visual property of the lenses is of no concern to the dispenser. One wonders if fashion spectacles are ever chosen just for the appearance on top of the head!

Light tints can serve as comfort tints, that is tints worn for the visual comfort effect. Just why a small reduction in light intensity reaching the eye is found to be more comfortable than with 'white' (untinted) lenses is not fully understood. Perhaps light pink and brown lenses, which tend to have good UV attenuation, reduce crystalline lens fluorescence caused by UV radiation, thereby improving image contrast by reduction of what is known as diffusive blur of the image.‡ If the effect of a light tint is to reduce the intensity of multiple reflections at the lens surfaces then a multi anti-reflection coating is likely to be more successful than the light tint. Light tints can be worn indoors and at night, the eye adapting over a much larger range of illumination levels than the 20% absorptance of the tint.

Photochromic lenses can act as cosmetic, comfort, fashion and sunlens tints all at the same time. Glass photochromics tend to retain a light tint during indoor wear whereas the plastic variety usually clear almost completely indoors and in the absence of UV radiation.

Sunglass tints

Why do people wear sunglasses? They rarely choose them because they know it is advisable to absorb UV radiation, the majority being unaware of the meaning of it. *They are seeking dark tints for comfortable vision in sunlight.* The effect of a dark tint is to reduce pupil constriction, which causes pain or a discomfort sensation in some people, and/or to reduce excess light which may be causing reduced image contrast by light scatter within the eye, especially in middle and old age where the crystalline lens scatters more light. Painful intolerance to bright light is called **photophobia**, whereas visual discomfort arising from reduced contrast sensitivity in the presence of excess light is more aptly called **dazzle**, the excess light usually being referred to as **glare**‡. Shading the eyes with a hat may be sufficient protection for some people in some cases, but sunglasses are a more direct 'eye shade'. Often, people will benefit from wearing both sunglasses and a hat.

As already intimated, sunlenses should have near complete UV absorption and a low Luminous Transmittance (less than 20%). This excludes some photochromic lenses at ambient temperatures of about 22°C and almost all photochromics at higher ambient temperatures. However, having said this the author has 'managed' with Transitions in Mediterranean sunshine. Nonetheless, dispensers should be aware of the fact that photochromics do not darken as well in warm climates and patients should be so advised.

Fixed sunlens tints should always satisfy the UV absorption and low Luminous Transmittance requirements. **When used for driving they must satisfy signal recognition standards too.** In this context, note that **lenses with ≤ 80% transmittance are unsuitable for night driving**. Table 6 shows UV absorbing tints, but one should also realise that on CR 39 lenses a UV blocker can be ordered with any tint.

Tints for dyslexia and migraine

It is fairly well established that a proportion of dyslexia sufferers benefit from the use of special tints. Symptoms such as 'words changing shape', 'words jumping about' and 'words wobbling or going wavy' are reported to be alleviated with a tint with a specific transmittance curve profile. In one study† where precision tinted lenses were provided to 55 subjects with visual discomfort and associated complaints, 40 presented with perceptual distortion of text and this was the one symptom more than any other which predicted continued use and helpfulness of the tinted lenses. Almost 90% of subjects reporting perceptual distortion with reading were still using the tinted lenses after about a year. Most tints prescribed in this study had blue hues, followed by yellowish-green, and fewest with purple hues.

Other research claims that 85% of dyslexics are helped by tinted lenses where 80% of these turn out to need blue filters and 8% red. The manner in which coloured filters alleviate perceptual distortion is not known although it may have something to do with their effect on visual nerve cells which respond differentially to different colours. For example, some cells fire more rapidly when stimulated by yellow light but reduce their discharge rate when illuminated by blue light. If some of these opponent colour cells are hyperexcitable by one colour it may be that the tint attenuating this colour is helpful in controlling the hyperexcitability thereby improving perception of form.

An alternative hypothesis involves one of the two processing systems for optical information. The two parallel processing systems are the transient (magnocellular – large cell) and sustained (parvocellular – small cell). The magnocellular system processes position, movement, shape and low contrast whereas the parvocellular system is responsible for perception of stationary images, colour, detail and high contrast. There is growing evidence for the involvement of the transient visual system in dyslexia: it is suggested that up to 70% of dyslexics have a transient system defect, the magnocells being smaller and having slower conducting rates than normal. The hypothesis is that, when reading, the sustained system processes the detailed information during a fixation and that the transient system suppresses the sustained system during eye movements between fixations. If there is a defect in the transient system this suppression does not occur properly and confusion occurs in the image processing. Just how tints allow the transient system to work better is unclear, especially since it is the sustained system which has the colour response.

---

* We often omit the word 'radiation' and simply say UV. Similarly, we would talk about IR instead of infrared radiation, even with patients, once having told them what UV and IR stand for!

‡ See *Introduction to Visual Optics*, A. H. Tunnacliffe, pages 390-1 for diffusive blur and page 359 *et seq* for a treatment of glare and related topics.

† Open trial of subjective precision tinting: a follow-up of 55 patients. Anne Maclachlan, Sheila Yale and Arnold Wilkins, Ophthal. Physiol. Opt.,13, 175-178 (1993)

Dispensing Tints

Cerium Visual Technologies markets an instrument called the *Intuitive Colorimeter* and the associated tints whilst the tint specialist firm BPI (Brain Power Inc.) markets a set of trial tints together with computer software for determining helpful tints in dyslexia cases. Despite the apparent success of tints in alleviating reading difficulties in some dyslexia cases, the prescribing of these precise tints must be regarded as experimental and the patient should be so informed. Nonetheless, tints are often very helpful and it is expected that their dispensing will continue so the dispenser should be familiar with them.

Research has found that many dyslexics have a personal or family history of migraine. The *Intuitive Colorimeter* should therefore prove useful in determining a patient specific tint in those cases where the condition may be triggered by light.

Contrast filters for sports and driving

Contrast filters have distinctive transmittance curve profiles. They transmit longer wavelengths and absorb shorter ones in the visible spectrum. This has two effects in the eye:

1. The retinal image is sharpened by reducing chromatic aberration. (See page 4.)
2. Some opponent colour visual nerve cells are hyperstimulated and present the wearer with an illusion of increased brightness.

Both of the above effects are often perceived by patients as improvements in their vision so that these lenses are readily accepted by some. Certainly, reducing chromatic aberration will increase visual acuity slightly and this is undoubtedly an advantage. The apparent increase in brightness of the 'environment' due to the increased firing rate of some of the opponent colour cells is seen by some patients as brightening their day! Indeed, BPI market a yellow contrast tint under the name *Winter Sun*, the express purpose being to make dull winter days less depressing.

Figure 17 shows the transmittance curves of Zeiss *Skylet* contrast filters which all have a brown colour. Figure 18 attempts to show the effect of *Skylet road* on image contrast.

The surface processes company, BPI, offers a number of sports tints where the object's contrast against the background is increased; see figure 19. For example, the *Golf Tint* absorbs mainly in the blue and green regions of the visible spectrum so that the white ball will have a higher contrast against the sky and the fairway, these appearing darker through the tint. A legend below each transmittance curve in figure 19 explains its use.

Night driving raises the problem of less but variable illumination due to use of headlights alone or in combination with street lighting. The German standard DIN 58216 *Spectacle lenses for drivers* states that filters for night driving should have over 80% transmittance. This will be satisfied by light coloured fixed surface tints (usually designated A or 1 by manufacturers) or by faded

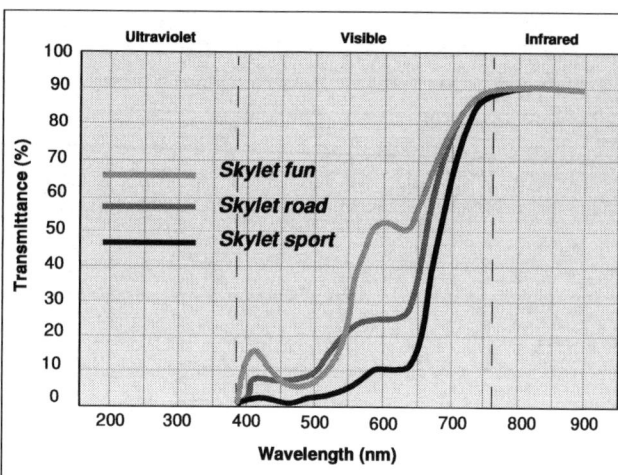

Fig 17 These are contrast filters known as *Skylet road*, *Skylet fun*, and *Skylet sport*. Because they stimulate the neural red and yellow on-effects, the scene does not appear as dark as the transmittance curves would suggest. The image is sharpened by the attenuation of the blue light and the consequent reduction in chromatic aberration in the eye and the spectacle lens. Traffic signals perception is not affected. Can be applied to Zeiss Clarlet (1.5 index) plastic lenses.

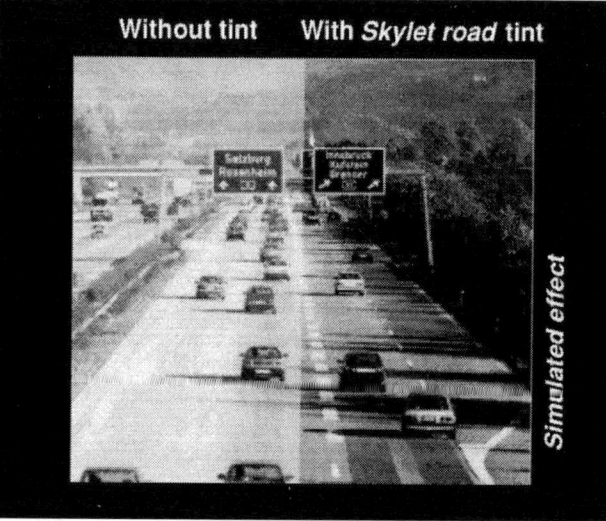

Fig. 18 Improved image contrast with the Zeiss *Skylet road* contrast filter. With the contrast filter the scene appears clearer. Note the clearer road markings.

photochromic lenses. Light solid tints may not satisfy this condition because the thickness affects the transmittance, thicker parts of the lens appearing darker. In plus lenses the centre is thickest and this must be considered whereas in minus lenses it is the periphery; if the tint is sufficiently light in the central 30 mm of a minus material tinted lens it would be satisfactory for night driving. Relatively few solid tints are worn nowadays with most tints being surface fixed or photochromic types.

Over the years yellow contrast filters, see curve 1 of Figure 16, have been marketed by non-professionals as night driving glasses. The evidence for their efficacy as night driving tints is equivocal but some people do find they help when faced with glare sources (oncoming vehicle headlights). It is a case of 'try-it-and-see'! The same yellow contrast filter almost always improves contrast sensitivity in photopic (daylight) conditions.

Dispensing Tints

Fig. 19 BPI Sports Tints

Ski Tint – reddish brown

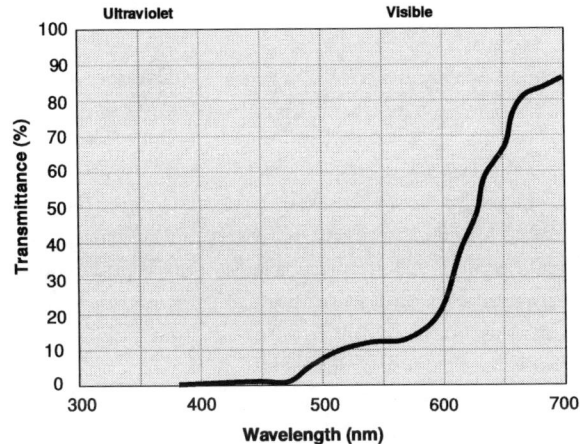

Absorbs in UV, blue and violet regions. Chromatic aberration is reduced and stereopsis increased.

Tennis Tint – yellow colour

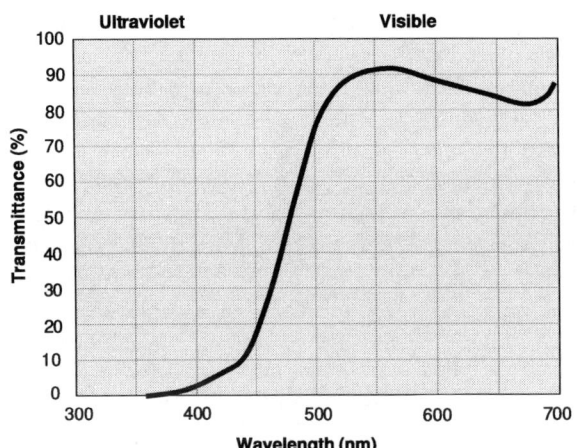

The contrast of a yellow tennis ball against the background is increased.

Golf Tint – Greenish Brown

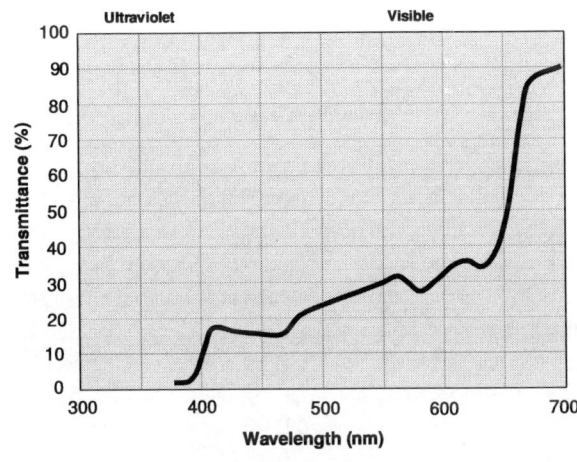

Designed to increase the ball's contrast against a blue sky and the fairway.

Skeet Tint – reddish orange

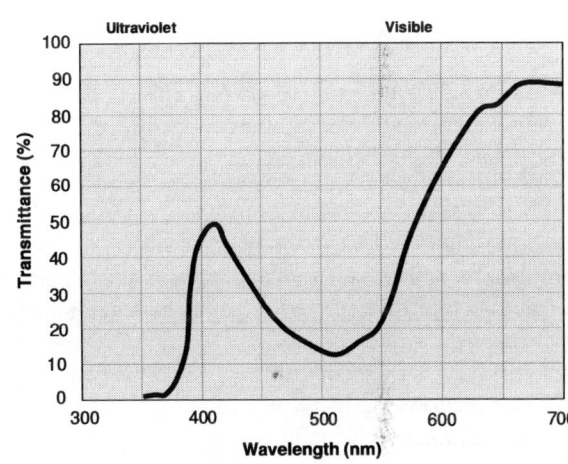

For clay-pigeon shooting.

Sport Tint – Brown

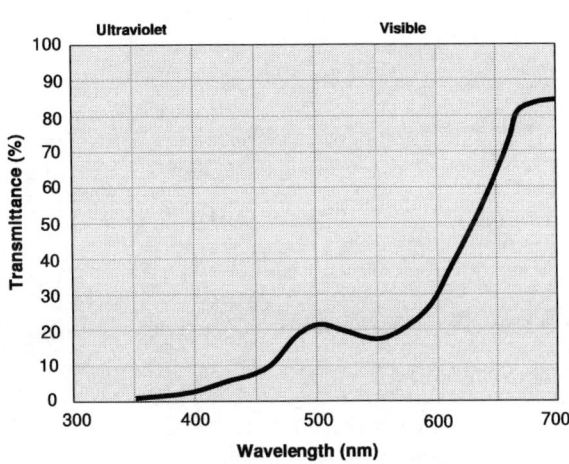

Designed to increase contrast. For boating and spectator use.

109

Industrial filters

Infrared radiation (IR), unlike ultraviolet (UV), can be sensed — it feels warm or hot. Hence we know when we are being exposed to it. It is generally only important to provide an infrared absorbing filter where a patient is exposed to it and cannot escape it. For example, glassblowers, furnace workers and users of infrared lasers. However, people undergoing these activities are provided with such protection as part of their job[†] and it is not very common to have to consider IR filters in routine ophthalmic dispensing. Infrared in the 760–1400 nm band (IRA) penetrates to the retina and in sufficiently high exposures can cause retinal burns. This is one reason why when viewing an admittedly rare solar eclipse one must view it through a totally IR (and UV) absorbing filter. Such filters are usually specially prepared for the occasion. IRA radiation can cause cataracts and retinal damage so it is important to wear an IR absorbing filter in the occupations referred to earlier. The transmittance curve for an industrial use IR filter must have a cut-off before the long wavelength end of the visible spectrum; see figure 20.

Filters for medical conditions

A number of tints have been designed to specifically absorb light in a large portion of the short wave visible spectrum as well as all the ultraviolet radiation. Because blue light is scattered more than longer wavelength light it reduces contrast sensitivity especially in ageing eyes. Such filters are used to alleviate visual symptoms with certain ocular pathological conditions such as developing cataract, macular degeneration, retinitis pigmentosa and diabetic retinopathy.

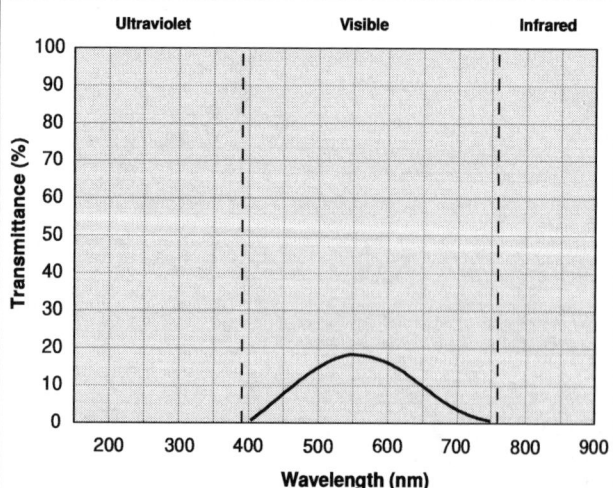

Fig. 20 Ideal transmittance curve of an infrared absorbing filter. Note that for industrial use the total transmittance will be very low, so the tint will be very dark. All ultraviolet should be absorbed since sources of infrared are often also sources of ultraviolet. For arc welding, for example, the total visible transmittance will be under 1%, some filters having a value as low as 0.003%, which should be compared with the minimum of 3% for very dark sunlenses. Incidentally, with peak transmission at 550 nm these tints will appear green.

Corning developed the CPF* glass photochromic lens in four forms, each with a different cut-off:

CPF 450, CPF 511, CPF 527 and CPF 550.

They are not recommended for night driving and may be prohibited under signal recognition legislation. CPF 450 is suited to indoor use with Visual Display Unit screens or for television viewing. It is lighter than the other tints but outdoors it darkens quickly from yellow to brown. The rest of the range comes in *Standard* (S) and *Design* (Dn) forms where the Standard form is lighter both in the faded and the darkened states. All are orange in the faded state darkening to brown on exposure to sunlight. CPF 550 is a very dark lens even indoors. Figure 21 shows the transmittance curves for the 511, 527 and 550 Standard lenses in the faded and darkened states, and also for the 511 and 527 Design lenses. Design lenses have a multilayer surface treatment which gives them a sunglass mirror look. They are available in 1.523, 1.7 and 1.8 index glasses in single vision, and 1.523 glass in a bifocal and a progressive form. The range, which is available from Norville Optical, is shown in Table 7. Table 8 on page 111 lists the CPF lens absorption characteristics.

Corning recommends the following choice of CPF lenses:

Condition	1st Choice	2nd Choice
Progressive cataract	CPF 511	CPF 527
Intra-ocular implants	CPF 511	CPF 527
Aphakia	CPF 511	CPF 527
Glare sensitivity	CPF 511	CPF 527
Photophobia	CPF 511	CPF 527
Optic atrophy	CPF 511	CPF 527
Macular degeneration	CPF 527	CPF 511
Diabetic retinopathy	CPF 527	CPF 511
Corneal dystrophy	CPF 527	CPF 511
Albinism	CPF 527	CPF 550
Aniridia	CPF 550	CPF 511

Zeiss produce a range of special medical filters which are dyes suitable for their whole range of CR 39 (Clarlet) lenses and can be supplied with hard and antireflection coatings. Like the Corning CPF lenses, these Zeiss tints are not suitable for driving because they upset traffic signal recognition.

Table 7 CPF range (maximum powers/cyls to 6.00):

Single vision Ø65 and Ø70
   1.523   −8.00 to +6.00
   1.7   −20.00 to −6.00 and +6.00 to +10.00
   1.8   −23.00 to −6.00 and +6.00 to +10.00

Bifocal Ø65/71 −8.00 to +6.00 Adds 0.50 to 6.00
          Ø70/76 −8.00 to +6.00 Adds 0.50 to 3.50

PAL   Ø70   −8.00 to +6.00 Adds 0.75 to 3.50

[†] For detailed coverage of this aspect of protective lenses see Rachel V. North, *Work and the Eye*, Oxford University Press, 1993.

* Corning Photochromic Filter.

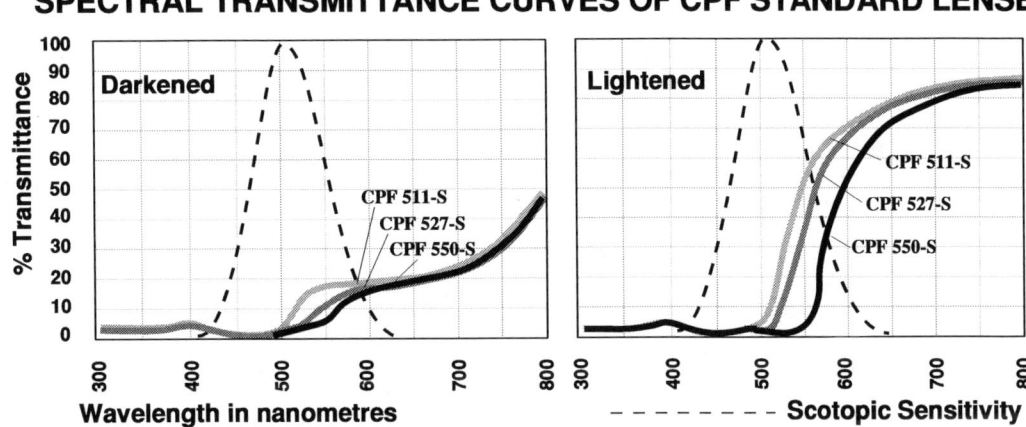

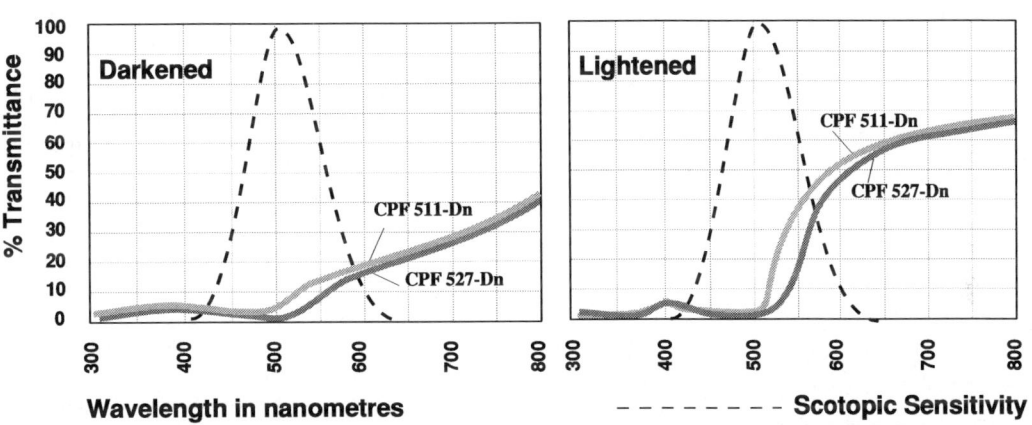

Fig. 21 UV and short visible wavelength glass absorbing filters originally with cut-offs at 511, 527 and 550 nm giving contrast enhancement and glare reduction. Later, a CPF lens with cut-off at 450 nm was added to the range. All prevent glare caused by scatter of short-wave visible light within the eye, hence they improve the retinal image contrast. CPF lenses are chemically tempered. *Design* (Dn) lenses are darker than the *Standard* (S) versions and are more suited to use by wearers who spend a high proportion of their time outdoors.

Zeiss' special medical filters come in three groups:

Brown coloured filters F60, F80 and F90 which were developed for use in cases of retinitis pigmentosa, achromatopsia (rod monochromatism) and advanced diabetic retinopathy. The colours are respectively reddish brown, brown and dark brown. The numbers refer to the absorptance. In figure 22(a), F540 (yellow), F560 (orange) and F580 (red) are contrast filters where the number is the cut-off wavelength in each case. They are used for the same the retinal conditions; see figure 22(b). Blue and dark blue coloured filters F451 and F452 are designed for blue monochromatism; see figure 22(c).

BPI have a range of therapeutic fixed tints for prescription lenses which go under the name of *Diamond Dye* and have similar shaped transmittance curves to those in figure 22(b). The numbers, shown in the following listing, indicate the cut-off wavelengths. There is also a range of 6 plano clip-ons with similar properties, the *BPI Designed Spectrum*

Table 8	CPF range lens absorption data							
	CPF	450	511S	511Dn	527S	527Dn	550S	550Dn
Visible cut-off (nm)		450	511	511	527	527	550	550
% absorption (faded)		27%	53%	66%	66%	74%	80%	92%
% absorption (darkened)		82%	88%	90%	91%	92%	95%	97%
% UVB absorption		100%	100%	100%	100%	100%	100%	100%
% UVA absorption		97%	99%	99%	98%	99%	99%	99%

Dispensing Tints

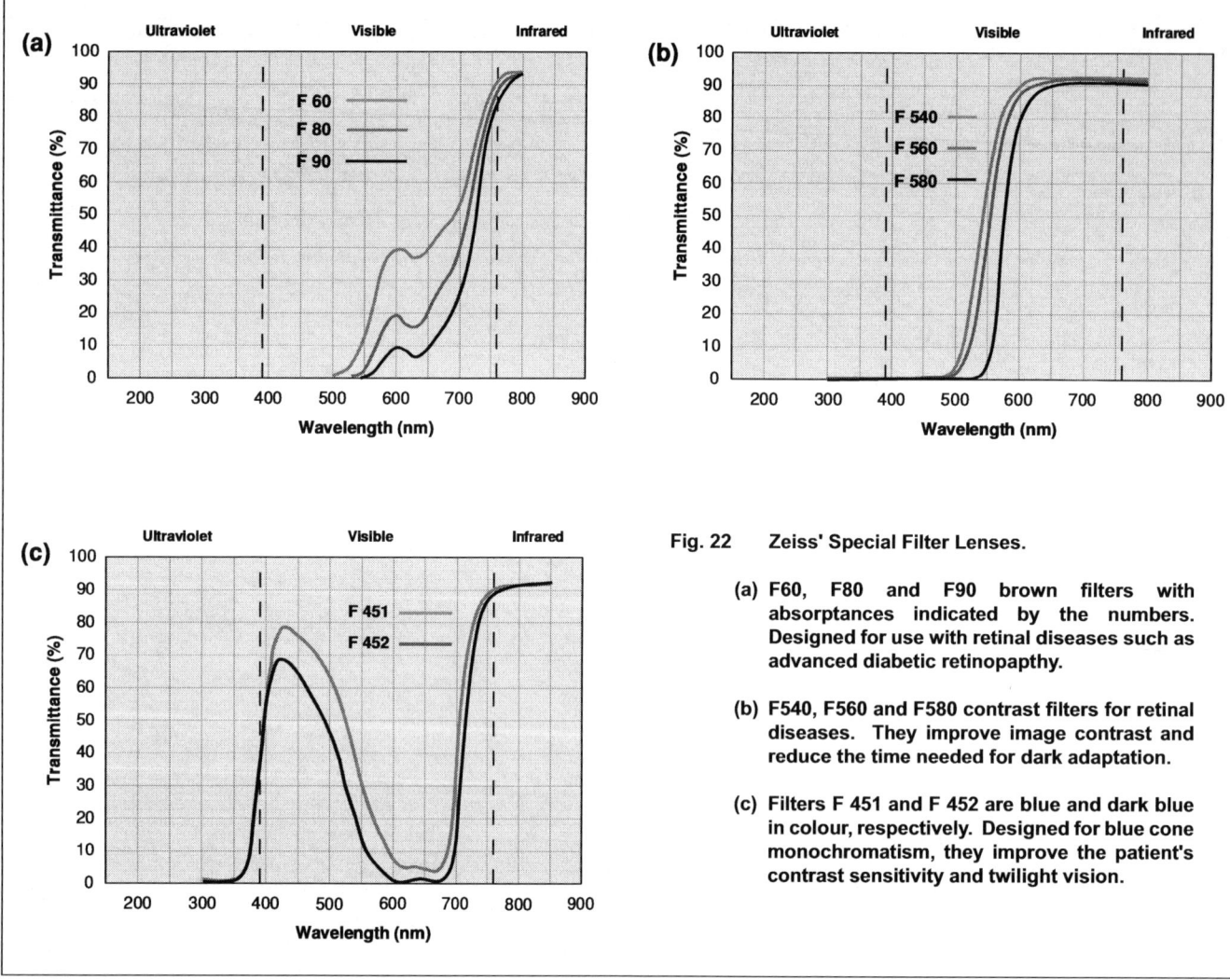

Fig. 22 Zeiss' Special Filter Lenses.

(a) F60, F80 and F90 brown filters with absorptances indicated by the numbers. Designed for use with retinal diseases such as advanced diabetic retinopapthy.

(b) F540, F560 and F580 contrast filters for retinal diseases. They improve image contrast and reduce the time needed for dark adaptation.

(c) Filters F 451 and F 452 are blue and dark blue in colour, respectively. Designed for blue cone monochromatism, they improve the patient's contrast sensitivity and twilight vision.

tints. This range includes additionally a purple tint, *Designed Spectrum 4/5/6*, with an absorption band in the yellow part of the spectrum.

BPI Therapeutic Tints

Name	Cut-off	Colour
Rx tints		
Diamond Dye 500	500 nm	Yellow
Diamond Dye 527	527 nm	Orange
Diamond Dye 540	540 nm	Brown
Diamond Dye 550	550 nm	Red
Designed Spectrum 450	450 nm	Yellow
Designed Spectrum 500	500 nm	Orange
Designed Spectrum 540	540 nm	Grey-Brown
Designed Spectrum 550	550 nm	Orange-Red
Designed Spectrum 600	600 nm	Brown

Special occupational filters

Patients with a need for this section's filters are met relatively infrequently and perhaps never by the majority of opticians in routine practice. Nevertheless, it is worth mentioning some of the lenses which can be seen in the literature and which may just crop up one day.

Lasers

The first laser was invented in 1960 and was initially referred to as an invention looking for an application. They are essentially parallel highly coherent beams of electromagnetic radiation which vary in power from almost harmless to absolutely deadly. Nowadays lasers are used routinely in cutting, measuring, printing, communications and surgical applications, not to mention military uses and many others. Pointers (laser pens), used by lecturers, and teaching laboratory lasers have a power of about 0.25 milliwatts (mW) and are safe unless one stares into the beam or its reflection from a shiny surface; just flashing the beam across the eyes will not cause any harm to the eyes although it may well cause temporary dazzle but even this is unlikely since the natural reaction is to avert one's gaze. If the laser has a power of less than 0.5 W (500 mW) no harm will come from an indirect flash on the eye. However, other types of lasers are more powerful; a focused carbon dioxide laser beam with a few kilowatts power can burn a hole in a 6 mm thick steel plate in just a few seconds! Lasers emit effectively monochromatic radiation either as continuous waves or pulses with a range of power densities from a few milliwatts to kilowatts per square centimetre. For comparison, a welder's oxyacetylene flame has a power density of about 1 kilowatt per cm^2. Depending on the type of material from which the laser is made, and there is a large number of solid state, gas, vapour and liquid lasers, lasers emit one or more monochromatic radiations in the UV, visible or IR. From what has been said about high powered lasers it is evident that safety absorbing filters should be worn by laser users who might sustain eye damage. Specialist protective goggles are not the sort of thing that opticians dispense in routine practice and laser users are subject to safety regulations and supply of protective goggles within their own work sphere anyway. Norville offer **Laser Protection Glass** in single vision only and having high absorption values at 694.3 nm and 1060 nm, where ruby and neodymium lasers have their outputs.

X-ray glass

Although lead shielding is the essential method of protection from X-rays, there is some evidence of risk of cataracts developing amongst those people working with X-rays. Norville supply single vision glass lenses with a cut-off at 300 nm in refractive index 1.8, $V = 25.4$ and $SG = 5.18$ which are opaque to X-rays.

Dentists' blue light filter

Dentists use a bright blue light to 'cure' ceramic fillings. Siltint and BPI have a tint which absorbs all the violet and blue in the spectrum. BPI call their version the *Blue Barrier 540* tint which only transmits light with wavelengths above 540 nm; the tint appears brown and is available in several shades. They suggest that in addition to use by dentists they could be recommended for pilots, lifeguards, sailors, skiers and sunbathers.

Didymium glass has a strong absorption band (90% absorptance) between 565 and 590 nm which is the yellow region of the spectrum. It is claimed to enhance red and green discrimination for red/green deficient patients and to be useful in aiding recognition of navigation lights at sea. It is light purple in colour with a Luminous Transmittance of 70%. Norville supply this tint in single vision lenses only.

Visual Display Unit (VDU) and fluorescent light filters

There is little evidence that tinted lenses designed to improve character/screen contrast are of any use with word-processors and drawing packages on modern computers since they use a full range of colours, unlike older systems in the early eighties. It is better to seek to remove reflections from screens by altering the screen position so that light sources cannot reflect in the screen and to ensure that glare sources do not appear within the field of view above and around the VDU. However, there may be one source of eyestrain (asthenopia) with VDUs in common with fluorescent lights.

Because an alternating current produces two brightness peaks per cycle in fluorescent tubes, these sources have a 100 Hz* pulsation in brightness. There is evidence that the 100 Hz variation in peak luminance affects the firing of neurons in subcortical visual structures and the retina[†]. When the pulsation was removed electronically, eyestrain in office workers was reported to be halved.

In the lateral geniculate nucleus of cat, neurons produce a response which is phase-locked to the 100 Hz luminance modulation and in humans there is evidence that this neural noise may affect eye movements. Wilkins[‡] (1986) found that there are small effects on the size of saccades (fixation movements) when reading text.

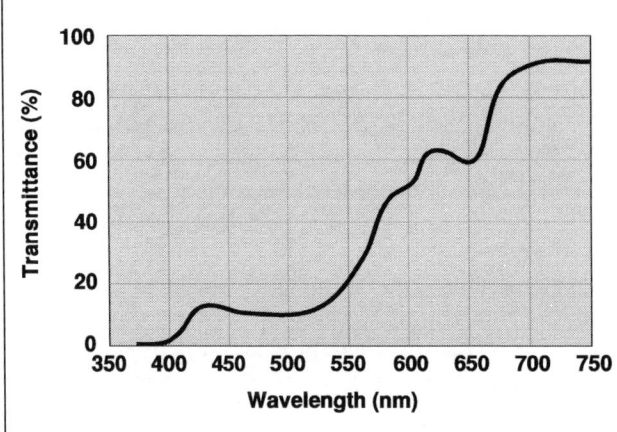

Fig. 23 Transmittance curve of Cambridge Optical's C41 tint designed for use by patients experiencing visual difficulty under fluorescent lights. The colour is brown and it acts like a contrast filter so the environment appears relatively bright.

Removal of the luminance modulation might be of benefit to those people who complain of headaches and eyestrain whilst working under fluorescent lighting. With this aim in mind, Wilkins and Wilkinson** reported the development of a tint devised to absorb light at those wavelengths where the luminance modulation was greatest. This tint, called C41 and produced by Cambridge Optical Company, is brown in colour and reduces the medium and long wavelength visible light modulation by about 25%. Figure 23 shows the transmittance curve for the C41 tint, which also acts like a contrast filter thus making the environment looker brighter!

Wilkins and Wilkinson also point out that fluorescent lamps vary in colour and the colour opponency neurons in the retina and lateral geniculate nucleus may contribute to interference with subcortical control of eye movements. Thus, other tints may prove beneficial to patients who complain of eyestrain under fluorescent lighting. This may account for anecdotal evidence for the efficacy of some light tints.

Siltint have produced a tint for use under fluorescent lighting and with VDUs. Available in light and dark bluish-green colours, they have called it **Tint X**; see figure 24. It is designed with the above research in mind.

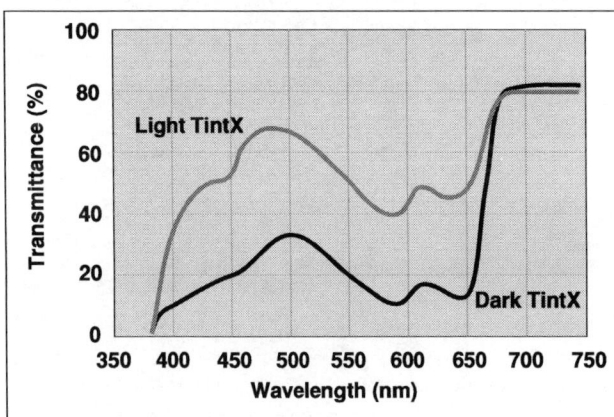

Fig. 24 Transmittance curves of Siltint's Tint X for use by patients complaining of asthenopia under fluorescent lights or when using a VDU.

---

* Hz = hertz, the unit of frequency; note the lack of a capital to commence hertz. 1 Hz = 1 cycle per second.
** Wilkins, A.J. and Wilkinson, P. (1991) A tint to reduce eyestrain from fluorescent lighting? Preliminary observations. *Ophthal. Physiol. Opt.* **11**, 172.
† Greenhouse, D.S., Berman, S.M., Bailey, I.L. and Raasch, T.W. (1988) Human electro-retinogram responses to visual display flicker. *Abstracts of Annual Meeting Association Research in Vision and Ophthalmology* **29**, 294.
‡ Wilkins, A.J. (1986) Intermittent illumination from fluorescent lighting and visual display units affects movement of the eyes across text. *Human Factors* **28**, 75.

Filters to assist colour deficiency

Abnormal colour vision occurs congenitally in 8% of the male and 0.5% of the female Caucasian population. Whites are reported to have a higher prevalence than non-whites, the Japanese, for example, being reported as having only 4% affected by colour deficiency. Congenital colour deficiency is attributable to the absence of or an anomaly in one or more of the three photopigments in the light receptors known as cones within the eye. Thus, the red, green or blue receptor mechanism may be affected. The condition in which only one photopigment is present is called monochromacy, two photopigments results in the condition dichromacy and three photopigments with one abnormal produces anomalous trichromacy. People with a red deficiency are called protans, since 'pro' is the first or red colour sensation. Those people with the second or third (green or blue) deficiency are known as deutans and tritans, respectively. The *monochromacies*, deficiencies in which only one photopigment is present, are much the rarest.

The common feature of all colour deficiencies is that the patient has some or considerable difficulty in colour discrimination. The first tinted lens made commercially available to assist the colour deficient patient was the X-chrom lens, in 1971, but this was available only as a contact lens. More recently the ChromaGen lens in 7 tints has become available in both contact and spectacle lens forms. A trial set and prescribing manual is supplied, see figure 25, but the tints are only available on licence to opticians and optometrists registered with the Corneal Laser Centre at the Clatterbridge Hospital in the Wirral.

Both eyes are involved, although one may be amblyopic and/or squinting, and the ChromaGen tint may be fitted uniocularly to the non-dominant eye. About 50% of patients are found to benefit from a Chromagen lens on the dominant eye, in addition to the one always fitted to the non-dominant eye, this second lens being determined by a trial assessing the quality of colour perception with the additional lens. Most cases end up with different right and left tints. In those cases who have spectacles with a uniocular prescribed ChromaGen tint, the other lens is tinted a neutral shade and the two lenses have a mirror coating added on the front surface so that they appear much the same.

Speculation as to how these lenses improve colour discrimination for colour defectives will be found in Appendix 5 in *Introduction to Visual Optics*, together with the transmittance curves for the tints.

4 Prescribing and dispensing tints

Some areas of prescribing can be held to be scientifically precise; that is, there is a defined filter or a defined range of filters from which a choice is to be made. Such areas would be UV absorbing filters, dyslexia tints, medical filters and special occupational filters. However, cosmetic and fashion tints largely come down to what the customer/patient desires with, perhaps, some counselling on possible needs for UV absorption, darkness of the tint, signal recognition constraints for drivers and colour perception fidelity for people who work in textiles, design, electronics, etcetera. Perusal of any tint supplier's range reveals a huge variety of tints available; consider once more Rodenstock's range in Table 5, page 104, for instance. The BPI catalogue is 32 pages long and claims more than 188 colours and 4000 products associated with tints (dyes, dye tanks, tint displays, photometers, etcetera not all of which needs to be available to the optometrist/optician but, nonetheless, a good deal does. So, the prescriber and dispenser must have a wide range of tints and related instrumentation to hand as listed below:

- Ranges of fixed tints – full and graduated, preferably in binocular demonstrators.
- Range of polarising sunlens filters.
- Photochromic tints and a demonstrator to show the change in transmittance on exposure, mainly to UV.
- Special purpose tints such as contrast filters, Zeiss *Skylet* range, Corning *CPF*, Siltint *Tint X*, BPI dyslexia tints, and so on.
- Spectral transmittance curves and Luminous Transmittance values for the lenses in the range held.
- Photometer for checking UV and visible transmittances.
- An Intuitive Colorimeter (Cerium Optical) for determining tints for dyslexics and migraineurs.
- BPI's Sunglass-Doctor for determining the density of dark tints (see figure 26).
- Zeiss-Humphrey lens analyser, which includes a spectrophotometer capable of producing a transmittance curve from 290 nm to 700 nm (see figures 27 and 28).

Dispensing UV blockers alone

The case against UVA as a cause of age-related cataract is well founded and certainly in countries with a lot of sunny

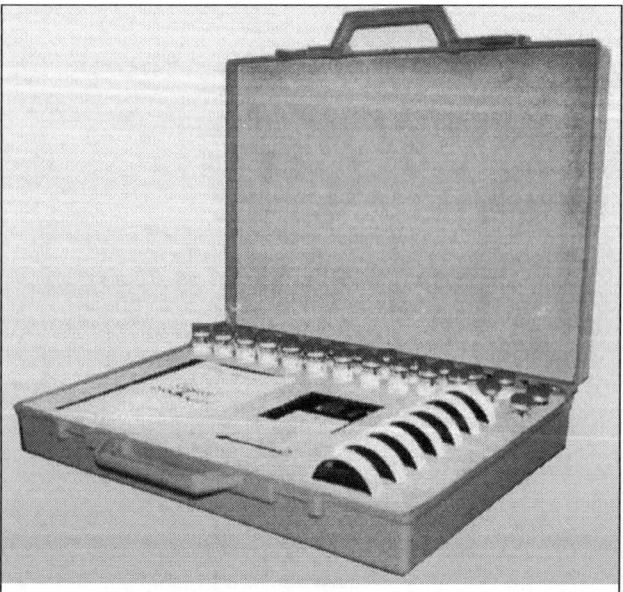

Fig. 25 The ChromaGen diagnostic set of seven filters and the contact lens fitting set.

Dispensing Tints

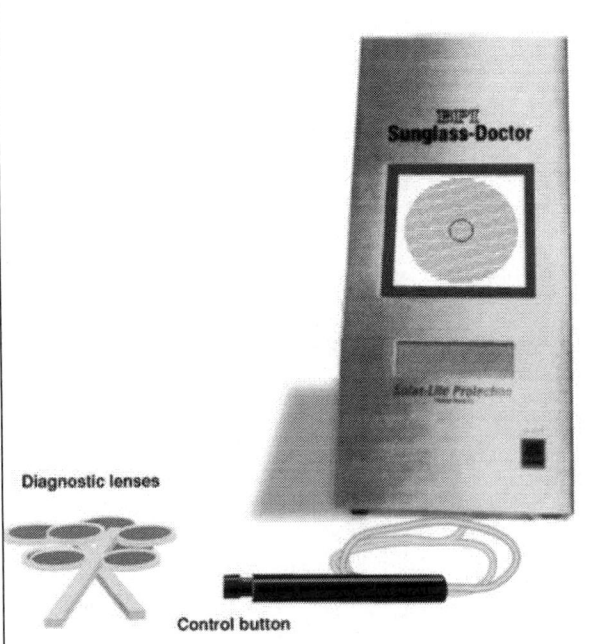

Fig. 26 BPI's *Sunglass-Doctor*, a device for checking the tint required by a patient to produce comfortable vision in bright light. The patient stands at about 1 m from the instrument and presses the button on the end of the cord (shown) which causes the light intensity to increase behind the target. This reduces the target contrast. When the lines in the centre of the circle can no longer be discerned he/she releases the button and the instrument indicates an initial tint density and a sensitivity reading. Pairs of diagnostic tints can then be used to determine the recommended sunglass tint density. At maximum intensity the instrument field of view represents full sunlight on white paper.

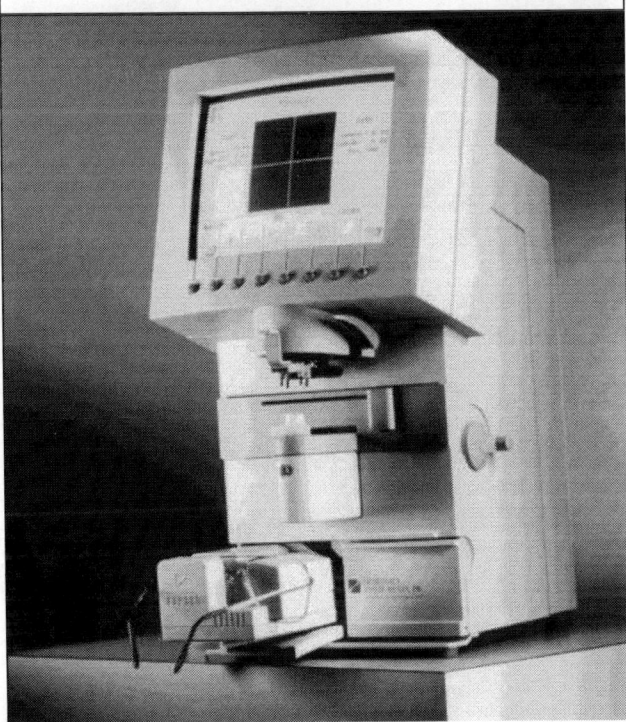

Fig.27 The Zeiss Humphrey Lens Analyser (HLA 360). A focimeter with a variety of monitor displays for lens measurement, one of which includes a spectrometer for displaying transmittance curves. Other displays are for progressive addition lens measurement, marking and setting, and measuring contact lens powers.

weather and with people working outdoors it might be well to advise a UV blocker on CR 39 lenses. Note that there is some absorption of the shortwave visible with these filters with the consequence that the lenses appear slightly yellow. If this is unacceptable cosmetically then the addition of a light brown tint will mask the objectionable yellow. Indeed, Zeiss counter this effect by including a 15% absorption light brown tint, as do Rodenstock.

Although aphakia (absence of the crystalline lens) is relatively rare now with the preponderance of intraocular lenses being the routine refractive treatment following cataract surgery, a UV blocker for an aphakic's lenses should be recommended. Intraocular lenses usually have a UV blocker within the material, but not all do so these patients should be told about the advisability for one on their spectacle lenses for outdoor use.

Dispensing light tints for cosmesis only

For those patients who simply want a tint which is fashionable and cosmetically pleasing, especially where the transmittance is not less than 80%, we can let them have free reign in their choice. One ought perhaps to ensure that colour discrimination is not going to be upset, as it would be with a yellow contrast filter even with an 80% Luminous Transmittance, although it is doubtful that a patient would choose such a lens for cosmetic purposes.

Dispensing light tints which have some other purpose

The prescriber should question the patient who complains of light sensitivity to determine the conditions under which it occurs. Where the light tint is for use with VDUs, or under fluorescent lighting, or a light tint combined with a UV absorber, the prescriber and dispenser must ensure that the filter meets the requirements — remember that colour alone does not indicate the tint's UV (or IR) absorbing characteristics so the dispenser will need to keep a set of transmittance curves for the range of tints he/she supplies. For measuring UV and visible transmittances the dispenser should possess a dedicated photometer such as those available from BPI or Hoya and the instrument should be used especially to confirm total UV absorptance where it has been prescribed.

Dispensing dark tints

Again, the patient should be questioned concerning any symptoms of light sensitivity because the problem is always to ascertain the tint which will resolve any visual problems associated with light sources in the work or leisure environment, perhaps at home and outdoors. Some people request medium-dark tints, LT in the range 60% to 30%, for purely cosmetic/fashion reasons but they may then use them for occasional sunlens purposes. In these cases it is advisable either to ensure the tint is UV absorbing anyhow or to advise inclusion of a UV blocker on CR 39 lenses. Rodenstock supply a UV blocker with all tints over 50% absorption on plastic lenses. Zeiss provide a UV protection to 380 nm on their CR 39 lenses with tints absorbing 30% or more. Note that some, though not all, mid-index plastic lenses are

Table 9 UV cut-off in white plastics lenses

Supplier	Material	Refractive index	V-value	Specific gravity	UV cut-off
PPGI†	CR 39	1.498	58.0	1.32	350 nm
PPGI (see Taylor)	Trivex	1.532	45.0	1.11	380 nm
Sola	Spectralite	1.537	47.0	1.21	370 nm
Signet Armorlite	RLX Lite	1.555	36.0	1.24	392 nm
Essilor	Ormex	1.561	37.0	1.23	350 nm
Signet Armorlite	Kodak Thin & Lite	1.562	36.0	1.24	392 nm
Nikon	Nikon Lite DXII	1.560	41.0	1.17	380 nm
Gentex	Polycarbonate	1.586	30.0	1.20	380 nm*
Essilor	Ormil	1.595	36.0	1.36	380 nm
American Optical	New Hi-index 1.6	1.600	42.0	1.22	380 nm
Sola	Finalite	1.600	42.0	1.22	380 nm
Zeiss	Clarlet 1.6	1.600	42.0	1.30	380 nm
Pentax	Mid-index	1.600	42.0	1.30	380 nm
Seiko	Super 16	1.600	42.0	1.38	370 nm
Hoya	Eyas 1.6	1.600	41.0	1.32	375 nm
Rodenstock	Perfalit 1.6	1.597	40.5	1.30	380 nm
Norville	Norlite	1.600	37.0	1.34	380 nm
Nikon	Nikon Lite III	1.600	36.0	1.34	360 nm
Zeiss	Clarlet 1.66	1.664	32.0	1.36	380 nm
Pentax, Rodenstock		1.67	32.0	1.35	380 nm
Nikon	Nikon Lite IV	1.67	32.0	1.35	380 nm
Hoya	Teslalid	1.71	36.0	1.40	390 nm
Nikon, Seiko, WLC	Very high index	1.74	33.0	1.46	380 nm

† Pittsburgh Plate Glass Industries.
* Polycarbonate is a very soft material and is hardcoated as standard. The coating contains an ultraviolet blocker.

usually inherently UV absorbing up to about 380 nm and the problem does not arise in those cases; see Table 9.

If these darker tints are to simply satisfy fashion whims then the patient has the final decision on the colour and the shade of the tint. Alternatively, where there is a sensitivity to bright light then the difficulty arises in trying to duplicate the lighting conditions in practice. BPI market a device called the *Sunglass-Doctor*, figure 26, where the patient views a target and the luminance increases until the target can no longer be detected, at which point the patient releases a button which records the reading and a recommended tint. The instrument comes with pairs of tints in different Luminous Transmittances so that the effect of the recommended tint can be subjectively assessed by the patient.

Even with fixed tint sunlenses the difficulty still exists in deciding what depth of tint to prescribe. Obviously, all sunlens tints must be supplied with UV absorption, but does one supply a category 3 or 4 tint (Table 1). As a general rule, for use in UK sunlight a category 3 would be satisfactory, but for use in the tropics and subtropics, for skiing and water sports, it would be better to recommend a category 4 tint.

Again, the patient's preferences will need to be addressed. Do not forget the possibility of clip-ons and flip-clips as sole or additional filters.

Certain activities lend exposure to more UV radiation than normally experienced outdoors. At high altitudes the atmosphere absorbs less UV so skiers and mountaineers are advised to have spectacles with total UV absorption and about 5 to 10% visible transmittance (very dark lenses!). Sailors and those engaged in on the water recreations are subjected to radiation reflected from the sea, plus light from the sky, and should again have a UV absorber plus a dark tint with 5 to 20% transmittance.

Dark tints will not be suitable for night driving and absorption may be further compounded by a tinted windscreen, a fact which should be brought to drivers' attention. Patients who wear dark tints habitually during the day will need to have a separate pair for night driving.

Fixed versus photochromic tints

Because photochromic tints change transmittance with increasing UV and shortwave visible light intensities, for many people they solve the problem of "just which shade of tint do I chose?" However, because they do not darken as much in hot weather as they do in cool/cold weather, the patient must be warned that they are not necessarily going to be suitable for that Mediterranean or Florida Disney World Holiday even though most patients find photochromics perfectly acceptable for use in the UK. Glass photochromics can be pretinted on the back surface to a greater absorptance in the faded state — a sort of combination of fixed and photochromic tints — but this is not recommended with plastic photochromics. Transitions XTRActive is available in a range of lenses from Norville and is somewhat more suited to sunlens use, in the sense that it never clears to more than 75% transmittance. Corning's Photobrown Plus and especially Photogray Dark are also more useful for bright sunshine.

Dispensing special purpose tints

Tints for dyslexia and migraineurs whose headaches are light-induced would benefit from prescription via the Intuitive Colorimeter although trial tint sets for dyslexia may suffice in some cases. The Zeiss-Humphrey lens analyser's spectrophotometer would be a useful piece of equipment to have in the practice for checking the spectral transmittance of specialist filters. The same instrument would provide a means of checking pairs of tints for a match, not only for precision tints but for other types in pairs or single replacement lenses.

Replacing a damaged tinted lens

There are certain caveats related to matching the tint:

- Plastic photochromics more than a year old may be difficult to match, so you may need to replace the pair.

- Fixed tints fade a little over time and the retained lens should be sent with the order to ensure a proper match is obtained for new lens.

- In the case of a solid tint it is essential that the centre thickness of the new lens matches the one being replaced.

Although this treatment of dispensing tinted lenses has implicitly assumed they will be prescription spectacles, plano sunlenses must also conform to the standards required especially with respect to UV absorption. Do read the manufacturer's literature and always request transmittance curves and Luminous Transmittance values.